The History
of American Homeopathy
The Academic Years,
1820-1935

PHARMACEUTICAL PRODUCTS PRESS®
Pharmaceutical Heritage:
Pharmaceutical Care Through History

Mickey C. Smith, PhD
Dennis B. Worthen, PhD
Senior Editors

Laboratory on the Nile: A History of the Wellcome Tropical Research Laboratories by Patrick F. D'Arcy

America's Botanico-Medical Movements: Vox Populi by Alex Berman and Michael A. Flannery

Medicines for the Union Army: The United States Army Laboratories During the Civil War by George Winston Smith

Pharmaceutical Education in the Queen City: 150 Years of Service, 1850-2000 by Michael A. Flannery and Dennis B. Worthen

American Women Pharmacists: Contributions to the Profession by Metta Lou Henderson

A History of Nonprescription Product Regulation by W. Steven Pray

A Social History of Medicines in the Twentieth Century: To Be Taken Three Times a Day by John K. Crellin

Pharmacy in World War II by Dennis B. Worthen

Civil War Pharmacy: A History of Drugs, Drug Supply and Provision, and Therapeutics for the Union and Confederacy by Michael A. Flannery

Federal Drug Control: The Evolution of Policy and Practice edited by Jonathon Erlen and Joseph F. Spillane

Dictionary of Pharmacy edited by Dennis B. Worthen

The Rexall Story: A History of Genius and Neglect by Mickey Smith

The History of American Homeopathy: The Academic Years, 1820-1935 by John S. Haller Jr.

John S. Haller Jr., PhD

The History
of American Homeopathy
The Academic Years,
1820-1935

Pre-publication
REVIEWS,
COMMENTARIES,
EVALUATIONS . . .

"**J**ohn Haller has written an outstanding internal history of professional homeopathy in America. It contains detailed information about leading homeopathic physicians, homeopathy in geographic regions of the country, homeopathic institutions, and lists of homeopathic journals and medical schools. It will become the primary source for general information and reference material on American homeopathy in the nineteenth and early twentieth centuries."

William G. Rothstein, PhD
Professor of Sociology,
University of Maryland, Baltimore County

"**I**n recent years John Haller has established himself as one of the leading historians of alternative medicine in nineteenth-century America. *The History of American Homeopathy* marks Haller's fourth book on American medical heterodoxy and equals his earlier volumes in depth of research, organization, and clarity.

In an eminently readable text, Haller explains Hahnemann's rejection of contemporary medicine and the development of homeopathic therapeutics. In successive chapters he narrates the emergence and growth of homeopathy in America, the public's perception of homeopathy's effectiveness, the bitter literary war that raged between allopaths and their homeopathic rivals, and, finally, the transformation of orthodox medicine into biomedicine that spelled homeopathy's doom. *The History of American Homeopathy* will remain the standard work on this subject for many years to come."

Christopher Hoolihan, MLS
Rare Books and Manuscripts Librarian,
University of Rochester Medical Center

The History
of American Homeopathy
The Academic Years,
1820-1935

John S. Haller Jr., PhD

ℐPPP

Pharmaceutical Products Press®
An Imprint of The Haworth Press, Inc.
New York • London • Oxford

For more information on this book or to order, visit
http://www.haworthpress.com/store/product.asp?sku=5405

or call 1-800-HAWORTH (800-429-6784) in the United States and Canada
or (607) 722-5857 outside the United States and Canada

or contact orders@HaworthPress.com

Published by

Pharmaceutical Products Press®, an imprint of The Haworth Press, Inc., 10 Alice Street, Binghamton, NY 13904-1580.

Cover images of Samuel Hahnemann and the Hahnemann Medical College and Hospital are courtesy of the National Library of Medicine and the Lloyd Library and Museum, respectively, and are used with permission.

Cover design by Lora Wiggins.

Library of Congress Cataloging-in-Publication Data

Haller, John S.
    The history of American homeopathy : the academic years, 1820-1935 / John S. Haller, Jr.
        p. cm.
    Includes bibliographical references and index.
    ISBN-13: 978-0-7890-2659-0 (hc. : alk. paper)
    ISBN-10: 0-7980-2659-7 (hc. : alk. paper)
    ISBN-13: 978-0-7890-2660-6 (pbk. : alk. paper)
    ISBN-10: 0-7890-2660-0 (pbk. : alk. paper)
    1. Homeopathy—United States—History—19th century. 2. Homeopathy—United States—History—20th century. I. Title.
    [DNLM: 1. Homeopathy—History—United States. 2. History, 19th Century—United States. 3. History, 20th Century—United States. WB 930 H185h 2005]

RX51.H34 2005
615.5'32'0973—dc22
                                                                        2004028187

For Robin

ABOUT THE AUTHOR

John S. Haller Jr., PhD, is a professor of history at Southern Illinois University at Carbondale, teaching courses in American intellectual history and the history of medicine. He is author of *Outcasts from Evolution: Scientific Attitudes of Racial Inferiority, 1859-1900; The Physician and Sexuality in Victorian America* (co-authored with Robin Haller); *American Medicine in Transition, 1830-1910; Farm Carts to Fords: A History of the Military Ambulance, 1794-1925; Medical Protestants: The Eclectics in American Medicine, 1825-1939; Kindly Medicine: The History of Physio-Medicalism in America, 1836-1911; The Making of a Medical Practice: An Illinois Case Study, 1885-1938* (co-authored with Barbara Mason); *A Portrait in Alternative Medicine: The Eclectic Medical College of Cincinnati, 1845-1942;* and *The People's Doctors: Samuel Thomson and the American Botanical Movement, 1790-1860.* He also served as past editor of *Caduceus, A Journal for the Medical Humanities.* Dr. Haller's current research involves nineteenth- and twentieth-century alternative medical systems.

The medical art stands in need of a thorough reform from head to foot. The evil has become so crying that the well-meaning mildness of a John Huss no longer avails, but the fiery zeal of a rock-firm Martin Luther is needed to sweep away the monstrous leaven.

Samuel Hahnemann, 1808

I am a sectarian in religion; by creed a Protestant, and yet I hope a Christian. I am a sectarian in politics; by creed a Republican, and yet I hope an American citizen. I am a sectarian in medicine; by creed a Homeopath, and yet I hope a physician.

William Tod Helmuth, 1889

CONTENTS

Foreword

Homeopathy entered the American medical landscape almost two centuries ago. Then as now, its essential principles, laid down by German physician Samuel Hahnemann, have engendered both ardent adherents and critics. In this superbly researched and well-written history, John S. Haller Jr. documents and explores the history of this philosophy of healing during the century and some when it loomed large among medical treatment options.

Homeopathy's early emphasis on the law of similars, the use of a single medication to treat all of the symptoms displayed by a patient, and an adherence to minimal doses was bound to bring it into conflict with allopathic medicine at a time when the therapeutics of the latter were not infrequently worse than the diseases from which people suffered. However, homeopathy began to lose ground in the late nineteenth century with the spectacular discoveries in chemistry, pharmacology, and microbiology that were to lay the foundations for twentieth-century scientific allopathic medicine. The triumph of allopathic biomedicine, as the author explains, increasingly cast homeopathy, with its roots deep in a range of old and scientifically unproven orthodoxies, as a movement without a rational basis.

The author thoroughly analyzes all aspects of homeopathy, including its essential principles, its early history in Europe and the United States, its quest to favorably compare its treatment outcomes with those of allopathic medicine, and its formal organization in local, state, and national professional societies. Equally important, he also details the establishment of homeopathic medical schools, of which there were a total of sixty-nine (chartered, unchartered, and reorganized) in the United States, and how a few, such as New York Homeopathic Medical College and Flower Hospital and Hahnemann Medical College and Hospital of Philadelphia, "had relinquished their homeopathic status and become regular medical schools" by 1936.

The decline of homeopathy was, as the author documents, gradual but inexorable, due to both steady advances in biomedicine and its inability to redefine itself in ways that could maintain credibility. Additional forces that advanced this decline included stricter state professional licensing standards and negative assessments of most homeopathic medical schools by Abraham Flexner, who conducted a national survey of medical schools in 1909-1910 for the Carnegie Foundation for the Advancement of Teaching.

By the midtwentieth century, homeopathy was but a vague memory for many. However, it continued to survive, albeit through residuary professional groups, a dwindling number of practitioners, a pharmacopoeia recognized by the Food and Drug Administration, and lay practitioners. My first contact with homeopathy was in fact with a woman who worked at my undergraduate college, and who, as a lay practitioner, enjoyed explaining homeopathy to premedical students. Memories of homeopathy were still vivid then among allopathic physicians, many of whom viewed it with either scorn or ridicule. I recall that my two physician uncles, both graduates of Weill Medical College of Cornell University, strongly advised me not to apply to those allopathic medical schools that had once been homeopathic, citing lingering negative reputations among medical practitioners and concerns about residual homeopathic teaching in the curriculum.

The revalorization of alternative medicine in the late twentieth century in the United States, and the creation of a National Center for Complementary and Alternative Medicine within the National Institutes of Health, slightly rekindled interest in homeopathy. Yet the halcyon days of this healing art have long past. It is this bygone era that is so thoroughly and objectively described in this excellent volume, and at a time when the flames of controversy surrounding homeopathy have dwindled to smoldering embers. The author brings to this study of homeopathy splendid research skills, a dedication to objectivity and understanding, and a reputation as one of America's most eminent medical historians. Engagingly written and admirably organized, *The History of American Homeopathy: The Academic Years, 1820-1935,* represents a landmark study of the history of a unique treatment art that prominently figured in American life for over a century.

Pascal James Imperato, MD, MPH, TM
Distinguished Service Professor and Chair
Department of Preventive Medicine and Community Health;
Director, Master of Public Health Program
SUNY Downstate Medical Center
Brooklyn, New York

Acknowledgments

Those to whom I am indebted include Dennis B. Worthen, Scholar in Residence at the Lloyd Library and Museum in Cincinnati; Pascal James Imperato, MD, Professor and Chair of the Department of Preventive Medicine and Community Health at the State University of New York Health Science Center at Brooklyn; Michael A. Flannery, Associate Director for Historical Collections at the Lister Hill Library of the Health Sciences, University of Alabama at Birmingham; homeopath Jay Yasgur of Van Hoy Publishers, Greenville, Pennsylvania; Director Kathleen Connick and staff members Carol Maxwell, Betsy Kruthoffer, Janet Keith, and Shauna Hannibal of the Lloyd Library and Museum; librarians Kathy Fahey, Mary K. Taylor, Barbara Preece, Kimbra Stout, and David Carlson of Morris Library, Southern Illinois University Carbondale; Connie Poole from the Southern Illinois University School of Medicine, Springfield, Illinois; and the librarians and support staff of the Newberry Library; Johns Hopkins University Library; Ohio State University; Yale Medical Library; University of Chicago Library; the Widener Library of Harvard University; University of California, Davis; Flower Veterinary Library of Cornell University; Health Sciences Library of the University of Washington; National College of Naturopathic Medicine; John Hay Library of Brown University; University of Pennsylvania; Kent State University Library; University of Maryland Library; New York State Library, Albany; Historical Society of Pennsylvania; Meadville Theological Library; and the Theodore Lownik Library of Illinois Benedictine College.

As always, I am grateful to my wife, Robin, who offered inspiration, encouragement, criticism, and substantial assistance, including the reading of numerous drafts and indexing the finished manuscript. It is to her, for her love and patience over many years, that this book is dedicated.

AUTHOR'S NOTE

There are four distinct spellings of Samuel Hahnemann's medical philosophy: *homöopathy, homœopathy, homoeopathy,* and the Americanized *homeopathy.* My preference was to use *homœopathy* or *homoeopathy* because they are the most historically accurate representations of the spellings used during the period covered by this book. However, for the sake of the reading audience, I have chosen the more Americanized *homeopathy.* No doubt this may trouble some readers, but my decision relies upon the preferred English usage as defined in *Webster's Unabridged Dictionary.*

Introduction

At the dawn of the nineteenth century, Western medicine sailed a precarious course between the lamentations of doubters and the siren calls of apostates. The structure of the human body—organs, nerves, bones, and muscles—had been determined with some degree of certainty, but the institutes of medicine and materia medica appeared to many as a confusion of "principles, conjectures, arguments, and testimony from a . . . thousand conflicting sources."[1] While the claim seemed inordinately rhetorical, it was no more or less than what many held to be true. As one of the century's more trenchant critics explained, medicine survived as "the shameless wreck of numerous exploded systems."[2] So much so that together doubters and apostates accused medicine of presenting a façade of authority that only incompletely hid centuries of error. Medical orthodoxy was not orthodox or monolithic at all, but a successive number of competing systems. Disregarding opposing doctrines, most systems offered patients a monotonous and repetitive fare of bloodletting, purging, puking, sweating, and blistering. The success of any one system of medicine elicited few marks of respect, fewer still of gratitude.

The school of medicine known as homeopathy trailed a long line of eighteenth-century system builders, each of whom held fast to an epistemology bent on discovering a universal law or principle that would explain disease causation. The years of its development paralleled successive waves of revolution, war, and social upheaval in Europe and the United States. Homeopathy was a system full of speculation and high hopes, maturing prior to the great advances in pathological anatomy, germ theory, laboratory science, and pharmacotherapeutics that so thoroughly revolutionized the medical sciences in the nineteenth century. Accordingly, any effort to understand homeopathy's historical and medical context requires an examination of not only the decades that preceded it but also the onrush of newer ideas that were beginning to pervade the landscape.[3]

As a philosophy, homeopathy fell among the group of schools that included Cullenism, Brunonianism, Rushism, and Broussaisism. Like

1

these predecessors, homeopathy's aim as enunciated by its founder was not to coexist with its competitors but to replace them with a new orthodoxy. Coming at the end of these theoretical systems, homeopathy had the good fortune to be the most benign of the group, a factor that served it well with the public—and with American society in particular, which viewed medical sectarianism as fully compatible with its Reformation-based religious culture. But rather than set out to destroy orthodox medicine, as had been the intent of its founder, American homeopathy sought instead to find a niche or an accommodation within standard medical practice, a distinctive place in therapeutics, and a recognizable professional identity.

Founded by the German physician Samuel Hahnemann (1755-1843) in the late eighteenth century, homeopathy continues more than two centuries later as a popular healing system. Staking claim to such ideologically charged words as *vitalism, succussion, vibrations, potentiation, provings, resonance,* and *structured water,* homeopathy enjoys a unique status within the health care marketplace. One hundred years ago, the school claimed as many as 10,000 academically educated practitioners in the United States. The term *academic* is loosely used to define those homeopaths who graduated from regular medical colleges or schools organized under their own auspices, or who had been licensed or otherwise legally recognized through apprenticeship, or a combination of these. Clearly, the line between qualified and unqualified practitioners did not hang on any one of these functions. As Motzi Eklöf explained,

> the laws about authorisation in the health care sector do not constitute a precisely formulated and unambiguous set of regulations . . . ; instead, they are generally rules that are drawn up and then subjected to negotiations, interpretations and judgments in applications of the law.[4]

The growth of proprietary colleges had certainly wrought havoc on state licensing and efforts to regulate competent medical practice. Nevertheless, the academic tradition in medicine, including the award of the medical degree, functioned however faintly to separate it from the domestic and lay traditions in medicine. Today, the academic side of homeopathy is barely discernable while domestic and lay homeopathy represents a robust business enterprise whose advocates hold an almost eschatological belief in the future and in their opposition to regular medicine. Arguably, homeopathy's present popularity has less to do with what homeopathy is than what certain elements in the population desire from health care and what, in their opinion, regular medicine has failed to deliver.

American homeopathy has been shaped by the same social, scientific, and philosophical forces as other schools of the healing art. It was, and is, the product of a very human endeavor—the treatment of disease based on the best knowledge of its practitioners and shaped by beliefs they hold to be true. As with regular medicine, the hopes and investigations of homeopathy's advocates, many of whom came from the ranks of regulars, led to both great ideas and flawed beliefs. That being said, homeopathy—both European and American—deserves closer scrutiny because the earliest historians of this healing system were too heavily biased in their assessment of its merits. Later historians, justifiably critical of medicine's "heroic" age of therapeutics, continued to underestimate homeopathy's influence on health and healing. In more recent years, with greater public acceptance of alternative and complementary therapies, and the openness of HMOs (health maintenance organizations) to cheaper options, historians have been less critical of homeopathy, promoting a friendlier and more integrative connection between its unconventional therapies and the rigors of scientific medicine. Currently, social and medical historians are seeking an even broader view of therapeutic change and professional identity by looking across cultural and national boundaries for signs of common healing practices. Some of these contemporary writings are case studies and anthologies rather than broad histories. Many are pathbreaking, opening new understandings of patient choices by social standing, class, and gender, and responding to Roy Porter's challenge to rediscover the patients' perspective in medicine. For Guenter B. Risse, the phenomenal rise of complementary medicine "is forcing a new global eclecticism in medicine with revolutionary implications for the future nature and shape of health care."[5]

I have sought to build on the contributions of past and contemporary scholarship by studying the manner in which academic homeopathy developed during medicine's introspective age of doubt and the emergent period of scientific reductionism. This history starts with the development of Samuel Hahnemann's ideas and their popularity in the United States. The growth of domestic and academic practice, the conflicts that ensued over dosage, and the claims and counter-claims based on the early use of statistics are recounted in later chapters. Academic homeopathy's evolving relationship with regular medicine, the migration of homeopathic ideas into other reform movements, and homeopathy's eventual accommodation with regular medicine conclude the study.

In my pursuit to understand how and why homeopathy flourished in American society, I have tried to avoid a strictly linear approach that portrays the rise of biomedicine as the sole determining factor. Such a view ignores the power and diversity of the medical market; the contextual boundaries between orthodoxy and unorthodoxy; and the role of gender, age, social class, religion, and even regional differences in the attraction of certain therapies. Although biomedicine was certainly important in marginalizing homeopathy for a culture increasingly bent on establishing an unambiguous definition of the practice and art of doctoring, homeopathy continued to claim a portion of the medical market. The epistemological effort to discriminate scientific truth from falsity succeeded in placing qualifications on homeopathic legitimacy but failed to break its network with various social elites whose wealth and power gave it continuous patronage. Unlike European homeopathy, which was predominantly eclectic in theory and practice, American homeopathy acted on a spiritual rather than material level, creating a distinct identity as well as a cadre of believers willing to nurture and promote its metaphysical traits against the claims of materialistic science.

It is perhaps relevant to note the convergence of several nonmedical tendencies that began in the 1830s and extended into the second half of the century. These included a steady erosion of Calvinism; the progressive secularization of thought, particularly with the impact of science and technology; the influence of European philosophy and literature; the emergence of a Unitarian and liberal Christian culture; and a more critical approach to conventional wisdom. Just as Christian rites, miracles, creeds, and theology were tested and rejected by liberal and orthodox Christians alike, so too did age-old axioms of medicine lose their relevance among an increasing number of families attuned to the newer forces of individualism and free inquiry.

Homeopathy met this crisis of faith by building a more personal and intuitive belief in healing that was urban, feminized, individuated, and spiritual. It presented itself as a new "romantic" medicine that healed the body as well as the soul; reassured Americans that the universe remained governed by laws; offered a cohesive worldview to offset the fragmentation of the body that came with the newer laboratory sciences; and reinforced habits of purity, benevolence, hygiene, and self-control. As a school or philosophy, homeopathy was optimistic, sympathetic, and respectful of personal and public restraint; it relieved fears and anxieties and restored faith in the natural order of things. It offered both an individual and a cosmic optimism that was far from static. Although laws were eternal and immutable, they gave life a spiritual energy capable of growth, adjustment, and survival. An ameliorative mood in homeopathic thinking stressed leadership by educated persons, fair-mindedness in their dealings, philanthropic stewardship, middle-class sensibilities, and good republicanism.

To be sure, populist medical sects such as the Thomsonians and eclectics had succeeded in challenging orthodox medicine's therapeutic superiority as well as its economic status through a series of anti-monopoly laws that removed the privileges of licensing. Nevertheless, the discordance evident in the orthodox medical journals of the day seemed not to capture the more rigorous medical training occurring abroad and the dismantling of medicine's rationalistic systems for a more empirically based system of therapeutics. Amid the cacophony of heightened competition, low standards of proprietary medical education, and professional disunity, regular medicine was shifting its professional identity to one based on clinical research, educational reform, the role of nature in healing, and a heightened appreciation of scientific knowledge. In other words, at a time when regular medicine was facing a decline in its power and status, it was also seeking to transform itself from a highly individualized "art" to a more standardized "science" based on objectified disease and statistical models that minimized differences among patients. What gave homeopathy its perceived strength during these tumultuous years was its image of heightening patient distinctiveness through symptomatology and highly individualized therapies and focusing on patient care and professional judgment. Homeopathy's message was simple: that alone among the schools of medicine, it had remained true to the needs of the patient.

Homeopathy had a particular appeal among middle- and upper-class American families. For one thing, being statistically among society's more educated, these families tended to be more cognizant of the expressions of doubt evident in the literature concerning the use of bloodletting, calomel, tartar emetic, and other depletive regimens. Among those of German, English, and French extraction, Hahnemann was someone who, in the respected tradition of Protestantism, had challenged orthodoxy with a simpler set of rules that were grounded in pharmacology and symptomatology rather than in the vagaries of "constitutional" therapeutics. Like Reformation religion, homeopathy carried within its belief system a degree of plasticity that allowed practitioners to find comfort at all points on the therapeutic scale. Those who were inclined to simple, uncomplicated beliefs could follow the basic homeopathic laws of *similia,* small (but not infinitesimal) doses, and single remedies. For them, healing became a matter of medical science and the superiority of a particular set of underlying materialistic rules and relationships. On the other hand, those who were more philosophical in nature and drawn to an idealistic worldview found Hahnemann's sojourn into vitalism a jumping-off point into a world of dynamization and the interplay of body, mind, and spirit. For them, homeopathy became a metaphysical healing system whose beliefs blended more easily with America's liberal religious tradition than with its medical establishment. Healing became a profoundly religious and philosophical experience that shunned the causal role of organic or material factors in the etiology of disease. The language of these high dilutionists conceptualized healing in terms of causal forces that operated on the frontier between physics and metaphysics where health, spirituality, immanence, healing, nature, nutrition, consciousness, and happiness were reconciled in a new reality. Ultimately, American homeopathy was not so much *ir*regular as it was *un*orthodox—a status that was wholly acceptable within the country's Reformationist tradition in that it represented a commitment to both science and spirituality.

This history of academic homeopathy attempts to answer a number of pertinent questions: How did the state of medicine in the early nineteenth century facilitate the acceptance of Hahnemann's theories? When and how did Hahnemann's theory of dynamization emerge from his earlier principles and how did it play upon the school's internal and external relations? How and why did Hahnemann's view of *vis medicatrix naturae* change over time? What was the special affinity between homeopathy and Christian religion, especially Swedenborgianism? How did homeopathy relate to other reform movements? What were the tensions between academic and domestic homeopathy? How did homeopathic medical schools emerge and what were their regional and philosophical distinctions? How different were the public and private images of homeopathy and regular medicine and how did they accommodate each other over time? What was the impact of scientific medicine on both homeopathy and liberal regular medicine? What accounted for the growing division between the liberal wing of homeopathy and the more conservative Hahnemannians and what effect did this have on the homeopathic movement?

Homeopathy was attractive to nineteenth-century Americans, due in no small measure to its compatibility with the culture's open-ended view of healing; the influence of unlicensed lay healers, family networks, and patient-to-patient recommendations; and its compelling explanation for a single set of governing principles and a nonmaterial cause of disease. The easy availability of home manuals, self-help guides, and self-medication, along with a cultural propensity to view sectarianism with a greater degree of acceptance, added to its popularity in American culture. Nevertheless, the focus of this study is on academic homeopathy that, until brought to its knees by Abraham Flexner's polemical *Medical Education in the United States and Canada* (1910) and the rigorous efforts of the Association of American Medical Colleges and the American Medical Association's Council on Medical Education, competed successfully with regular medicine by assembling numerous national, regional, and local societies as well as an impressive array of journals, schools, hospitals, and dispensaries. When, in the early decades of the nineteenth century, regular medicine shifted from an emphasis on rationalistic system theories to clinical and laboratory science, academic homeopathy held back, choosing instead a bifurcated course that took many of its members far afield. Divided by ideological differences over the spiritual-versus-material definitions of vitality and force, and dogged by internecine feuds (including the definition of science and the importance of dogma in an increasingly undogmatic medical environment), academic homeopathy eventually defaulted on its educational mission and was forced to turn over to regular medicine its remaining schools and, in essence, its future.

Chapter 1

The Sage of Cöthen

Although most of medicine's critics stayed within the boundaries of orthodoxy, a few chose routes that took them far from the medical mainstream. Typically, these individuals placed greater value on making a break from the past than holding to its threads, however fragile. Samuel Christian Friedrich Hahnemann (1755-1843), the founder of homeopathy, was just such an apostate, born in Meissen, a small village northwest of Dresden in the state of Saxony. Little is known of his grammar education, but by the age of twelve he was identified as a pupil with exceptional abilities, particularly in languages. Informed that Samuel was a gifted student, his father, at first hesitant, eventually allowed him to further his studies at a private school under the gratuitous instruction of rector Magister Müller, a teacher in languages and German composition.[1]

In 1775, at the age of twenty, Samuel Hahnemann left home with a proficiency in eight languages and his father's blessing to pursue the study of medicine in Leipzig. He supported himself during his two-year residence by teaching German and French. This, plus income from translating medical and philosophical works into German, paid his expenses. During this time, Hahnemann translated John Steadman's *Physiological Essays* (*Physiologische Versuche und Beobachtungen,* 1777), Christopher Nugent's *An Essay on Hydrophobia* (*Versush über die Wasserschaden,* 1777), and John Ball's *Modern Practice of Physic* (*Neuere Heilkunst,* 1777-1780), among others.[2]

Since the University of Leipzig provided no clinical training, and given the freedom students had in their learning *(Lernfreiheit),* Hahnemann transferred to Vienna in 1777 where medical education was taught on a model developed by Gerhard van Swieten (1700-1772). German universities would later undergo a massive transformation in the inductive sciences, but the early postings of academic freedom and autonomy and the breakdown of rigid curricula were already under way in the early decades of the century.

Enhanced by an intellectual climate that was highly philosophical and speculative, Hahnemann experienced a sense of freedom and excitement in his disciplines that translated easily into a temperament conducive to asking big questions (e.g., the nature of disease) and challenging tradition and authority.

At Leipzig, Hahnemann worked under the guidance of Dr. Joseph von Quarin (1733-1814), physician to Maria Theresa and the Emperor Joseph of Austria. Quarin adopted the young student as his protégé and Hahnemann practiced at the hospital of the Brothers of Charity. "To him," admitted Hahnemann, "I owe my claims to be reckoned a physician. . . . He loved and instructed me as if I had been his only pupil."[3] Because of his persistent financial difficulties, Hahnemann used Quarin's friendship to obtain an appointment as medical attendant and librarian to Baron von Bruckenthal of Hermannstadt, governor of Transylvania. This sinecure afforded him sufficient leisure to continue his studies, practice medicine, and improve his language skills. Here he became a deist and Freemason, joining the Lodge of St. Andrew of the Three Lotuses. Hahnemann left Hermannstadt for the University of Erlangen where he continued to attend lectures, defended his dissertation titled "A Consideration of the Etiology and Therapeutics of Spasmodic Affections," and, at the age of twenty-four, took his doctor of medicine degree on August 10, 1779.[4]

Following three years residence in Gommern, and several more in Leipzig, Hahnemann wrote an account of his experiences as a practitioner, beginning with reflections on his medical education and the absence of any overriding principle to guide practice. Scanning the literature, he was struck by the falseness of existing medical systems and grew increasingly troubled over the type of medicine practiced by himself and his peers, concluding correctly that contemporary medicine was too uncertain to be scientific. He also directed his attention to the known medicines that had been handed down from one generation of doctors to another and concluded that they were too ineffective to cure patients of their ills. Moreover, remedies were little understood and frequently left pernicious results. Hahnemann confessed years later to Christoph Wilhelm Hufeland (1762-1836), a reform-minded teacher, professor, physician, and publisher:

It was painful for me to grope in the dark, guided only by our books, in the treatment of the sick. . . . To become in this way a murderer or aggrevator of the sufferings of my brethren of mankind, was to me a fearful thought.[5]

Hahnemann became so obsessed with the poor state of medical therapeutics that he abandoned practice and moved to Dresden where he made his living translating books and writing medical essays on such subjects as syphilis, scrofulous sores, wine purity, and the toxicology of arsenic. He also tried his hand at producing proprietary medicines.[6] In 1790, he translated the 1789 edition of William Cullen's popular *Materia Medica,* originally published in 1773.[7] Fascinated with Cullen's description of the virtues of Peruvian bark or cinchona *(Cortex peruvianis)* but finding unsatisfactory the explanation for its power in checking intermittent fever, Hahnemann decided to experiment with the medicine on himself, taking four drams of the bark twice a day. Such experimentation was common practice among botanics and empirics as well as among medical teachers; Danish surgeon Georg Ernst Stahl (1660-1734), physiologist Albrecht von Haller (1708-1777) of the University of Gottingen, and Anton Stoerck (1731-1803) of Swabia were known to test medicines on themselves before prescribing them to avoid the error of confounding pathological with mere medicinal symptoms. Nor was it unusual for Hahnemann to include the results of his experiments within the text of the books he translated. His translations typically contained scores of footnotes giving further perspective on the text, its author, and his own observations.[8]

Remembering cases in which the symptoms produced by taking certain poisons in health were similar to the symptoms of certain diseases, Hahnemann wondered whether a medicine that produced an artificial disease in a healthy person could have the power to cure a disease with similar symptoms. If this could be demonstrated, he reasoned, then it might be possible to remove the uncertainty and empiricism that for so long had dominated medicine and provide the missing principle or law he had been seeking since his days in medical school. Curious by nature and anxious to improve the practice of medicine, having studied the systems of Thomas Sydenham (1624-1689), Friedrich Hoffmann (1660-1742), Hermann Boerhave (1668-1738), Hieronymus Gaubius (1705-1780), Georg Ernst Stahl (1660-1734), William Cullen (1710-1790), and Anton de Haen (1704-1776), Hahnemann found himself lured by the prospect of somehow finding another of nature's great secrets—like the discoveries of Sir Isaac Newton (1642-1727) and Galileo (1564-1642).[9]

Proceeding on this hypothesis, Hahnemann administered repeated doses of the bark (later known as "China" in the homeopathic lexicon) on himself and discovered that it produced symptoms similar to those of malarial or intermittent fever *(Wechselfieber)* he had observed eight years earlier. He described the symptoms in great detail and recorded them in special notebooks—a procedure that became known as *provings.* Hahnemann chose the word to demonstrate that he was providing the truth, in other words what actions a substance could produce. From this he surmised that diseases might be most safely cured by medicines capable of inducing in healthy persons symptoms similar to those of the disease. It is important to note that, like many of his contemporaries, Hahnemann ridiculed nature's healing power, believing the self-help efforts of the organism to be insufficient, crude, irrational, and inappropriate.[10] Hahnemann discounted the body's inherent forces as not only dubious but also injurious to health. By itself, nature could not effect the body's own cure. Disease could only be displaced through another artificial disease that provoked a symptom complex similar to the original disease. According to Hahnemann,

> The pitiable and highly imperfect efforts of the vital force to relieve itself in acute diseases is a spectacle that should excite our compassion and command the aid of our rational mind, to terminate the self-inflicted torture by a real cure.[11]

Setting aside the self-help efforts of nature, or *vis medicatrix naturae,* Hahnemann acted on the principle that when two similar diseases met in any individual, the weaker would give way to the stronger. Hence, by imitating nature and substituting a stronger medicinal disease for that which had arisen from common cause, a physician could repulse the weaker and return the body to health.[12] Cinchona became Hahnemann's first homeopathic remedy, and over the next six years he and friends continued with experiments on fifty different medicines, confirming what Hahnemann had discovered from his original test, namely that cinchona's power resided in its ability to produce symptoms similar to disease in a healthy person. Before long, he began to suspect that he had discovered a law which might revolutionize therapeutic practice.[13] The conjunction of Hahnemann's agnostic feelings concerning orthodox medical practices and his newfound faith in symptoms caused him to put aside the incomplete findings of anatomy, physiology, and pathology, and strike a bargain between symptomatology and medicaments. For the new reform physician, the symptoms of diseases were all that were to be regarded; and of remedies, only specifics were to be employed. He thus rejected nosology, or the classification of diseases, and instead placed his faith in treatments based on the patient's most prominent symptoms.[14]

In 1796, six years after his experiment with cinchona, Hahnemann used Hufeland's *Journal of Practical Medicine* to announce his further objections to current practice. In his "Essay on a New Principle for Ascertaining the Curative Power of Drugs, with a Few Glances at Those Hitherto Employed," Hahnemann took issue with mixing more than one medicine in prescriptions because doing so prevented the ability to determine the efficacy or force of a particular substance. "Let us make a brotherly compact and all agree to give our patients but one substance at a time," he urged on his colleagues, "and then we shall see with our eyes what medicine can do, and what it cannot." In the meantime, Hahnemann dissented from the popular view that the living body was little more than a chemical laboratory and objected as well to building medical systems from the "chance hits" of "uncertain empirical experiments." Neither medicine nor the health of the individual should be "so precariously established." Instead, he stressed the importance of "design" in perfecting the institutes of medicine.[15]

Hahnemann used Hufeland's journal to caution against adding to the number of remedies before learning the virtues and exact powers of the existing materia medica. Nor should doctors waste their time searching for specific remedies for diseases. Instead, they should pay attention to the characteristics of the morbid action itself, and when they had identified all of the observable symptoms of the disease, they had, in fact, discovered the disease itself.[16] "Although there are not specific medicines for individual diseases," he reasoned, "yet for every particular phase of disease there is a specific remedy." For too long, doctors had determined to fight disease by suppressing the existing symptoms with the use of medicines that produced an opposite condition, better known as *contraria contrariis curantur.* In situations of acute disease, these remedies were often proper; but when

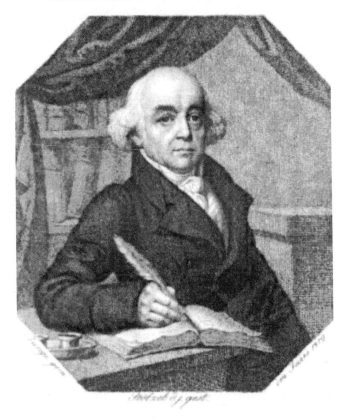

Samuel Hahnemann (1819). (*Source:* Courtesy of the National Library of Medicine.)

doctors prescribed these same means to address chronic disease, Hahnemann deemed them irresponsible. "I hesitate not to call it— palliative, dangerous, destructive," he wrote. Such was the road to ruin of many a "proud empiric."[17] Better for doctors to undertake a rational understanding of medicines, leaving little to empiricism and chance discoveries. True, much had been achieved through accidental discovery; however, physicians should take a more methodological approach: not empirical trials made in hospitals using sick patients, but trials using healthy individuals. Physicians should not only learn the effects, or drug force, of each medicine (and in what dosage) on a healthy person but also determine what practical implications could be drawn from these observations. From this effort, "a complete collection of such [drug] histories . . . would form the grand code of our Materia Medica."[18]

Every medical substance was a form of poison that produced in the human organism a peculiar kind of disease; and the more powerful the substance, the more violent the disease. To discover the appropriate medicine for a specific disease, it was first necessary to find the specific *artificial* disease it created in the healthy human organism and then employ the medicine for a similar morbid condition. Having earlier observed that large doses of Peruvian bark produced a "true attack of fever, very similar to the intermittent fever," Hahnemann deduced that the same medicine "overpowers, and thus cures" the intermittent fever. This became Hahnemann's principle of *similia similibus curantur,* or like cures like.[19]

With this principle of similars, to which he gave the name Nature's Law, Hahnemann claimed the key to the true art of healing. The creation of a similar, more powerful artificial disease overpowered or displaced the disease in the sick patient. None of this was new, or even revolutionary, except Hahnemann's provings of medicines on the healthy body. The assumption that an artificial disease would extinguish the diseased condition in the body was one of several a priori principles held by earlier theorists in Western medicine as justification for their bleeding, blistering, puking, purging, and sweating regimens. But here, too, was the breakthrough Hahnemann needed to understand how a specific medicine affected disease.[20] He urged colleagues to abandon the principle of *contraria contrariis curantur* in diseases, arguing that it was "the deceitful by-path in the dark forces that lead to the fatal swamp."[21] Not surprisingly, when Hahnemann announced the Galenic principle of *contraria contrariis* to be in error and *similia similibus* to be the *only* true therapeutic law, his reputation fell among many of the very people who had once admired his reform zeal. Nevertheless, those who supported Hahnemann's principle regarded it as equal in stature to Newton's Law of Gravity, Harvey's demonstration of the circulation of the blood and the nonexistence of air in the arteries, and Jenner's principle of vaccination.[22]

Hahnemann's contributions came at a time when German medical education had been heavily sedated with the ideological, metaphysical, and highly romantic notions of the nature-philosophers *(Naturphilosophen).* Whether addressing the imaginative speculations of the transcendental naturalist and philosopher Lorenz Oken (1779-1851), the scientist and philosopher Carl Gustav Carus (1789-1869), or the philosopher Friedrich W. J. Schelling (1775-1854) who studied at Leipzig and taught at the universities of Erlangen, Munich, and Berlin, the views of Germany's scientific community were remarkably consistent. Far from savoring objective science, they sought to devise laws or principles that would explain and compel an all-controlling unity in nature. In this idealistic philosophy, a correspondence between nature and mind ensured a timeless and unchanging coherence to the diversity of organic creation. Ideal archetypes, not unlike Plato's eternal ideas, stood as guideposts amidst the play of nature's forces, offering to reconcile any passing discrepancies. This dynamic, spiritual, and vitalistic view of nature and its postulate of an overarching "force" remained in place for nearly a half century before succumbing to the rigid reductionism of Germany's newer generation of investigative scientists.[23]

Between 1797 and 1801, Hahnemann published several additional articles in Hufeland's *Journal of Practical Medicine*. Reflective of the notions expressed by the nature-philosophers, Hahnemann explained the dangers of large doses, noting that the Creator operated his grand designs by the "simplest machinery." Surely, remedies were part of God's design in that "each possesses a certain power, through the right employment of which in small doses, great and many cures might be effected."[24] Strong medicines and mischievous measures only blinded the eye of the physician to the true needs of the patient. Just as nature worked by eternal laws and simplicity, so doctors should imitate nature by simple principles and faithful adherence to laws. This meant giving one medicine at a time and withholding additional doses or other medicines until the effects of the first had manifested.[25] Since symptoms most often proceeded from a single cause, physicians should proceed with a single drug that would encompass most symptoms.[26]

In 1801, Hahnemann used Hufeland's *Journal of Practical Medicine* to critique John Brown's *Elements of Medicine*, poking fun at the author's polypharmacy and his boast of having reduced the art of medicine to an exact science. Hahnemann accused Brown of being a "scholastic pedant" who "plume[d] himself . . . on his logical forms." Brown's theory of sthenic and asthenic diseases captured Europe's attention for a quarter century but, according to Hahnemann, Brown had looked only to the initial action of his favorite remedies (opium and alcohol) and ignored their aftereffects. This characteristic, so hotly criticized by Hahnemann, became the basis for his use of the shibboleth "Old School" to identify orthodox medicine.[27] Hufeland, who published Hahnemann's critique and joined in attacking Brown's therapeutic ideas and methods, praised Hahnemann as "one of the most distinguished of German physicians"—a physician of "matured experience and reflection."[28]

In 1805, the same year botanic entrepreneur Samuel Thomson (1769-1843) introduced his patented medical system into New Hampshire, Vermont, and Massachusetts, the German medical profession and public were being drawn to Hahnemann's method of treatment through the publication of two major works: the pamphlet *Aesculapius in the Balance,* and a two-volume *Fragmenta de Viribus Medicamentorum Positivis Sive in sano Corpore Humano Observatis.* In *Aesculapius in the Balance,* published at Leipzig, Hahnemann reported that, having discovered the errors of earlier medical teachers, he became disgusted with the study of medicine and resolved to address it forthright. He began once again by reasoning a priori that the Divine Spirit would not have permitted disease to exist without providing the means for lessening or removing it. To this end, the records of nearly every physician, including the "most egregious blockheads," recounted instances of rapid and effectual cures, even in some of the most difficult cases where death seemed imminent. Knowing great cures were possible, the challenge was to learn how, and by what power, physicians could accomplish their feats.[29]

Most cases for which a physician was called were acute diseases that ran a short duration before terminating in recovery or death. Some patients died from acute diseases whether they took medicine or not. In truth, argued Hahnemann, numerous patients had been cured "not only by refusing the physician's medicine, but by secretly transgressing his artificial and often mischievous system of diet."[30] Chronic diseases were more of a challenge. Here, argued Hahnemann, Old School physicians demonstrated the true ineffectiveness of their medical systems. "How does it happen that, in the thirty-five centuries since Aesculapius lived, this so indispensable art of medicine has made so little progress?" Hahnemann asked. "What the physicians have already done is not one-hundredth part of what they might and ought to have done." Medicine was never nearer to true science than when Hippocrates saw and described diseases with the faculty of pure observation. The only thing he lacked was the knowledge and application of medicines. Since the days of Hippocrates, however, medicine had embraced all manner of postulates and succumbed to the wiles of the system builders with their harmful regimens.[31]

In his two-volume *Fragmenta de Viribus Medicamentorum Positivis Sive in sano Corpore Humano Observatis,* published in 1805, Hahnemann provided a useful index, identifying each symptom produced by medicines on the healthy body. This first collection of provings included *Aconitum napellus,* acris tinctura, *Arnica montana, Atropa belladonna, Laurus camphora, Chamomilla matricaria, Cinchona officinalis, Digitalis purpurea,* Ipecacuanha, *Helleborus niger,* and *Veratrum album.* Later, in 1834, Dr. Frederick H. F. Quin (1799-1878), a pupil of Hahnemann and England's first homeopath, would condense the work into a single volume.[32]

A year later, in a pamphlet titled "The Medicine of Experience" (1806) published in Berlin (and a forerunner of his later *Organon of the Healing Art*), Hahnemann laid down his first maxim: when two dissimilar diseases acted on the body, the action of the weaker would be suppressed by the stronger for a time; on the other hand, when two similar diseases acted on the body, the weaker disease, together with its effects, were extinguished by the stronger. Doctors could never attain complete knowledge of the internal changes on which diseases depended; they could only identify through observation the external exciting causes or symptoms. Only by producing in the healthy body a series of morbid symptoms could they know which medicines would extinguish a specific disease.[33]

For several years, Hahnemann had talked of using specific remedies for specific symptoms. This belief, viewed as gross empiricism, incurred the wrath of Old School doctors who typically prescribed their medicines on the basis of effecting change over the patient's *general* constitution. Dissatisfied with his own reasoning, Hahnemann looked to vitalism to find the answer. Disease, he argued, represented a derangement of the body's vital principle or force, which itself was invisible but verifiable by the body's morbid disturbances. This explained why it was so important to analyze symptoms; however, it was equally important not to confuse symptoms with the disease itself. What we understand of life, explained Hahnemann in

1809, can only be obtained empirically from its phenomena and manifestations. No conception of it could be reasoned a priori. What life really is, in its essential nature, "can never be ascertained nor even guessed at, by mortals." Life was in no respect regulated by physical laws; rather, it was regulated by laws "peculiar to *vitality* alone" (italics mine). It followed, therefore, that the exciting causes of disease acted in a dynamic manner on the body's state of life (vital force) and health. Diseases were "dynamical derangements" of the organism's vital force, and the power to remove them came only from agents that were capable of producing a similar derangement of the healthy body. Diseases were cured only by those active substances that dynamically altered the body in its healthy state. It stood to reason, then, that "the same power of the medicine that cures the disease in the sick [gave] rise to the morbid symptoms in the healthy."[34]

Convinced of his newfound principle, Hahnemann disregarded the ordinary treatments of medical practice—purgatives, cooling drinks, solvents, antispasmodics, sedatives, narcotics, general stimulants, general diuretics, diaphoretics, rubefacients, leeches, cupping glasses, issues, and other general therapeutic appliances.[35] He had at last begun to see his principle in a larger light. For too long medicine had operated on opinions, with each physician acting in accord with the manner he was taught or "as his fancy dictates," and each found an infinite number of opinions and authorities on whom to base his decision. "The medical art stands in need of a thorough reform from head to foot," he proclaimed. "The evil has become so crying that the well-meaning mildness of a John Huss no longer avails, but the fiery zeal of a rock-firm Martin Luther is needed to sweep away the monstrous leaven."[36] Rather than regard his work as an alternative to medical orthodoxy, he saw himself as the defender of true medicine. At long last, Hahnemann had found his vocation.

ORGANON *AND THE* MATERIA MEDICA PURA

Organon

Hahnemann carried out his provings over a period of twenty-five years, but not until 1810, at the mature age of fifty-five, did he give a full exposition of his principles in 271 aphorisms (later increased to

294). He chose the title *Organon of the Rational Art of Healing (Organon der Rationellen Heilkunde)* after English philosopher Francis Bacon's *Novum Organum* (1620), which replaced the deductive logic of Aristotle with the inductive method of ascertaining truth. Subsequent editions were titled simply *Organon of Medicine, Organon of Homeopathic Medicine,* or *Organon of the Healing Art.* To be sure, Hahnemann's *Organon* was no attempt to reconcile with his critics. Although regulars viewed it as the cant of German mysticism and treated it with silence, the book represented Hahnemann's boldest effort yet to set forth his beliefs. With revolutionary intent, he wrote as a true protestant, bitter in his persecution and inflammatory in his denunciation of Old School doctors and apothecaries.[37]

The *Organon* represented the best thinking of Hahnemann's earlier writings and provided a fuller explanation of his general law of similars; gave directions for the use of medicines, the amount of dose, and the propriety of their repetition; and instructed physicians on how they might detail their cases, paying strict attention to symptomatology. He also challenged the imperfect manner in which orthodox medicine had approached disease. Although founded initially on scientific principles, he accused Old School medicine of having formed an "obscure and imaginary picture" of disease.[38] Convinced that the human body contained a plethora or superfluous quantity of blood, doctors had prescribed bleeding, cupping, and leeching regimens that deprived patients of the essential vitality necessary for existence. Instead of administering small doses of aconite to reduce an inflammatory condition, they bled until syncope. Similarly, they produced artificial ulcers (issues and setons) or blisters (cantharides) to draw off morbid or peccant matter from the chest and lungs. "But the essence of diseases, and their cure," Hahnemann reasoned, "will not bend to our fancies and convenience." The true causes of disease were not material but "dynamic aberrations" in the body's state of health.[39]

Hahnemann identified three distinct systems of medical treatment: (1) *allopathic* or *heteropathic;* (2) *antipathic, enantiopathic,* or *palliative;* and (3) *homeopathic.* The *allopathic* (from the Greek *alloion,* meaning "different"; and *pathos,* meaning "suffering") system, in use from the earliest times to the present, employed derivative, revulsive, and counterirritant methods for attacking disease by creating a dissimilar artificial disease in the healthy parts of the body (usually on the body's surface), and drawing the disease from its original source to the skin where it could be treated topically. Thus, an allopath could attack an internal pain, fever, or oppression with the application of a warm poultice or mustard plaster on the body's surface. In the *antipathic* mode, the physician prescribed a medicine known to produce an opposite effect *(contraria contrariis curantur)* from the original symptom. Examples included administering opium for pain; purgatives for constipation; or cold water for burns. Hahnemann surmised that the antipathic method had been the first system tested by humankind, guided by experience, primitive reasoning, and the principle of antagonism. But after a short spate of relief, the patient's condition invariably worsened, leaving the body in a more desperate condition. This was particularly true of electricity and galvanism, which doctors had recently begun using to restore feeble and paralyzed limbs. These temporary palliatives ended with the destruction of muscular irritability and even paralysis.[40]

Other Old School doctors tried to imitate the self-help aspect of nature, or *vis medicatrix naturae,* by applying what they termed *derivatives* thought to imitate nature by forcing a *crisis* in the disordered system and then allowing the powers of nature to take control.[41] Notwithstanding the theoretical differences between the derivative and counterirritant schools of medicine, both applied the same regimen of forced evacuations that weakened and often destroyed the powers of life. By themselves, Hahnemann explained, nature's inner resources brought only temporary relief to a diseased organ by exciting the appearance of an external local symptom, thereby removing the danger from organs that were deemed indispensable to life. These actions were nothing more than nature's palliatives, which stopped short of cure. Everything that nature performed to relieve acute or chronic disease was "highly imperfect."[42] That was because the vital power in a healthy or diseased organism was without intelligence. Therefore, doctors were to avoid following it as a guide in the cure of disease. "What reflecting man," Hahnemann asked rhetorically, "would copy the efforts of nature in curing disease?"[43]

Despite these failed systems, certain earlier physicians stood apart from their peers by proposing the use of medicines that excited symptoms on the healthy body resembling those of the disease. Notable examples included John Hunter (1728-1793), Georg Christoph Detharding (1671-1747), Anton Stoerck, and the Danish physician Georg Ernst Stahl, who suggested that diseases were most effectively subdued by agents which produced a similar affection: treating burns with heat, frostbite with cold water, and inflammations with alcohol and other spirituous applications.[44] For this mode of treatment, Hahnemann introduced the term *homeopathy* (from the Greek *homoios,* meaning "similar" or "analogous"; and *pathos,* meaning "feeling" or "suffering") to distinguish from *allopathy.* The former used medicines that produced effects analogous to the disease (i.e., purgatives in diarrhea) while the latter prescribed medicines that produced effects contrary to the disease (i.e., cold to burns, blisters to local inflammations, or acid to correct an alkali).[45]

When dealing with the particulars of a disease, Hahnemann responded no differently than regular physicians by taking into consideration the patient's constitution, disposition, occupation, mode of life, age, and habits. But unlike Old School physicians, he argued that the totality of symptoms constituted "the true and only form of [the disease] that the mind is capable of conceiving." Since it was impossible for the physician to see or understand the immaterial "spiritual essence" or "vital power" that produced the disease, it was enough to know its outward signs or symptoms and to treat them accordingly. Thus, physicians were to direct the power of their art at the totality of symptoms ("symptom complex") visible to the patient and physician.[46] This was the outward expression of the disease, perceptible to the senses. The precise manner in which the vital principle produced these symptoms was irrelevant to Hahnemann. Such questions "will forever remain unanswered." To the watchful eyes and senses of a physician, however, no curable disease failed to make itself known through certain discernable symptoms. Once again, this was an a priori assumption that Hahnemann held to be consistent with the Creator's infinite goodness. Although he did not attribute to diseases a metaphysical explanation, he did insist that, except for those belonging to surgery, diseases were due solely to spiritual or dynamic changes to the vital principle and not to any mechanical or chemical changes in the organism. Therefore, insofar as the injured vital principle that animated the living body was itself immaterial, it required a spiritual or dynamic agency to restore the body's health and harmony.[47]

In choosing an appropriate medicine, Hahnemann instructed physicians to identify the one whose effects on the healthy body most closely resembled the disease symptoms. Believing that no two substances acted exactly the same on the healthy body, he encouraged doctors to learn the peculiarities of each medicine by experimenting on themselves and on other healthy individuals. The medicine thus chosen would "inoculate" the patient with an artificial disease ("counter-disease") resembling the natural one, affecting the same parts of the body that had been affected by the natural disease. Because the artificial disease created by the remedy was supposedly more intense, it substituted itself for the natural disease, which disappeared. After the vital or spiritual principle was activated to repel the invader, the medicinal disease disappeared, leaving the body free from the debilitating effects of the natural disease.[48]

Hahnemann urged doctors to administer their medicines in simple, unadulterated form, in powder, alcoholic tincture, or in water. Infusions of plants in water were to be prepared and administered without delay to avoid fermentation. Every drug was to be given in its purest form, alone, and without the addition of any other substance. Healthy persons were to take it on a strict diet and pay close attention to its effects.[49] A materia medica that left little to conjecture required many observers accounting for each and every symptom complex. Only then would the art of medicine "no longer be mocked as an art of conjecture lacking all foundation."[50]

In his doctor-patient relations, Hahnemann not only expected his more educated patients to have read the *Organon* but also required them to assume a significant degree of personal responsibility in the treatment phase of their illnesses. The role played by the patient was more active than passive, characterized by an obligation to fulfill specific functions before, during, and after treatment. For example, Hahnemann placed great importance on diet during treatment to ensure that foods did not adversely influence the effect of the medicine. To accomplish this, he forbade intake of coffee, spices, and carbonated waters during treatment, as well as use of perfumes. Patients should eat and drink only that which sustained life. Each acute disease had its own specific dietetic rules, while chronic diseases had more general ones. For chronic disease, patients avoided all foods of a stimulating character. Foods allowed included beef, mutton, lean ham, venison, chicken, fresh fish, mild cheese, raw or soft-boiled eggs, bread, biscuits (except soda biscuits), puddings, noodles, rice, oatmeal, tapioca, farina, potatoes, turnips, carrots, tomatoes, dried peas, fresh or dried fruit, water, jelly, milk, ice cream, and moderate amounts of salt. Forbidden foods included smoked meat and fish, rancid butter or cheese, duck, turtle, catfish, lobster, crab, and clams; any foods prepared with blood or large amounts of animal fat; sausages; spicy sauces and soups; pastries and all kinds of confectioner sugar products; radishes, celery, onions, garlic, parsley, cayenne pepper, mustard, vanilla, bitter almonds, cloves, cinnamon, fennel, anise, coffee, green tea, and spiced chocolate; all spirituous liquors, mineral waters, and herb teas; tooth powders with aromatic substances; and inhaling the vapor of sulfur matches. Hahnemann even directed patients to avoid excessive labor, "debauches," and "mental excitement."[51]

Coffee posed a particular challenge and, in an article on its effects published in 1803, Hahnemann explained that the drink was purely medicinal. "No healthy person ever drank unsugared black coffee for the first time in his life with gusto," he argued. The results were immediate and obvious. This example, he felt, should have been warning enough not to transgress the laws of health. However, when coffee became fashionable, it lost its medicinal properties.[52] Coffee initially brought strength and "nobility of mind," but it soon turned to debility, nervous affections, melancholy, irresolution, cowardly acts, and malicious envy. Every coffee imbiber faced the prospect of "degeneration" in mind and body. Indulgence led eventually to leucorrhoea, impotence, sterility, onanism, acute pains, caries of the bones, destruction of the teeth, rickets, imperfect sleep, stammering, and a multitude of other problems and impediments.[53] If coffee were allowed during homeopathic treatment, it was only on the assurance that the patient would drink it in "great moderation," and only for those who had consumed it over a long period of time. The same held true of snuff, chewing, and smoking tobacco; hemp leaves and opium; and several kinds of stimulating drinks, including brandy, beer, and tea.[54]

With respect to the homeopathic remedy itself, Hahnemann pointed out that "even the very smallest dose" always caused an "aggravation" in the first hours of its administration. For that reason, he allowed no second dose until careful consideration had been given to the effects of the first. "Every improvement in an acute or a chronic disease, however small it be, . . . is a condition which absolutely forbids any further administration of any medicine as long as it lasts," he wrote. Some remedies exhausted their power in hours; others took days and even weeks to complete their full effect. In some chronic diseases of many years standing, repeat doses were not to be given for three to six months, and each successive dose was to be smaller than that which preceded it. Nevertheless, every true homeopathic dose surpassed, in some degree, however small, the intensity of the disease. When the homeopathic medication took effect, its causative action subsided or displaced the natural disease.[55]

Interestingly, Hahnemann claimed the diseased body was so extraordinarily sensitive that the smallest dose of an appropriate homeopathically prepared remedy could overcome the disease. In fact, a single drop of a tincture added to ninety-nine drops of water and shaken vigorously produced a greater effect on the disease than a single dose of the tincture—so much so that he called the action upon the human body "spirit-like" in its rapidity and completeness. As yet, however, Hahnemann had not begun using the infinitesimal doses with which his reform movement would later be identified. This change in his thinking became evident only in later revisions of his *Organon*.[56]

Following the publication of the *Organon,* Hahnemann's system of medicine spread across Europe through the writings of Moritz Mueller (1784-1849), Johann Ernst Stapf (1788-1860), Gustav W. Gross (1794-1847), Gottlieb Ludwig Rau (1799-1840), and others.[57] The *Organon* went through five authorized editions (1810, 1819, 1824, 1829, 1833) during Hahnemann's lifetime and was translated into French, English, Italian, Spanish, Hungarian, Dutch, Polish, Russian, Danish, and Swedish.[58] The fourth German edition was translated into French and published in Paris and London in 1833 and 1834 by A. J. L. Jourdan, a member of the Academie Royale de Médicine. These editions made their way to the United States and mark a significant period in homeopathy's expansion. An unauthorized edition, published by Ernst Arthur Lutze in 1842, became the focus of serious differences among homeopaths. A sixth authorized edition was finally published in 1921 in Germany and a year later in the United States by Boericke & Tafel of Philadelphia.

Materia Medica Pura

With the *Organon* at last bringing him recognition, Hahnemann returned to Leipzig for the third time, enjoying both fame and notoriety.

It was there that he perfected his *Materia Medica Pura,* publishing the first volume in 1811. Between 1811 and 1821, Hahnemann remained in Leipzig where he published five additional volumes (the second and third volumes in 1816; a fourth in 1818; a fifth in 1819; and his last in 1821), and a second edition of his *Organon.* In all, Hahnemann proved sixty-one remedies himself or under his specific directions.[59] In the third volume of his *Materia Medica Pura,* Hahnemann took up his pen against those who had criticized his first two volumes. "The sophisms of my opponents," he wrote in 1817, "remind me of the squibs which mischievous boys send off to tease people." He insisted that the truth of homeopathy would not fail to "kindle into a flame" the spark of common sense that "still glimmered in the gentlemen of the opposition." This fact, he observed, was evident from "the moanings and lamentations with which they fill their halls and journals about the approaching downfall of their orthodox delusions."[60]

Meanwhile, Hahnemann arranged the pathogenetic symptoms of his medicines into fifty-nine different categories, based upon how those substances affected the body, building a bond between his medicines and the organism. Categories included the face, lips, teeth, throat, taste, genital organs, breath, neck, thighs, complaints in the open air, spasms, fever, changes occurring in the feelings, and affections of the soul. Hahnemann considered every symptom, whether internal or external, whether affecting the mind or the body, essential to proper diagnosis. It was equally important to know when the feeling or symptom occurred—whether in the morning, afternoon, or evening; before or after meals; when walking or at rest; in or out of bed.[61]

Critics found much merriment in the moral symptoms created by the homeopathic materia medica. *Aconitum napellus* left a healthy subject with a sense of peevishness "as if she had no more life in her"; "a desire to sing and dance"; "inconsolable anguish and piteous howling"; "dread of men"; and "apprehension of approaching death."[62] *Ambra grisea* produced "lewd fancies, even when dreaming"; "anxious thoughts"; "great sadness"; and "an indifference to joy or grief." Belladonna produced "weeping and extreme ill humor when waking up from sleep"; "violent quarrelsomeness"; "rage with gnashing of teeth and convulsions"; "wants to bite those around him at night"; "afraid of an imaginary black dog"; and lasciviousness.[64] In the genital organs, chamomile produced itching and "excited sexual desire,"

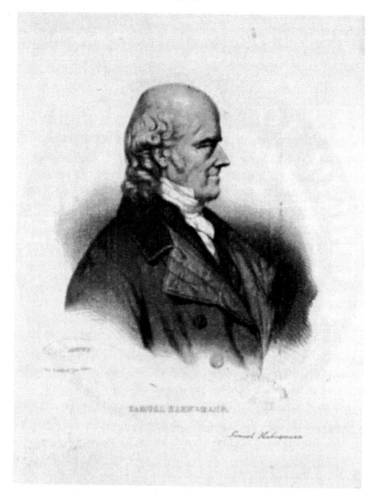

Samuel Hahnemann (1755-1843) by A. Maurir. (*Source:* Courtesy of the National Library of Medicine.)

nightly emissions, and morning erections. Similarly, *Menispermum* produced "itching of the scrotum"; "violent pains in both testicles"; "excitation of the genital organs and desire for an embrace"; and "nightly emission of semen."[65]

Hahnemann realized the convenience of looking upon medicines as "unpolished levers and sweeping machines" rather than as dynamic curative substances. "I cannot reasonably expect that men, accustomed to the routine of materialism, should look upon disease as an immaterial disturbance, and upon medicinal powers as dynamic, or almost spiritual substances," he wrote.[66] But knowing that a single spark from a Leyden jar could shake the strongest man, he reasoned that material notions of substances could not, in themselves, account for the electric and mesmeric powers exercised over a healthy person. Working with an iron bar eight inches in length and placed in contact with a healthy person, he reported symptoms that included anger, aversion to tobacco, burning of the tongue, cold hands, diarrhea, erections, flatulence, headache, indolence, itching of the eyelids, nightly emissions, nose bleeds, ulcers on the lower lip, vertigo, and whistling in the ear. Here could be found a force far more powerful than ordinary material medicinal substances.[67]

In 1813, Hahnemann wrote "The Spirit of the Homeopathic Healing Law" for *Allgemeine Anzeiger der Deutschen* that explained the effects of remedies prescribed according to his law of similars. In 1825, Dr. Hans Burch Gram translated this article to introduce homeopathy to American physicians.[68]

From 1821 to 1835, Hahnemann lived in the relative seclusion of Cöthen. In his senior years, he ceased to enjoy the verbal battles that now distracted a younger generation of followers. Having completed much of his life's work, gaining international recognition for his doctrines and provings, he retired to a peaceful life in a rural village where he carried on extensive correspondence with disciples, patients, and friends.[69] During this time, many of Hahnemann's former pupils stepped forward to lead the reform movement. These included Carl Haubold and Moritz Mueller in Leipzig; Carl F. Trinks, Wilhelm Lux, and Paul Wolf in Dresden; Gossner in lower Austria; Marenzeller in Prague; S. Vieth in Vienna; George Necker and Francis Koller in Naples; and Frederick H. F. Quin and Paul F. Curie in England. They experimented in drug treatments, enriching the record with new provings, clinical cases, and practical information, and began advancing their own ideas and methods.[70] At this time, too, the Leipzig authorities granted homeopathic physicians the right to dispense medicines, a sign of the reform movement's increased power and recognition.[71] Doctors Gustav W. Gross and Johann Ernst Stapf, two able converts and provers for Hahnemann, published and edited *Archives of Homeopathic Healing (Archiv für die homöopathische*

Heilkunst) from 1822 until 1843. This publication, which took home-opathy beyond the bounds of its inventor and theoretician, was until 1830 the only German journal dedicated to the theory and methods of Hahnemann.[72]

DYNAMIZATION, OR LESS IS MORE

Although preferring the comfort of Cöthen to the strenuous life of a public champion, Hahnemann was by no means inactive; in fact, he now began some of his most controversial work. Between 1825 and 1830, Hahnemann published articles explaining his interest in po-tentization. During this time he also revised the *Organon,* adding sub-stantially to his original principles and contributing significantly to differences among his followers, not to mention to an even greater di-vide between homeopathy and regular medicine.

Early in his practice, Hahnemann, like rival allopaths, prescribed large doses of drugs. Over time, however, his views changed as he ob-served that larger doses often made patients worse, not better. As early as 1813 he began testing gradually reduced amounts by taking the juice of a vegetable substance which he mixed with an equal amount of alcohol, forming what he called a *tinctura fortis.* He then took two drops of the tincture and added ninety-eight drops of alco-hol. After shaking the mixture ten times, he called it the first centesi-mal *potency.* Of this potency he took one drop and put it into another vial with ninety-nine drops of alcohol, shook it, and produced a sec-ond potency; he then repeated the process to achieve still higher po-tencies. With dry substances, he took one grain of a juiceless plant, metal, or mineral, and for one hour vigorously triturated it in a mortar or dish with ninety-nine grains of powdered sugar, and called it the first potency (or first trituration). He repeated this through the third potency, after which he took one grain, dissolved it in ninety-nine drops of a mixture of alcohol and distilled water, and shook it, pro-ducing the fourth potency.[73] Hahnemann claimed that instead of re-ducing the effectiveness of the medicinal substance, the attenuated medicine acquired a pathogenetic or symptom-producing power as well as a disease-curing power many times more effective than the original grain. This led to his pronouncement of the principle of *potentization* or *dynamization*—terms given to effects that could not be understood in chemicophysical terms.[74] At each dilution medicines acquired a new degree of power from the rubbing or shaking they underwent, thereby developing "inherent virtues" heretofore unknown. So energetic were the virtues of these medicines that Hahnemann reduced the number of shakes from ten to two.[75] There was a world of difference, he explained, between a quantity of medicinal substance mixed imperfectly and one that was made "intimately" by means of "a rapid motion by a single powerful stroke of the arm descending." Hahnemann applied the term *succussion* to explain the physical process used to change crude substances into spiritually dynamized medicinal agents.[76]

Like Georg Ernst Stahl before him, Hahnemann formed a spiritualistic conception of disease, regarding it as "the outward expression of an interior derangement of the vital force." This explained Hahnemann's interest in the process by which a substance's medicinal powers were developed in a menstruum, or "neutral medium," where its energy was conserved and then transmitted to the organism.[77] If shaken properly, a neutral menstruum such as water, alcohol, sugar of milk, and even lard could be "medicinalized" by a single drop or grain of medicine. In fact, the true virtues of medicines were obtained only through the "minute mechanical division of their particles." Just as the vital force of a body could be affected by the introduction of a single smallpox pustule, so through chemical, electrical or magnetic forces a vial of alcohol could be medicinalized by a single drop or grain. Doses scarcely thought to be material could exert an impressionable effect on the organism.[78] Homeopaths guaranteed no specific ratio of drug to inert substance, believing that ratios differed with each medicine.[79] For his part, Hahnemann settled on the thirtieth (decillionth) attenuation as the most appropriate dosage in most cases.

From where had this idea of sugar globules and potentization come? Although Hahnemann was very much the product of the eighteenth-century Enlightenment, he was also impressed by the vitalistic ideas of the Romantic school of *Naturphilosophie*. He interpreted the immaterial and dynamic virtues of his medicinal substances as entirely new and unique. Even substances that in their natural or crude state showed no signs of medicinal power could become "penetrating," "operative," and "remedial." He thought it possible to obtain their full virtue in doses of four or six globules of sugar of milk impregnated with a thirtieth dilution of the substance. The globules, he advised, should be mixed with water and given in the morning, and only if there were no apparent effects should the physician consider increasing the dosage.[80]

Hahnemann distinguished between a true dilution, which consisted of adding water to a medicinal substance until it lost its power, regardless of how much it was shaken, and a dynamization, in which the latent powers in a crude substance were excited and set free to act spiritually upon the body's vital forces. "I have been the first to discover and to promulgate this awakening of the latent dynamic properties of medicinal drugs," he explained. He considered it improper to use the term *dilution* even though every new potency of drug had to be mixed with alcohol or sugar of milk to set free "the very inmost power of the drug, which could not be done by simply triturating or shaking the original substance, were we to do it for ever so long a period." He reasoned that when homeopaths failed to obtain the desired effects from their higher potencies, either the doctor or the manufacturer had erred in the potentializing of the drugs. However, by employing vigorous shakes and proper care in the preparation of the potencies, even a fiftieth potency became so powerful that a pellet dissolved in a large quantity of water had to be taken in small doses to prevent an overpowering effect.[81]

CHRONIC DISEASES

Hahnemann divided diseases into two classes: *acute* and *chronic*. Acute diseases were either of an individual or epidemic origin, of moderate duration, and characterized by rapid loss of vital power. Chronic disease, while hardly distinguishable from acute at first, gradually diminished vitality to the point that the body was unable to defend itself against ultimate destruction. Concerned that he had failed to treat successfully a number of patients suffering from chronic diseases, Hahnemann examined the possible reasons and observed that many of the chronic maladies of his day had developed following an attack of scabies and its suppression by some external treatment.[82]

Hahnemann had been thinking about this phenomenon as early as 1816 but refrained from telling all but a few of his closest disciples.

"The Homeopathic system as till now promulgated by me, however much it can do, has not by a long way reached that perfect healing which has become possible only since this new discovery," he wrote to a close friend in Berlin in 1823. Not until 1827 did he explain his newest theory to Stapf and Gross, when he asked each to test the effectiveness of certain antipsorics (cures for itch) on their patients. He also sought support from Duke Ferdinand to establish a hospital at Cöthen for the treatment of chronic diseases.[83] Between 1828 and 1830, Hahnemann published his *Chronic Diseases, Their Peculiar Nature and Homeopathic Cure.* He regarded this work as his crowning achievement, offering the key to the treatment of humankind's most ancient diseases.[84]

In explaining his theory on chronic diseases, Hahnemann reported that most ailments enumerated in pathological works under very distinct names were really the products of three separate miasms: *psora, syphilis,* and *sycosis.* When individuals lived in an unhealthy state, eventually one of the chronic miasms would surface. Psora, the "oldest, most universal and most pernicious" of the three, had existed for thousands of years, slumbering in the inner recesses of the human organism, infecting all of humankind, and representing seven-eighths of all chronic maladies.[85] In earlier ages, it visited humankind in the form of leprosy and malignant erysipelas (St. Anthony's fire). Later its cutaneous eruptions produced any number of so-called fixed diseases (e.g., deafness, dropsy, epilepsy, gout, hysteria, impotency, insanity, jaundice, melancholy, nervous debility, paralysis, rickets, sterility). In 1493, *syphilis,* the second miasmatic disease, emerged, followed by milder forms of psora. In the last three centuries, the psoric miasm had manifested itself in the common itch, although it often disappeared as a result of some physical or moral impression on the body.[86] Unlike psora and syphilis, the third chronic miasm, designated by the term *sycosis,* had existed intermittently over time and had given rise to a number of chronic diseases that spread through Germany between 1809 and 1814. Often misdiagnosed as syphilis, sycosis's cauliflower excrescences on the genital organs were treated internally with mercury and externally by cauterization and cutting.[87] These allopathic treatments had caused the disease to return in more dangerous and disagreeable manners.[88]

In acute diseases, homeopathic medicines usually resulted in the subsidence of the disease in a matter of hours or a few days. In treating them, Hahnemann recommended doses every twenty-four, twelve, eight, or four hours, and sometimes every five minutes, depending on the nature and violence of the disease. With chronic diseases, patients could expect a longer time for treatment and recovery. For these, Hahnemann recommended medicinal doses at intervals of fourteen, twelve, ten, eight, and seven days. In instances where the patient was extremely weak or irritable, he suggested the momentary whiff of a moistened globule of medicine.[89]

Hahnemann did not claim to be the discoverer of the miasmic theory of chronic disease, pointing out that it had been suggested by numerous figures in ancient Israel, by the Greeks and Arabians, and even by Europeans in the Middle Ages.[90] Despite being documented in earlier history, the theory did little to advance the spread of homeopathy and even checked its popularity among the very individuals Hahnemann hoped to win.[91] In part, this was due to Hahnemann's efforts to stifle the very freethinking that had brought him fame. Those followers who were dubious of his miasm principle asked for further investigation, clarification, and a rethinking of homeopathic theory and practice. Exemplary of this position was P. W. Ludwig Griesselich (1804-1848) of Baden who, as one of the young new leaders of homeopathy in Leipzig, chose to weigh the importance and relevance of each of Hahnemann's several principles. While accepting the spirit of homeopathy in the law of similars, and in the experimentation of medicines on the healthy organism, he treated the theories of potentization and psora as secondary concepts that homeopaths were free to accept or reject.[92] Lamenting the fact that homeopathic medicine appeared in the public press as a caricature, he used the pages of his journal *Hygea* (1834-1848) to correct and expose inaccuracies. Griesselich supported homeopathy but remained defiantly critical of Hahnemann's more questionable claims.[93]

To some, it seemed that Hahnemann had become unnecessarily dogmatic, even bitter, in his old age: spiteful of opponents, suspicious and overbearing in his relationship with colleagues, and anxious to keep his system undefiled by revisionists.[94] Hahnemann himself said:

> He who does not walk on exactly the same line with me, who diverges, if it be but the breadth of a straw, to the right or to the left, is an apostate and a traitor, and with him I will have nothing to say.[95]

The aging leader made frequent references to "crypto-Homeopath-ists," "vile medical changelings," and "eclectics."[96] Not surprisingly, these hostile remarks led to a rupture between Hahnemann and the Leipzig homeopaths who objected to his authoritarianism and in-sisted that scientifically educated doctors should follow their own convictions when practicing medicine. True scientific medicine could not be held in check by "personal anathemas."[97]

In the midst of these intrigues, Hahnemann surprised his followers by taking a second wife and leaving for Paris to begin a whole new epoch in his career. Hahnemann's move to Paris was welcomed by friends and foes alike since it allowed him to become more of a fig-urehead for the reform movement in Germany. Homeopathy had de-veloped any number of "parties" and even Carl George Christian Hartlaub, a strong supporter of Hahnemann and author of *Katechis-mus der Homoopathie* (1824), agreed in 1837 that "the time has passed when every one who takes an interest in [homeopathy] must accept it as infallible and take Hahnemann's word as the gospel."[98]

PARIS

In October 1834, several years after the death of his first wife, Hahnemann was visited at his home in Cöthen by Marie Mélanie d'Hervilly (1800-1878), an emancipated young artist. After suffering several years from abdominal pain, she learned of Hahnemann's sys-tem of medicine and traveled from Paris to seek his advice. Following her cure, the doctor and patient became close confidants and married on January 28, 1835. Mélanie was then thirty-five and Hahnemann was about to celebrate his eightieth year. Hahnemann's friends and disciples reacted with surprise at the announcement, but those who knew Mélanie recognized little out of character. A woman of particu-lar tastes, she was much taken by Hahnemann's medical attainments and breadth of mind. She was also fond of dressing in male attire, and even after marriage preferred traveling in the disguise of Hahne-mann's son. She excelled in shooting, riding, swimming, painting, and poetry, and was sometimes compared with contemporary French author George Sand (1804-1876).[99] Wealthy in her own right, she took charge of the household, bid good-bye to Hahnemann's daugh-ters, and moved with her octogenarian husband to an elegant mansion in Paris.[100]

Once in Paris, Mélanie promptly brought her husband out of retirement and into high society where, for the next eight years, he basked in a lucrative practice and enjoyed an international reputation. There too he vied for public favor with the likes of François Broussais, who had introduced leeches as a substitute for bleeding to treat inflammation.[101] Although Hahnemann was known to have treated all classes, the French bourgeois and nobility paid dearly for a consultation, and Mélanie, who was always at his side, not only learned the rules of homeopathic practice but soon began practicing medicine under her husband's tutelage.[102] Their home at No. 1 Rue de Milan became an oasis of homeopathic treatment where carriages queued in long lines outside the gates, waiting for the opportunity to deposit their occupants for a visit with the two doctors. So active was Mélanie in the practice that Hahnemann wrote Constantine Hering at the North American Academy of the Homeopathic Healing Art in Allentown, Pennsylvania, requesting a diploma for his wife.[103]

In his final years, Hahnemann found himself continually defending the strength and effectiveness of his attenuated medicines. Over and over again, detractors devilishly compared his dilutions to the power of a drop of tincture in various lakes and oceans.[104] Defending himself, Hahnemann explained that the analogies failed to account for the *process* of succussion and trituration. In other words, a drop of medicine in a body of water such as Lake Geneva failed to make even a superficial mixture since the drug only slightly mingled with the water. Besides, the decompositions taking place in the lake would have destroyed the power of the medicine in the course of a few hours. Only by using the succussion and trituration methods would there ensue "not only the most intimate mixture" but a "higherto unknown and undreamt of change, by the development and liberation of the dynamic powers of the medicinal substance so treated, as to excite astonishment." Despite this ratiocination, critics remained unconvinced.[105]

Hahnemann died at his home on July 2, 1843, in his eighty-ninth year, following a six-week illness. He died a wealthy man, having earned nearly 4 million francs during his eight years in Paris.[106] His disciples compared him to Hippocrates because of his close observation of diseases and honored him as the founder of the Rational School or New School of Medical Sciences. But those who knew Hahnemann best compared him to Martin Luther because of his unwillingness to allow the hierarchy of older authorities and dogmas to dictate men's consciences.[107]

Following her husband's death, Madame Hahnemann continued to practice medicine, even conducting a clinic for the poor. In 1847, the dean of the Medical Faculty of Paris brought charges against her for practicing without a license. Although she claimed title of doctor of medicine from the Allentown Academy (see Chapter 5), her diploma had been awarded after the school closed, and she was fined for practicing medicine and pharmacy without a license. Unrepentant, Mélanie continued practicing for several more years.[108] In 1876, she donated a bust of Hahnemann, created by a well-known sculptor, Pierre-Jean David, to Hahnemann Medical College of Philadelphia.[109] When she died in 1878, she was buried with Hahnemann at Montmartre. In 1898, the bodies of both Mélanie and Hahnemann were moved to a new site at Père-Lachaise.[110]

SUMMARY

Beginning in the 1830s, one observes a gradual separation between the founder and many of his most ardent followers. Old age, pride, obtuseness, deep-seated suspicions, and ingrained stubbornness may explain Hahnemann's intense disdain for any sentiment that sought to question his wisdom or otherwise blur the distinctions he had codified between New School reform and medical orthodoxy. But other forces were at work as well. Those who were enamored with the new Paris Clinical School and who had tired of the burdens Hahnemann had imposed on their ideas and inductive methods sought to redress the balance between Hahnemann's metaphysical temperament and the development of clinical medicine. Just as in previous years American students had flocked to London and Edinburgh to provide a proper finish to their medical studies, now they gathered at the feet of Auguste François Chomel, Jean-Nicolas Corvisart, Pierre C. A. Louis, Gabriel Andral, Pierre François O. Rayer, Jean Baptiste Bouillaud, Pierre Adolphe Piorry, Léon Rostan, and others where they witnessed the combination of clinical anatomy and medical statistics triumph over medicine's past attentiveness to speculative rationalism. At Charité, Hôtel Dieu, Hôtel Vénérienne, La Pitié, Enfans Malades, and elsewhere, American students witnessed the emergence of hospital or clinical-based medical education from Europe's newest and most influential teachers. The Paris Clinical School's contribution to orthodox practice was the establishment of rigorous postmortem examinations of tissues (and organs) and their correlation with specific diseases determined through prior clinical descriptions of a patient's illness and systematic record keeping. Motivated by both statistics and skepticism, the French clinicians kept detailed records and discovered in the process of their work the extent to which diseases were self-limited, the relative value of orthodox medicine's materia medica, and the correlation of localized pathology with specific remedies. The Paris school, which Erwin Ackerknecht and Michel Foucault examined and which Caroline Hannaway and Ann La Berge later documented in all its complexity, was an important turning point in modern scientific medicine. To be sure, disagreements lingered on among inquiring doctors, but the Enlightenment's ethos of reason dominated their pathological studies. Lying beneath their many disagreements was a more enduring pattern of empirical research that became the foundation for clinical medicine and a demarcation line between old and new medicine.[111]

As a consequence of the Paris Clinical School, homeopaths were faced with two competing forms of their own medicine: one increasingly nonideological and evincing unequivocal confidence in the scientific method; the other, exuding an eccentric, religious, and meandering disposition, intent on preserving homeopathy's more speculative and apocalyptic spirit. Together, they formed a tapestry of homeopathic beliefs expressing the bipolar nature of medicine's last great system.

Chapter 2

The American Diaspora

Through most of the nineteenth century, three groups practiced homeopathy in America: licensed physicians, lay practitioners, and self-care advocates. Their strongest adherents were in New York, Pennsylvania, and the Midwest due principally to the proselytizing effectiveness of Hans Burch Gram and his followers; the influence of German immigrant doctors; the support given by the social, intellectual, and business elites; the advocacy role taken by clergy and other lay advocates; and the cultural affinity of homeopathy to theological perfectionism and America's liberal sectarian tendencies.[1] Homeopathy also proved popular because it was cost-effective, a factor not lost upon elected officials since it proved kind to municipal coffers. Together, these elements provided homeopaths with entrée into many communities and won them equity before the law. Of the three groups that practiced homeopathy, lay practitioners and self-care advocates held ancillary roles to the more authoritative academics. Lay voices gave homage to the principles of homeopathy, but because their theories and practices were often idiosyncratic, they tended to operate on the fringe, tempting homeopaths with the siren appeals of their more extreme positions. Not until the eclipse of academic homeopathy in the early twentieth century would these adherents move as pseudo-professional activists into leadership roles within the movement.

HANS BURCH GRAM

In New York and New England, homeopathy spread initially through the influence of Hans Burch Gram of Boston who at the age of eighteen sailed to Copenhagen where, following a failed attempt to claim his father's share of a family inheritance, he received from relatives a classical education, and studied medicine at the Royal Medical and Surgical Institute. Upon graduation in 1814, he joined the Royal Military Hospital and during the Napoleonic wars rose to the rank of assistant physician to the king. After leaving the military, he opened a lucrative practice in Copenhagen and by the age of forty enjoyed the respect and friendship of the country's most eminent physicians and scientists.[2]

In 1823, Gram learned of the views of Samuel Hahnemann from a Dr. Hans Christian Lund and tested the principle of similars on himself and friends.[3] After he was satisfied with the results he began using the method on patients. In 1824, as a result of local prejudices, he gave up his practice and sailed for America, moving in with his brother on Broome Street in New York City, and resuming his medical practice. In 1829 he was elected president of the New York Medical and Philosophical Society.

To introduce homeopathy to his new patients and peers, Gram prepared a twenty-four-page translation of Hahnemann's *Geist der homöopathischen Heillehre,* which he retitled *The Characteristics of Homeopathy.* He dedicated the translation to David Hosack (1769-1835), president and professor of the theory and practice of medicine at the New York College of Physicians and Surgeons, and distributed it to members of the medical profession.[4] Gram's translation was so poor that few read or understood its meaning. Nevertheless, it was the earliest homeopathic material published in English in the United States. Unfortunately, the pamphlet did little to educate other physicians, showing the limitations and flaws of translated material.[5]

Determined to preach the benefits of homeopathy, Gram used his membership in the Freemasons to attract loyal supporters. His first two colleagues (and patients) were Dr. Robert B. Folger, who opened a practice in New York City in 1824, and Ferdinand L. Wilsey, a wealthy merchant and manufacturer, and master of a Masonic lodge. Both permitted Gram to treat them homeopathically in 1826. Folger, of Hudson, New York, was an early critic of homeopathy; after reading the German texts of Hahnemann's *Organon* and *Materia Medica Pura* with the help of Gram, he converted his practice in 1827.[6] Wilsey was so taken by New School reform that he assumed the title of lay doctor and practiced without charging fees. He was Gram's first true disciple and became his companion during his final months. Wilsey eventually earned the doctor of medicine degree in 1844 from the College of Physicians and Surgeons in New York City and built a lucrative practice based on homeopathic principles.[7]

With the support and assistance of Folger and Wilsey, Gram nurtured a loyal circle of disciples who met frequently to discuss Hahnemann's writings as well as explore topics such as mesmerism, craniology, psychology, physiology, and the spiritual levels of the soul. The fact that Gram was a devout member of the Swedenborgian faith no doubt colored the group's choice of subject matter and, in particular, their interest in spiritual matters. The group members remained loyal to one another and were willing to risk customary courtesies among physicians, consultations, patronage, memberships, as well as loss of practice, by remaining faithful to Hahnemann's teachings. As John F. Gray (1804-1882), one of the circle members, commented:

> *Aude sapere* was our motto; at least we shut our eyes to the light of no fact in God's universe, nor did we refuse to listen to any earnest man's inferences from real phenomena, howsoever they might conflict with our own.[8]

Gray, originally from Sherburne, New York, had studied medicine with Peter B. Havens, MD, of Hamilton, New York, and later with Ezra Williams, MD, of Dunkirk. In 1824, he became the pupil of doctors David Hosack and John W. Francis at the College of Physicians and Surgeons. He received his license to practice that same year, and at twenty was appointed assistant surgeon in the Navy. Hosack helped him obtain an appointment as assistant surgeon in the New York Hospital and he later opened a lucrative practice on Carlton Street. Through Wilsey, Gray met Gram in 1828 and a lifelong friendship formed between the two men. Wealthy and well liked within the medical profession, Gray opened an office at the corner of Hancock and Broadway and welcomed students interested in learning homeopathic medicine. Gray was one of Gram's most influential converts and a major factor in the spread of the reform practice.[9] He later edited with Amos Gerald Hull the *American Journal of Homeopathia* and the *Homeopathic Examiner;* worked with Charles Hempel in preparing Jahr's *Symptomen Codex;* and authored several pamphlets related to homeopathy, including *Homeopathy in New York: And the Late Abraham D. Wilson, A.M., M.D.,* published in 1865.[10]

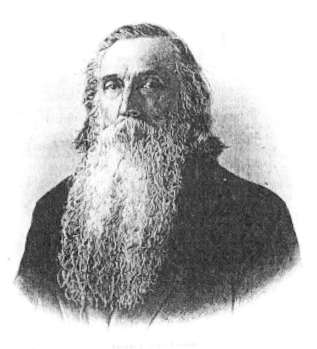

John F. Gray (1804-1882), pupil of Hans Burch Gram and co-editor of the *American Journal of Homeopathia* and *Homeopathic Examiner*. (*Source:* Courtesy of the Lloyd Library and Museum, Cincinnati.)

Another member of the circle was Amos Gerald Hull (1810-1859) from New Hartford, New York, a graduate of Union College in Schenectady in 1826. Following two years of postgraduate work in chemistry and anatomy with Dr. Benjamin F. Joslin (president of the college and a convert of Gray), he entered Rutgers Medical College in 1828 where he studied under Hosack, Valentine Mott, William J. Macneven, John W. Francis, and George Bushe. While there, he took daily instruction in botany and anatomy from Gram and became the first student of homeopathy to undergo a public recorded examination by the Medical Society of the County of New York. Hull practiced for twenty-seven years, during which time he helped edit the

American Journal of Homeopathia and served as editor of the *Homeopathic Examiner.* He also edited several editions of Jahr's *Manual of Homeopathic Medicine,* assisted in the publication of the *Symptomen Codex,* and edited the American editions of Thomas R. Everest's *Popular View of Homeopathy* (1842) and Joseph Laurie's *Domestic Homeopathic Practice* (1846). He served as corresponding secretary and president of the New York County Medical Society, and in 1835 became one of its censors. Both Hull and his brother-in-law, John Gray, were personal friends and physicians to poet and journalist William Cullen Bryant.[11]

Abraham D. Wilson (1801-1864), another gifted disciple, joined Gram's circle in 1829. A graduate of Columbia College in 1818, he received his MD from the College of Physicians and Surgeons in 1822, and reportedly maintained one of the larger practices in New York City. When he converted to homeopathy, Wilson lost many of his patients. Although a person of considerable talent, he could not read German, a handicap that faced many other American homeopaths. Wilson relied on Gram to oblige him with German translations.[12]

Other members of Gram's circle included Daniel E. Stearns, MD, of Hinesburg, Vermont, who met Gram in 1829, a year after graduating with a medical degree from the University of Vermont.[13] In addition, William Channing (1800-1855) converted from regular medicine during the cholera epidemic of 1832, and Joseph Thomas Curtis, MD (1815-1857), of Danbury, Connecticut, entered Gram's office as a student in 1833. Well versed in the sciences, Curtis helped edit James Lillie's *An Epitome of Homeopathic Practice* (1843), and in 1852, was elected president of the Hahnemann Academy of Medicine.[14] Another of Gram's friends was Stephen R. Kirby, MD (1801-1876), who, like Abraham Wilson, found himself at a disadvantage because of his inability to read German. After the English translation of the *Organon* in 1836 and *Materia Medica Pura* in 1846 were available, Kirby became more vocal in his advocacy. He formally embraced homeopathy in 1838 and helped organize the first homeopathic dispensary in the United States under the auspices of the New York Homeopathic College and the Women's Medical College in New York. He also served as editor of the *American Journal of Homeopathy.*[15] A final disciple was Federal Vanderburgh, MD (1788-1868), of Dutchess County, New York, who studied medicine in New

Milford, Connecticut; attended lectures in New York City; and practiced in Geneva, New York, before moving back to New York City in 1838 where he authored *The Geometry of the Vital Forces* (1865) as well as several essays on homeopathy.[16]

The small circle of physicians around Gram had either known how to read German or had learned to translate Hahnemann's writings with the help of colleagues. The group kept the information to themselves and chose not to disseminate it for fear of being accused of quackery. Gray cautioned:

> The propounder of a reform of any kind, which jostles the immemorial usages of society should be very careful . . . otherwise he may do more harm, even with a valuable truth, than other men do in striving to bolster up existing errors.[17]

During these early years, homeopaths made little effort to openly challenge regular medicine. At most, they sought recognition as a nonthreatening option within orthodox practice. As a result, the Medical Society of the County of New York even made Hahnemann an honorary member in 1832, and in 1834 a number of homeopaths and patrons formed a society in New York City. This, in turn, served as catalyst for various county medical societies. However, given growing Old School hostility to homeopathic ideas and practices, and, in particular, to its popularity among affluent patrons, the detente between the two groups of academic doctors showed visible signs of stress—signs that soon turned to hostility, ridicule, and retaliation. Not until April 13, 1857, were homeopathic medical societies extended the same rights and privileges as regular societies. The first license to practice homeopathy was granted in 1858 by the Homeopathic Medical Society of the County of New York.[18]

Gram's health failed just as New School practice was being more generally accepted. He died February 18, 1840, tended in his last days by a close circle of friends. After Gram's death, his cause of reform practice was carried by other homeopaths, many of German extraction, who had left Europe to settle in the United States. In 1833, Joseph Birnstill (1809-1867), a native of Germany, took homeopathy into Chautauqua County, New York. Later a Reverend Dr. A. W. Gray, who resigned his pastorate during an epidemic of scarlatina, went into homeopathic partnership with William S. Hedges; together, they enjoyed an extensive practice. By 1876, the Chautauqua County Homeopathic Society had sixteen members.[19]

Homeopathy moved into Albany County in 1837, with Dr. Augustus P. Biegler and the Reverend Dr. Myers who brought with them a number of homeopathic books and remedies, followed by Henry Paine and Charles Hoffendahl who were both homeopaths and mesmerists, an early sign that homeopathy carried a broader metaphysical appeal among those with more progressive views on health and personal behavior. As in other regions, these early practitioners of homeopathy were converted physicians, lay practitioners, or recent immigrants from Germany. By 1876, thirty-seven homeopathic physicians were practicing in the city of Albany, twelve having begun before 1850. The Homeopathic Medical Society for the County of Albany formed in January 1860.[20]

Dutchess County's first homeopathic physician was Federal Vanderburgh, who introduced the system in 1838. Homeopathy moved county by county, first into the Hudson Valley, and then turning west into Queen's County in 1839; Columbia County in 1838; Schenectady County in 1840; King's County in 1840; Cayuga, Lewis, Jefferson, Schuyler, and Onondaga in 1842; Oneida in 1843; and in Herkimer and other counties in subsequent years. By 1876, some 830 homeopathic physicians were actively practicing in New York.[21]

NEW ENGLAND STATES

Samuel Gregg (1799-1864) was the first homeopathic practitioner in New England. A graduate of Dartmouth College in 1825, he established a popular practice in Medford, Massachusetts. There he learned of homeopathy through the socially prominent Thatcher Magoun family on whose recommendation he consulted with Federal Vanderburgh regarding his daughter's advanced consumption. Although she soon died from the disease, the relief given by Vanderburgh's treatment inclined Gregg to study New School therapeutics, and he subsequently adopted homeopathy in 1838. Rather than lose patients, as did most announced homeopaths, Gregg's practice flourished. He moved to Boston in 1840 where he became one of the founders of the American Institute of Homeopathy in 1844 and of the Massachusetts Homeopathic Society in 1856. He also helped found the Massachusetts Homeopathic Hospital in 1855 and the Homeopathic Medical Dispensary in 1856. He remained in practice until his death in 1872.[22]

Others quickly followed in the steps taken by Gregg, including Josiah F. Flagg, MD (1789-1853), son of a Boston dentist and a student of Dr. John C. Warren of Harvard. After graduating in 1815, Flagg practiced in Uxbridge before moving to Boston where he invented numerous instruments and became involved in the legal disputes surrounding the discovery and patenting of ether. In 1838 he was drawn to homeopathy and recorded 300 successfully treated chronic cases. There was also William Wesselhoeft (1794-1858) of Saxe-Weimar, Germany, who first learned of homeopathy in 1828, and with the help of Johann Ernst Stapf began a series of experiments with the materia medica. His early work took place at the North American Academy in Allentown, but he moved to Boston in 1841 and began a practice that included transcendentalist Theodore Parker among his many patients. His brother, Robert Wesselhoeft, moved to Boston in 1845, and from there to Brattleboro, Vermont, where he established a practice and, with his brother, founded a hydropathic asylum, better known as the Brattleboro Water Cure, frequented by many of New England's perfectionists, temperance reformers, and Swedenborgians. Clearly, New Englanders were enamored with alternative healing systems that promised greater personal responsibility while demonstrating willful obedience to nature's laws.[23]

Other early Massachusetts homeopaths included C. M. Weld, MD; William Ingalls, MD, former professor of anatomy and surgery in Brown University; John A. Tarbell, MD, who took his degree at Bowdoin and later authored *Homeopathy Simplified* (1856); David Osgood, MD; Hiram L. Chase, MD, a graduate of Harvard Medical School; and Joseph Birnstill, MD. By 1852, sixteen homeopaths were practicing in the Boston vicinity; by 1861, the number had jumped to thirty, and by 1876, to seventy. Outside Boston, the numbers were equally impressive, with homeopaths establishing practices in Medford, Andover, Waltham, and Worcester in 1840; New Bedford in 1841; Newburyport, Plymouth, and Norton in 1842; Salem and Lowell in 1843; Westfield and Springfield in 1844; Fall River in 1845; Taunton and Egremont in 1846; Pittsfield and Roxbury in 1847; Lynn and Woburn in 1848; Stockbridge in 1850; Lee in 1851; and Fitchburg in 1855.[24]

At a Christmas Eve party in 1840, three homeopathic members of the Massachusetts Medical Society (J. F. Flagg of Boston, Charles Wilde of Brookline, and J. P. Spooner of Dorchester), met to discuss Hahnemann's methods for prescribing drugs. Two weeks later, they gathered again in the company of several additional members (Samuel Gregg, Milton Fuller, and C. M. Wilde) and a lay practitioner (Mr. Robinson of Brookline). On February 2, 1841, they held a third meeting and resolved to form an association to investigate "the doctrines and practice of the new system of Therapeutics called Homeopathy." Within weeks, the group had approved a constitution, seven articles, and three by-laws for their association, which they named the Homeopathic Fraternity. Of particular note was Article II requiring participants to also be members in good standing in the Massachusetts Medical Society or at least be eligible for membership. By 1852, the society had grown to fifty-seven members. Among the members were William Wesselhoeft, Robert Wesselhoeft, Charles Beck, and Charles Follen.[25]

The early meetings of the Homeopathic Fraternity functioned similar to the Friendly Botanic Societies of Samuel Thomson (1769-1843), the founder of the American botanical movement known as Thomsonism, in that the members gathered to share experiences, seek counsel, and reinforce their common interests. After 1856, the society devoted its work to the study of the materia medica and the findings of clinical medicine.[26]

In July 1851, the members of the Homeopathic Fraternity voted to change their name to the Massachusetts Homeopathic Medical Society. Four years later, the society petitioned the state to charter a homeopathic hospital in Boston. In 1856, the society received a charter of incorporation from the Massachusetts General Assembly and, at the same time, a charter for a dispensary. The first hospital of sixteen beds opened in Burroughs Place on January 23, 1871. It grew to 400 beds by 1911, with construction under way for eighty-two more in maternity. The legislature also authorized a hospital for the insane in Westborough, operated exclusively on homeopathic principles. In 1886, this hospital opened with a staff of three and an initial population of forty-four patients. By 1915, it had expanded to a staff of ten physicians and a patient population of 1,237.[27]

On April 10, 1855, Boston's homeopathic community celebrated the centennial birthday of Hahnemann at the Tremont Temple, one of the city's largest public halls. William E. Payne of Maine gave the inaugural address, followed by Henry C. Preston of Rhode Island who wrote a poem for the occasion. Representatives from five states were present. Participants included Dr. Samuel Gregg of Boston; the mayor of Boston; anatomist Jeffries Wyman of Harvard Medical College; and Winslow Lewis, president of Boylston Medical School. The banquet at Faneuil Hall included the lieutenant governor, numerous members of the Massachusetts General Assembly, clergy, editors, and several regular physicians.[28]

Boston homeopaths, like those in many other larger cities, used homeopathic fairs to support their dispensaries. Along with the sale of baked goods, paintings, wax fruit, and flower baskets, they displayed cabinets of curiosities; offered demonstrations of their system of medicine; sold raffle tickets for watches, carved tables, sewing machines, domestic kits, and other donated merchandise; and gave readings and vocal performances.[29]

Elsewhere in New England, Dr. Louis Parlin, a graduate of Bowdoin College, introduced homeopathy into Rhode Island in 1839. Gram's student, Dr. William Channing, was another frequent visitor to the state between 1839 and 1841 and did much to popularize the system there.[30] The Rhode Island Homeopathic Society formed in 1849 with ten members, its membership doubling within three years.[31] The Hahnemannian Medical Society of Rhode Island formed at Providence in 1854 with A. Howard Okie as president. The society met monthly with seventeen active and nine honorary members. By 1876, fifty homeopaths were practicing in the state.[32]

In Connecticut, the first case treated homeopathically occurred in 1837 when Dr. Federal Vanderburgh of New York successfully treated the wife of Dr. Charles Taylor, who then began a course of study and converted to the new system. The Connecticut Homeopathic Medical Society formed in 1864 after a false start in 1851; by 1876, the state claimed seventy-two homeopathic practitioners and two pharmacies.[33]

As in many states, homeopathy entered Maine by way of graduates of regular colleges[34] and only later relied on graduates from homeopathic schools. Recalling the history of homeopathy in his home state, William E. Payne (1815-1877) of Bath reported that the practice had been unknown prior to 1840. During his own medical education which began in 1833, he remembered having read about New

School reform in the medical journals, but such references were little more than caricatures of its theory and practice. In September 1840, an itinerant homeopath named D. F. Sandicky came to Bath from Eastport and set up an office in the hotel where Payne boarded. "Regarding him as an adventurer, and influenced by preconceived opinions of homeopathy," Payne consciously avoided meeting him. Nevertheless, "We occasionally came in contact at meal time, where his gentlemanly deportment unconsciously engaged my attention." Gradually, as their confidences in each other grew, Payne found himself less reserved and engaged in conversation that eventually touched on medicine. Realizing that homeopathy was other than how it had been represented to him, Payne accepted a copy of the *Organon*. Discovering the rule of similars that held good in all diseases, he soon felt that an "oppressive burden" had been lifted from his shoulders. Reading facts gathered from ancient as well as modern authorities, Payne concluded that he must settle the issue to his own satisfaction by making a practical test of the theory. To do this, he borrowed Sandicky's copy of Jahr's *Symptomen Codex* and purchased a few medicines.[35]

Payne's first opportunity to test homeopathic theory came a few weeks later, on a child sick with pneumonia. He selected belladonna, employing it according to the rules laid down in the *Organon,* and the child's condition improved immediately. This was the first recorded homeopathic treatment by a resident practitioner in Maine. On this auspicious note, Payne became more familiar with homeopathic practice and began consciously to practice what he had learned. He noted that many of his colleagues, upon learning of his conversion, "blazed [with] ridicule, sarcasm, derision, and misrepresentations." Nevertheless, Payne held to his beliefs and practiced for nearly twenty years without a professional ally. In 1859, M. S. Bing, MD, abandoned allopathic practice and joined homeopathy. He was followed by Payne's son, F. W. Payne, MD, who received his medical degree from Harvard, and entered practice in 1866.[36]

Dr. Sandicky, the itinerant homeopath, moved on to Portland where he interested resident physicians E. Clark, Albert Rea, and John Merrill in studying the system. In 1841, each renounced regular practice and embraced homeopathy. All of these early converts came by way of regular medicine, which they had been practicing between fifteen and forty years.[37]

In 1843, a Dr. Snell of Bangor opened a homeopathic practice with the aid of a domestic book and a box of remedies. This became a popular route taken by many to the new healing system. During the cholera epidemic of 1849, homeopathy gained added popularity from its less invasive therapy and its perceived superiority over regular treatment. In the aftermath of the epidemic, homeopathy assumed a more prominent standing, particularly among the community's wealthier and more educated classes. In 1867, Bangor citizens elected homeopath J. M. Blaisdell, MD, to the office of city physician.

Another Maine convert from regular medicine was Richard Bradford, MD, of Auburn, a member of the so-called Bowdoin Banner Class of 1825, which was distinguished for its graduates: poet Henry W. Longfellow, novelist Nathaniel Hawthorne, the Reverend George B. Cheever, and Congressman Jonathan Cilley. After graduating from Maine Medical School and practicing some fifteen years, Bradford abandoned regular practice in 1845 and devoted himself to New School therapeutics.[38]

Conversions from regular medicine often followed the ravages of epidemics. After losing his first child to scarlet fever, H. B. Eaton, MD, of Rockport, who earned his degree at Maine Medical School in 1845, left medicine, convinced he was unfit to practice. After visiting schools and hospitals in New York and Philadelphia, he decided to test the homeopathic theory. When his second child contracted dysentery and was "sinking under the disease," he treated her successfully using a domestic book on homeopathy and a box of medicines. Eaton subsequently resumed practice as a staunch homeopath.[39]

Similar stories of regulars who despaired of the failures of their medicine and converted to homeopathy occurred all over Maine—from Auburn and Augusta, to Brooks, Calais, China, Ellsworth, Kennebunkport, Lewiston, Montville, Vassalboro, Winthrop, and Yarmouth. By 1850, homeopathic physicians were practicing in each of these towns and influencing ever larger regions of the state. By 1862, homeopathy had reached the towns of Damariscotta, Farmington, Rockland, and Waterville.[40]

New Hampshire's first homeopath, Dr. Moses Atwood, settled in Francistown in 1840 and later moved to Nashua, Concord, Manchester, and finally to New Boston where he died in 1850. Others settled in Antrim, Bedford, Canterbury, Dover, Exeter, Keene, Laconia, Lake Village, Lyndeborough, Milford, Portsmouth, Weave, and Wilton during the mid-1840s and 1850s. In 1850, Dr. D. White of Keene published *The Homeopathic Advocate,* which lasted for one year. By 1876, forty homeopaths were practicing in the state.[41]

In Vermont, homeopathy was first introduced by a Dr. Baird who, though not himself a graduate of a medical college, was nonetheless a person of ability who attracted patients to his practice in Troy. Others soon followed, including converts from regular medicine and graduates of homeopathic colleges.[42]

The numbers of well-educated regulars in New England who traded allegiance during this period suggest that the canon of medical literature was neither complete nor closed to new theories and interpretations. To be sure, a healthy skepticism prevailed through the ranks of the medical profession as winds of change blew through the halls of learning. It was not just the influence of Parisian medical schools and the use of the stethoscope that challenged dogmatic thinking but a pervasive attitude among Old School students and their teachers that the practices which defined medicine were open to change. The combination of failed "intake" and "outflow" therapeutics, a recognition of self-limited diseases, and the determined belief in personal responsibility conspired to attract increasing numbers to the diluted doses and less invasive therapies of homeopathy.

MID-ATLANTIC STATES

Any history of homeopathy in the United States must mention Philadelphia and Lehigh counties in Pennsylvania as among the pioneer regions for the establishment of Hahnemann's doctrines. Lehigh County was home to the Allentown Academy (1836-1842) and Philadelphia County was home to the earliest homeopathic pharmacy in 1835 and the first hospital in 1850. The city's first homeopathic physician was Carl Ihm, a native of Frankfort-on-the-Main and a graduate of Würtzburg in Bavaria. Encouraged by William Geisse, a Philadelphia merchant, Ihm adopted homeopathy shortly after opening his practice in 1829. Another early homeopath was Charles F. Matlack, MD, a graduate of the University of Pennsylvania, who experimented with homeopathy in 1832 and practiced in the city until 1851 when he relocated to Germantown.[43]

The most prominent of the city's homeopaths during these early years was Constantine Hering (1800-1880), considered the father of American homeopathy, who studied medicine at the Surgical Academy of Dresden and the University of Leipzig, and graduated with a medical degree from the University of Würzburg. He wrote several articles for Johann Ernst Stapf's *Homeopathic Archives* before immigrating to the United States in 1833. In 1834, he published *Domestic Physician* (1834) which went through six editions and was translated into several languages. Hering spent his first several years at the Allentown Academy before moving to Philadelphia, where he continued his provings. His years in Philadelphia were devoted to the establishment of the Homeopathic Medical College of Pennsylvania (see Chapter 5) where he held the chair of materia medica and served as editor of the *American Journal of Materia Medica*.[44]

Prominent Philadelphia homeopaths in the 1840s included Matthew Anderson, Samuel R. Dubs, Samuel Freedley, Richard Gardiner, Jonas Green, H. F. H. Hoffendahl, Gideon Humphreys, Jacob Jeanes, James Kitchen, Jacob Lentz, George Lingen, Caleb B. Matthews, Charles Neidhard, G. S. F. Pfeiffer, J. G. Rosenstein, Frederick Schaeffer, Henry Schmoele, Alvan E. Small, and Walter Williamson.[45] By 1852, sixty homeopaths were engaged in practice in the city and county, and out of a population of approximately 450,000, an estimated one-sixth to one-fourth were patients and supporters of New School reform.[46]

American homeopaths began early to form societies and associations but, unlike their German cousins, showed little sentiment toward cutting themselves free of the majority profession. Most retained memberships in their local medical associations "and quietly pursue[ed] their calling—content to abide by the verdict of time and experience in establishing the claims of [their] art as a great advancement upon previous or existing modes of cure."[47] They did not see themselves as Hahnemann intended (i.e., destroyers of orthodoxy) but as a school within a school—one devoted to fostering change from past traditions. Only when forced by allopathy's refusal to fraternize did American homeopaths seek to invest their societies with the same legal powers as regular medical societies and to establish colleges to teach New School reform.[48] In defense of this position, Benjamin F. Joslin, himself a graduate of Union College in New York, observed that almost every academic homeopath had gone through a course of study under the direction of regular professors and allopathic boards of examiners, and had been declared qualified to practice medicine. To now disqualify them for the knowledge and experience attained since their medical education, and the judgment they had made regarding majority medicine, seemed petty, if not "monomaniac" in its suspicions and jealousies. Converts to homeopathy were not recruited from undergraduates still dependent on their professors; nor were they enticed from among newly licensed practitioners "still fortified against new truth by undue reverence for the dogmas of the schools, and inexperienced in their practical fallacy at the bed-side of the patient." Instead, explained Joslin, the disciples of Hahnemann were advocates of Francis Bacon in their pursuit of the truth and in their use of the inductive method to build the basis for their beliefs. They were, in fact, experienced physicians who "aimed to do their duty and promote the welfare of man under the best lights."[49]

In April 1833, physicians Carl Ihm, George Henry Bute (1792-1876), Charles F. Matlack, Constantine Hering, and William Wesselhoeft (1794-1858), along with several lay friends of Hering, formed the Hahnemannian Society, the first formal organization dedicated to the principles of homeopathy in the United States. In one of its first official actions, the society published Hering's address, "A Concise View of the Rise and Progress of Homeopathic Medicine," the second homeopathic publication in the United States after Gram's.[50]

The involvement of lay practitioners in these early societies was due partly to the temper of the time and partly to the popularity of the Friendly Botanic Societies that formed around the self-help medical system of Samuel Thomson. Intending to make every person his or her own physician, Thomson had authorized agents to sell family rights to his patented botanic system for twenty dollars. Along with the right to treat themselves and family members, purchasers were also entitled to membership in the Friendly Botanic Societies to share information. This democratic health system appealed to farmers, mechanics, and housewives, and it quickly spread across the American landscape. In time, however, the laypeople's influence over these societies conflicted with trained botanic practitioners (physiomedicals) who saw their future in more professional terms. The experiences of homeopathy were similar: its early history reflects a continuing struggle between the interest and power of the lay practitioner and self-help advocate, and the increasing pressures brought by academic homeopaths to control the system of New School therapeutics.

Five years after the formation of the Hahnemannian Society, the Homeopathic Medical Society of Philadelphia formed, holding monthly meetings at the Academy of Natural Sciences on Arch, between Front and Second Streets. Although the organization got off to a good start, including the preparation of "diet cards" for patients during treatment, there remained no clear criteria for admission. As a result, a number of lay practitioners joined the association, a situation that caused considerable dissension within the society. Unable to resolve the internal differences, the society dissolved in the early 1840s.[51]

Elsewhere in Pennsylvania, Henry Detwiller (1795-1887) was another pioneer of homeopathic theory and practice. A native of Switzerland and a naturalist, Detwiller moved to Allentown in 1817 and a year later to Hellertown in Northampton County. In 1828, he investigated the doctrines of Hahnemann and, along with William Wesselhoeft, a young physician and German immigrant, adopted homeopathic principles. Six years later, Detwiller visited Hahnemann, who was then living in Paris, and returned with renewed interest in the reform practice. Detwiller was a member of the faculty of the North American Academy of the Homeopathic Healing Art.[52]

Allegheny County became a particularly strong center for homeopathy as Germans flocked to Pittsburgh at the confluence of the Monongahela and Allegheny Rivers. Doctors such as the strict homeopathist Gustavus Reichhelm (1837), C. Bayer (1841), Charles Hoffman (1848), and H. H. Hoffman (1849) were among those who emigrated from Germany. Others were native Pennsylvanians, many of whom graduated from the Homeopathic Medical College of Pennsylvania, the Homeopathic Medical College of Cleveland, Union College, Bowdoin Medical College, University of Pennsylvania, and Jefferson Medical College. While Pittsburgh was a favored location for homeopaths, others chose Allegheny City, Sewickley, and McKeesport—all in the Pittsburgh vicinity and under the auspices of the Allegheny County Medical Society that founded the Homeopathic Medical Society of Pennsylvania in 1866.[53]

Homeopathy entered New Jersey around the same time it began in New York, first in Newark, and then in other towns and cities. Several graduates of Jefferson Medical College practiced as regulars before converting to homeopathy, including Walter Ward and J. R. Andrews, who graduated in 1840 and 1841 respectively. As in other regions of the country, patients came from among the wealthiest and most influential citizens. By the 1860s, many of the newest practitioners were graduates of the Hahnemann Medical College of Philadelphia, and by 1876, nearly 200 homeopaths were practicing in New Jersey.[54]

Homeopathy was introduced into Delaware in 1839 when J. C. Gosewich, MD, a graduate of the Allentown Academy, settled in Wilmington, a city of about 40,000 people. Although initially prevented from obtaining a license by the three-member state medical society, Gosewich profited by an 1840 act of the legislature exempting those who practiced medicine according to the Thomsonian, botanic, or homeopathic systems. By 1876, twenty homeopaths, including nine in Wilmington, were serving the 120,000 citizens of Delaware. In 1903, there were only thirty, a number that remained constant for the next fifty years.[55]

In 1829, seven years after botanic entrepreneur Samuel Thomson introduced his system of botanic medicine into Baltimore, Dr. F. R. McManus brought the practice of homeopathy to the city. McManus learned the system from a Dr. Matlack of Philadelphia who encouraged him to purchase several German texts on the subject, including Constantine Hering's *Domestic Physician* and its accompanying box of forty-five medicines. McManus spent his mornings with patients, taking careful notes of their symptoms, and in the afternoons and evenings, selected appropriate medicines that he then sent around to his patients. By 1876, there were thirty-two homeopaths practicing in Baltimore alone, and a branch pharmacy of Boericke and Tafel served the city's needs. Outside of Baltimore, some twenty-one homeopaths were practicing in the state by 1876.[56]

J. R. Piper, MD, of Baltimore, introduced homeopathy into the District of Columbia in 1844. By 1858, four homeopaths were practicing in the city; by 1876, there were twenty-five. In 1866, Tullio S. Verdi, MD (1829-1902), a graduate of the Homeopathic Medical College of Pennsylvania and personal physician to former Secretary of State William Seward, opened the Homeopathic Medical Dispensary of Washington. In 1870, the Washington Homeopathic Medical Society organized with Dr. Verdi as its first president. A year later, President Grant appointed Verdi to the city's board of health; in 1873, he was sent to investigate the sanitary laws in Europe and to report his findings so that the federal government might improve sanitary conditions in the nation's capital. In 1879, President Rutherford B. Hayes appointed Verdi to the National Board of Health.[57]

In April 1870, the Washington Homeopathic Medical Society announced the approval of a bill of incorporation passed by the U.S. Senate and House of Representatives. The bill gave the members of the society the power to practice medicine and surgery; to collect fees as the members of other medical societies did; and to examine all candidates for membership, including those of color.[58] As reported in the *New York Tribune* of May 9, 1870, white physicians in the District of Columbia opposed the bill's recognition of African-American candidates and resolved to break ties with any of their number who attended a meeting to which African Americans were admitted. The newspaper editorialized, if "a negro physician . . . is such a horribly

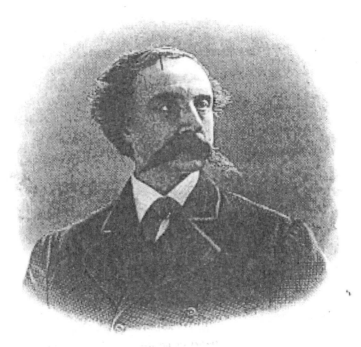

Tullio Verdi (1829-1902), physician to Secretary of State William Seward. (*Source:* Courtesy of the Lloyd Library and Museum, Cincinnati.)

objectionable person," then why not break ties with any of their members who accepted African-American patients? "If a sound darky is so bad, a sick one must be a great deal worse," reasoned the paper's editor.[59]

SOUTHERN STATES

Unlike the North, homeopathy made slow progress in the upper South. The impediments were due largely to local prejudices; the lack of urban centers; economic and demographic circumstances; sectional differences; support by noted northern homeopaths of liberal causes, including abolitionism; and the Civil War. Although introduced into Norfolk, Virginia, as early as 1830 by a lay practitioner named Kuper, homeopathy made few inroads except in Richmond.[60] In Tennessee, Dr. Philip Harsh, a student of Joseph H. Pulte in Cincinnati, introduced a mixture of eclectic and homeopathic practice in Nashville in 1844. Not until 1853 did the next homeopath, George Kellogg, MD, of New York, open a practice, remaining less than two years before moving on. By 1876, homeopathy stretched through most of Tennessee, with seven physicians practicing in Memphis and Nashville; three each in Chattanooga and Knoxville; and one each in Camden, Clarksville, Columbia, Hollow Rock, Jackson, Sweetwater, and Trenton.[61]

Homeopathy entered Kentucky in the medical practice of I. G. Rosenstein, MD, of Louisville, author of *Theory of the Practice of Homeopathy* (1840). Rosenstein lamented that homeopathy had made great progress in New York, Philadelphia, and Boston, but the entire West and South remained a "barren field."[62] From then, there was a steady stream of homeopathic doctors to Louisville, and by 1870, they claimed "a fair proportion of the wealth and intelligence of the community." Louisville also was home to the Homeopathic State Medical Society, formed in 1872.[63]

Kentucky's homeopaths were graduates of both regular and reform medical schools. One of the early converts was Jonathan R. Paddock, MD, a graduate of Worthington Medical Department in 1827 and later one of its professors. Worthington, the first chartered sectarian medical school in the United States, represented the western branch of the unchartered Reformed Medical School of New York, founded by eclectic Wooster Beach. Until it closed in 1842 after a resurrection riot and the subsequent rescinding of its charter, Worthington graduated numerous reform doctors, several of whom converted to homeopathy. By 1876, approximately seventy-five homeopaths were practicing in Kentucky, a number significantly less than the state's 1,600 regulars.[64]

In the lower South, homeopathy entered Savannah, Georgia, in 1842 when James B. Gilbert, MD, a graduate of the College of Physicians and Surgeons, started his practice. By 1875, twenty-five homeopaths were practicing medicine, most of whom were graduates of allopathic schools. However, only a few younger homeopaths settled in the state after the war. The depressed economy and diminished patronage forced many doctors who had previously depended on plantations for their livelihood to move to the cities. As a result, Atlanta, with a postwar population of 35,000, supported nearly seventy doctors of various types. No homeopathic societies existed in Georgia; nor were there any homeopathic institutions, although several pharmacies offered homeopathic departments. Most homeopaths dispensed their own medicines, ordering their supplies directly from distributors in the North.[65]

Introduced into Alabama by lay practitioners about 1843, homeopathy was not represented professionally until two years later when German physicians Ulrich and Schafer started a practice in Montgomery. By 1850, after their success during a typhoid fever epidemic, two more homeopaths opened practices in Montgomery. In Mobile, homeopathy was introduced in 1846 by G. W. Belden, MD. In 1850, the legislature authorized the State Homeopathic Medical Society, but it languished for lack of members. As late as 1876, only seven homeopaths had established practices in the state: three in Mobile; and one each in Huntsville, Montgomery, Opelika, and Selma.[66]

Dr. Joseph Martin of the French Navy is credited with introducing homeopathy into Louisiana, having visited New Orleans while in the service and immigrating there in 1836. Another early pioneer was a layman and former French soldier named Formel who practiced "with more zeal than discretion." Other pioneers in the system included Robert Glass, MD, of Kentucky, who spent his winters in New Orleans; Gustavus M. Taft, MD, who moved to New Orleans from Connecticut; and doctors James G. Belden, Alexis Leon, Alexander H. Burritt, Adolphe Cartier, L. V. M. Taxil, Louis Caboche, and William H. Holcombe. Originally from Virginia, Holcombe earned his medical degree at the University of Pennsylvania and then moved to Cincinnati where he embraced homeopathy in the wake of the cholera epidemic of 1849. Along with other orthodox physicians, he despaired of regular medicine's failed efforts to save lives and contain the pandemic. During this same period, he was attracted to the New Church of Jerusalem (Swedenborgian) and he began to bridge his New School thinking with his spiritual views. He later moved to Natchez where he opened a practice.[67]

Two early papers advocating the principles of homeopathy and published in New Orleans were *Le Practicien Homeopathique* (1857-1858) and *L'Homoion* (1859-1860). Both proved popular among French-speaking physicians, while the latter was touted as the most influential medical periodical in the city.[68] By 1876 the city supported twenty physicians, three pharmacies, and one dispensary. In addition, the city had placed the Protestant Half Orphan Asylum under homeopathic management for eighteen years. Outside New Orleans, however, few homeopathic physicians practiced due to the plantation system and scattered population.[69]

In April 1848, Henry C. Parker, MD, of Mississippi, brought homeopathy to Houston, Texas. It entered Galveston in 1850; Huntsville in 1858; Dallas in 1874; and Austin, San Antonio, and Sherman in 1875. The State Homeopathic Medical Association, which organized in 1874, had a membership of fourteen. Because of its small numbers, the association had no hospital, dispensary, pharmacy, college, or journal.[70] As late as 1876, there were no reports of homeopaths practicing in Arkansas, Florida, Mississippi, or North and South Carolina.[71]

In 1885, Southern homeopathic physicians meeting in New Orleans formed the Southern Homeopathic Medical Association. Its goal was to

> disseminate the Homeopathic system throughout the South, to meet annually for the reading of papers and discussion of medical topics, to guard Homeopathic interests in the Southern States, and to oppose all unjust and sectarian legislation as regards the right of different schools to engage in the practice of medicine.[72]

MIDDLE WESTERN STATES

Homeopathy entered Ohio around 1836 in the medical bag of a little known itinerant German physician, Dr. Cope, who practiced near Plymouth and was known as a "high dilutionist." Within ten years, homeopathic converts from regular medicine opened practices in Akron, Bainbridge, Burton, Cincinnati, Cleveland, Columbus, Oberlin, Painsville, and Ravenna. In 1846, Dr. B. H. Bartlett opened the first homeopathic pharmacy in Cleveland which, by then, had witnessed the influx of several additional practitioners and was fast becoming a center for homeopathy in northern Ohio.[73]

Besides the chair of homeopathy held by Storm Rosa (1791-1864) at the Eclectic Medical Institute in Cincinnati, the city had also been favored by William Strum, MD, whose practice lasted from 1839 to 1876, and the town's most famous homeopathic pioneer, Joseph H. Pulte, MD (1811-1874). A graduate of the University of Hamburg, Pulte opened a private dispensary in 1840 for treatment of the poor. In 1848, he partnered with Benjamin Ehrmann, MD, and together they treated 1,100 cases of cholera in 1849, reportedly losing only 50 of their patients. Their success caused the desertion of many regulars from orthodox medicine and gave homeopathy a much-garnered reputation in the Queen City.[74]

Homeopathy entered Indiana via Indianapolis in 1840 when Dr. Isaac Coe converted from regular medicine. By 1867, four homeopaths were practicing in the city. Elsewhere in the state were smaller numbers, most having come in the 1860s and 1870s. By 1876 there were 120 practicing in the state, with 24 towns outside of Indianapolis having 1 to 3 homeopathic practices. The Homeopathic Institute of Indiana organized in 1867 but floundered soon afterward due to internal bickering; it reorganized in 1870 as the Indiana Institute of Homeopathy, with a membership of thirty-four.[75]

The city of Chicago, Illinois, had fewer than 10,000 inhabitants in 1840. Within a decade, the population had risen to 30,000; to 120,000 by 1860; and more than 500,000 by 1875. Homeopathy showed similar growth. David S. Smith, MD (1816-1891), introduced homeopathy into the state in 1838 but did not proclaim himself a homeopath until 1843. Soon afterward, he was joined by doctors R. E. W. Adams, Aaron Pitney, J. F. Temple, A. R. Bartlett, and E. A. Guilbert. Nine homeopaths were practicing in Chicago in 1850; 15 by 1860;

and 115 by 1875. According to Alvan E. Small and Reuben Ludlam, the secular press of Chicago added much to the reputation of the new system. The editors of the *Western Citizen*, the *Democratic Press*, and the *Chicago Tribune* were all zealous supporters of homeopathy and used their columns to give a fairer representation of the system against the claims and recriminations of regulars. Besides support from the secular press, homeopaths gained in popularity as a result of their public service during the Great Chicago Fire of October 1871.[76]

In November 1864, German homeopaths practicing in the northern suburbs of Chicago formed the Society of German Homeopathic Physicians of the Northwest.[77] The United States Association of Homeopathic Physicians (German) gathered regularly in the lecture room of Hahnemann College at 168 South Clark Street. There, the delegates passed a resolution recommending the establishment of a monthly journal, written in the German language, and devoted to homeopathic theories.[78]

The state capital of Springfield, which had a population of 25,000 in the early 1850s, was served by R. E. W. Adams, MD, who labored among the wealthiest of the city's families. By 1876, four homeopaths were practicing in the city, and some of the strongest advocates of New School reform included the governor, the state treasurer, the attorney general, the assistant state auditor, and members of the state's congressional delegation and general assembly. By the late 1870s, nearly 500 homeopathic physicians were practicing across the state.[79]

At its fifth annual session of the State Homeopathic Medical Association in Jacksonville, Illinois, in November 1859, Dr. Marco Reed proposed an amendment to the association's constitution which, in effect, permitted membership for both homeopathic and nonhomeopathic physicians. Reed's intent was to open the association's doors to partial converts. Those who supported the amendment felt the time had come for the followers of Hahnemann to drop the term *homeopath* from their title. However, opposition was strong and forceful, with critics arguing that the amendment, if approved, would "fatally injure" the cause, lower standards, and encourage a reign of "mongrelism" in medicine by giving favor to the more liberal "*eclectic* element" within the school. As a result, the Illinois State Homeopathic Medical Association rejected the amendment, holding that it did not want members who would be "sometimes on one side of the field and sometimes on the other."[80]

The "Dean of Springfield Physicians" was Wilber Price Armstrong (1860-1940), who received his medical degree in 1884 from the Homeopathic Hospital College in Cleveland and practiced for over fifty years. In 1894, Armstrong was one of fifty-four physicians listed in the city directory. By 1897, he was among the original sixteen-member medical staff of the Springfield Hospital and Training Center, the forerunner of Memorial Medical Center. He delivered the hospital's first baby and introduced the first trained nurses to the city. A trendsetter, Armstrong was the first of the city's physicians to replace his horse and buggy with an automobile. He introduced several different electrical devices, including heat lamps; regularly attended meetings of the Illinois Homeopathic Medical Association and the American Institute of Homeopathy; and developed a sizable clientele from Springfield's more affluent citizens, treating this "carriage trade" in the privacy of their homes rather than in his office. He later brought his son, Wilber Price Armstrong Jr., into the practice, a regular educated in the early 1920s at Harvard Medical School. Together, they treated the city's blue bloods, one offering homeopathic treatment, the other, regular. The Armstrong practice makes clear that historians chose to make more of the differences between regular and homeopathic medicine than did the public at large. Although state licensing boards and the American Medical Association took official positions against homeopathic practice, patients determined their choice of physician more on the basis of word-of-mouth, reputation, location, and availability.[81]

St. Louis, a city of 40,000 in the early 1840s, became the portal for homeopathy into Missouri and the West. John T. Temple, MD, a native of Virginia, a graduate of the University of Maryland in 1824, and a private student of George McClellan, MD, of Jefferson Medical College, practiced in the District of Columbia until 1833, then moved to Chicago. In 1843, he turned to homeopathy, and a year later arrived in St. Louis where he opened a flourishing practice. He also served as dean of the Homeopathic Medical College of Missouri where he held the chair in materia medica and therapeutics. In 1848, Temple started the *Southwestern Homeopathic Journal,* which he published for two years. Other early pioneers to St. Louis included doctors Spaulding and John Grainger from New York; Ira Vail, MD, from

Kentucky; J. D. Stinestel, MD, from Germany; and Thomas W. Vastine, MD, from Pennsylvania.[82]

One of the more notable events in the history of homeopathy in Missouri was the trial and expulsion of G. S. Walker, MD, from the St. Louis Medical Society for practicing "the quackery of homeopathy." A graduate of Jefferson Medical College in 1852, Walker served in the United States Army as a surgeon from 1861 through 1863. In 1864, he embraced homeopathy and was appointed professor of obstetrics in the Homeopathic Medical College of Missouri.[83]

By 1876, forty homeopaths were practicing in St. Louis. Throughout the state were approximately 150, principally in Boonville, Hannibal, Hartford, Kansas City, Lexington, St. Joseph, Sedalia, Springfield, and Warrensburg.[84]

Elsewhere in the Midwest, Michigan saw its first homeopath between 1841 and 1843 when S. S. Hall, MD, a Detroit regular, converted to New School reform. The earliest lay citizens who practiced homeopathy included the Rev. Mr. Kanosh, the Rev. J. N. Reed, and Hon. H. C. Knight.[85]

In Wisconsin, an Episcopal clergyman's wife introduced homeopathy in 1842. Four years later, two practitioners moved from the east to Milwaukee. One left shortly afterward, but James S. Douglas from New York became one of the state's leading homeopaths, founding the *Homeopathic Medical Reporter,* a pharmacy, and a medical society devoted to New School reform.[86] The Wisconsin State Homeopathic Medical Society organized in 1858 and later reorganized in 1865. By 1874, 21 homeopaths were practicing in and around the city of Milwaukee and 162 others were practicing in 44 different counties in the state, although 14 counties had none.[87]

In 1870, when homeopaths accounted for 5.9 percent of the medical profession in the United States, they numbered 14.9 percent of Wisconsin practitioners, the highest of any state, followed by Rhode Island and Michigan.[88] Interestingly, only 70 of the state's 183 practitioners in 1874 had graduated from medical schools. Of that number, the majority were educated at regular medical schools and converted to homeopathy. The balance of the state's homeopathic practitioners were without degrees, having attended medical school for only a single session; learned under the supervision of a mentor physician; or were self-taught with the help of domestic texts and kits of medicines.[89]

Homeopathy arrived in Iowa in 1851 when a Dr. Beck located in Dubuque. He left two years later, forced out by the machinations of regulars and the prejudices of the public. Soon afterward, other homeopathic practitioners made their way into the state, including doctors P. L. Hatch and G. J. Wagoner in Dubuque, and Isaac and Zebulon Hollingworth in Keokuk. By 1876, approximately 240 homeopaths were practicing in the state, including a dozen or more women. It was estimated that half of the educated population were proponents of New School reform.[90]

WESTERN STATES AND TERRITORIES

Homeopathy entered the Minnesota territory with the first practitioner, a Dr. Sperry, arriving in St. Paul in 1852. Two years later George T. Hadfield, MD, settled in the same area and remained until 1859. Many of the earliest practitioners were lay practitioners, including the Reverend Clement Staub, rector of the German Catholic Church in St. Paul, who prescribed for hundreds of parishioners.[91]

The first homeopath in Nebraska was A. S. Wright, MD, who came from Indianapolis in 1862 and practiced in Omaha until 1874, then moved to California. Four years later, Dr. J. H. Way and a Dr. Hemingway located in Nebraska City. Others settled in Headland, Lincoln, Palymra, Seward, and elsewhere in the state. By 1876, twenty-six homeopaths had located in Iowa, of whom twelve continued to practice.[92]

The Colorado territory was home to a scattered population of miners in the 1860s and 1870s. The earliest known homeopath, a Dr. Luther J. Ingersol, practiced in Denver City for several months in 1863 before moving away. Three years later, M. L. Scott, MD, of Vermont, relocated to Denver and remained two years. In 1869, A. O. Blair, MD, from Cleveland, opened an office in one of the Denver hotels and practiced for several months before leaving. By 1876, 18 homeopathic physicians were located in Denver, which then had a population of 16,000. The city's first homeopathic dispensary opened in 1871, but the only source of homeopathic education came through preceptorships in the offices of physicians.[93]

Homeopathy arrived in California along with the wave of forty-niners during the Gold Rush. In July 1849, Dr. Levi E. Ober arrived and practiced in San Francisco until his death in 1867. He was followed in succeeding years by Moritz Richter, John N. Eckel, John J. Cushing, Charles G. Bryant, David Springstead, and F. Kafka. Nearly twenty-five homeopathic physicians practiced in San Francisco in the 1870s, eighty-eight in 1890, and about ninety in 1904. Other homeopaths settled in Oakland (eight); Los Angeles (four); San Jose (four); Sacramento (two); San Diego (one); Santa Barbara (two); and Stockton (two). Interestingly, the majority of California's German homeopaths converted to New School therapeutics after leaving their native homeland, and of that number many were graduates of East Coast homeopathic colleges.[94]

As late as 1876, no reports were found of homeopathic practitioners in the Dakota and Wyoming territories, Kansas, Nevada, New Mexico, Oregon, or Utah.[95]

SUMMARY

In 1851, the nation's population was 23.5 million with 40,564 doctors, of whom an estimated 600 were homeopaths. By 1880, an estimated 6,000 homeopathic physicians were practicing in the United States. By 1901, the population had increased to 76 million and the number of homeopaths had increased to 9,664 out of a total of 123,553 physicians. This was one homeopath for every sixty-eight physicians in 1851, and one for every thirteen in 1901. Interestingly, while statistics showed that female physicians made up a small proportion of the medical population, according to Anne Taylor Kirschmann women homeopaths "were equal or more numerous than women regular practitioners," a factor that brings into question the so-called marginality of homeopaths at the turn of the century. In 1851, homeopaths had formed 8 local societies, 10 state societies, and 1 national society, the American Institute of Homeopathy (AIH), with a membership of 250. By 1880, there were twenty-three societies, seventeen of which had been incorporated by acts of state legislatures. A regional society had also been established: the Western Academy of Homeopathy, with 150 members from the Western and Northern states. By 1901, membership in the AIH had increased to 2,002, and 7 other national societies were devoted to homeopathy. By this time, too, there were also 116 local organizations and 35 state societies. In 1851, there was one homeopathic hospital, located in Philadelphia. By 1880, there were thirty-four hospitals and twenty-nine dispensaries. By 1901, there were 92 public and 52 private hospitals, holding 16,037 beds, and ascribing to homeopathic principles and practices. Similar comparisons existed for medical journals: in January 1851, fourteen journals existed, compared to thirty-nine some fifty years later (see Appendix A).[96] Finally, in 1851, two medical colleges were in place—one in Philadelphia, and the other in Cleveland—devoted to the principles of homeopathy. By 1901, twenty-one schools were scattered from Massachusetts to California, three of which were departments in state universities. Homeopathic graduates numbered 13,517 while annual matriculants numbered 1,545 and graduating classes averaged 383. Attached to these colleges were 11 alumni associations, 6 of which were supported by 4,711 alumni.[97]

Several factors contributed to the growth and spread of homeopathy. For starters, the cholera pandemics of 1832 and 1849 had led to a wholesale migration of regular doctors over to New School reform as well as to other sectarian groups who had successfully exploited regular medicine's failure to provide an effective treatment. For another, the 1833 French translation of Gottlieb Jahr's *Manual of Homeopathic Medicine* brought added disciples, something that German editions had failed to achieve. English translations followed in quick succession as faculty of the Allentown Academy and other homeopathic colleges busily spread the word. Before long, American homeopaths had available a wide variety of books and periodicals that connected them with homeopathic thinking in Europe. More significant, perhaps, was the focus of Hahnemann and his followers to a more metaphysical view of matter and spirit. As historian Joseph F. Kett explained,

> homeopathy appealed to a wide segment of the American intelligentsia in the forties, not in spite of its vagueness but because of it. Disillusionment with the tidy categories of eighteenth century empiricism, nurtured by the influx of German idealistic philosophy, was creating a desire for a more profound approach to the mind-body problem.[98]

This also explains the compatibility of homeopaths with other vague but appealing mind-body movements of the period, including phrenology, mesmerism, Grahamism, and Swedenborgianism. All of these movements reinforced a spiritlike activity within the healing process that won the endorsement of many Americans.[99]

FAMOUS HOMEOPATHIC PATRONS

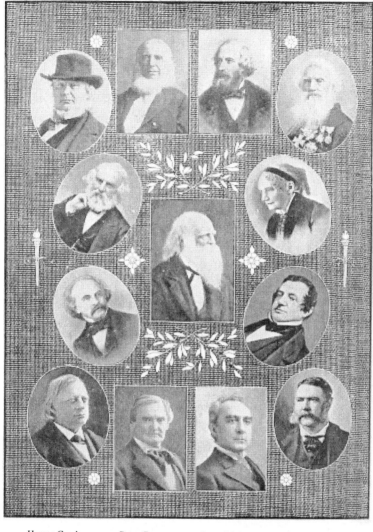

Horace Greeley   Peter Cooper   Cyrus W. Field   Samuel F. B. Morse
    Henry W. Longfellow   Harriet Beecher Stowe
             William Cullen Bryant
    Nathaniel Hawthorne   Washington Irving
Henry Ward Beecher   Joseph Jefferson   Edwin Booth   Chester A. Arthur

Famous homeopathic patrons. (*Source:* Courtesy of the Lloyd Library and Museum, Cincinnati.)

Chapter 3

The High Dilutionists

Believing that it was as hard for patients to rid themselves of their medicines as their maladies, homeopaths accused allopaths of forcing new acute and chronic drug-induced diseases upon their patients. Allopathy, so went the homeopaths' argument, taught that unless a medicine "inflicted" itself on the patient, there was no assurance that it worked. The more violent the effect, the more convinced doctors and patients could be of certain cure. This rationalistic thinking led patients to expect harsh side effects as signs of a medicine's power and efficiency. Thus, that a medicine caused purging, sweating, vomiting, or otherwise excited the secretions or excretions was a good indication that it could cure. But as homeopath Benjamin F. Joslin observed in 1850, "We might as well estimate the power of a steam-engine by the jarring of the boat . . . as that of medicine by the evacuations. Every motion is not progression; every accident is not proper action."[1]

Joslin's viewpoint is at odds with historian Charles E. Rosenberg's opinion that therapy "worked" within a holistic doctor-patient relationship which paralleled social and cultural attitudes and expectations. For Rosenberg, traditional therapeutic modalities reflected the outcomes of expected physiological consequences that were part of regular, domestic, and sectarian medicine. Yet while it is true there was widespread agreement in the doctor-patient relationship that spanned therapeutic modalities, Rosenberg's analysis failed to do justice to the high dilutionists within homeopathic circles who did much to challenge the conventional therapeutic worldview. True, the low dilutionists chose to minimize differences that existed between their therapeutics and the culture's predominant physiological assumptions by choosing dosages which more or less paralleled the predictable responses of regular medicines. Such compromises ensured a modicum of continuity with traditional practices. The high dilutionists, on the other hand, divested themselves of the culture's conventional view of disease and, with it, the older modes of therapeutics. Their sugar of milk tablets, attenuated with infinitesimal amounts of medicine, did more than reduce aggressive therapeutics; rather, they substituted a system that was strikingly similar to the drug regimens of today that, except for a few discrete medicines, give the patient little or no feeling of physiological change.[2]

Not surprisingly then, Hahnemann's principle of infinitesimal doses jarred against a culture that expected medicine to produce a forceful effect upon the body to confirm its healing powers. If patients did not purge, vomit, blister, or salivate, they questioned whether they had received any benefit from the medicine at all. Not having been made worse by it, was there any assurance they could be improved by it? In response, homeopaths argued that true medicine worked by small "imperceptible degrees" and not by shock. Was it not more reasonable to subdue fever, overcome congestion, or obviate arterial excitement with a minute dose of aconite than to abstract pints of blood? Was it not preferable to address constipation with a few attenuated doses of nux vomica or lycopodium than to drench the intestines with cathartics? And was it not more expedient to restore the stomach's tone than to force it "to perform a violent labor"?[3] Hahnemann regarded his system as occupying the high ground of common sense against the extremes of Old School rationalism and rank empiricism.

MATTER OF DEFINITION

To determine with greater certainty the power of his attenuations, Hahnemann recommended as early as 1824 that each part of a dry medicinal substance be pulverized and mixed with twenty parts of alcohol, shaken several times a day, and kept in a room of moderate temperature in a stoppered bottle, with the clear liquid (tincture) drawn off after six days. These tinctures were to be guarded against light by pouring them into bottles painted black or placing them in tin or wooden boxes. Every drop of tincture prepared in this manner equalled one-twentieth of a grain of medicinal substance. Physicians would then prepare their attenuations from the tincture by adding one drop to 500 drops of alcohol, and so on, to reach the desired attenua-

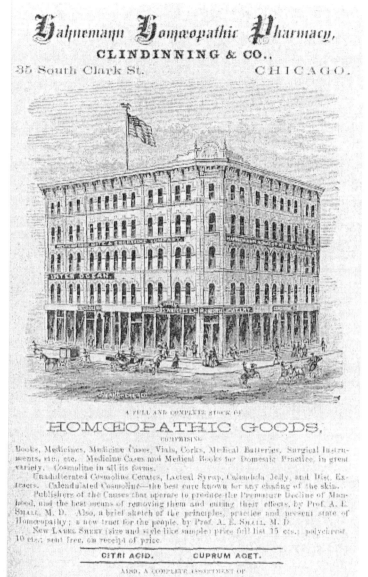

Advertisement for the Hahnemann Homeopathic Pharmacy, Chicago, 1874. (*Source:* Courtesy of the Lloyd Library and Museum, Cincinnati.)

tion. Dilutions were typically prepared using a factor of ten and indicated by the Roman numeral X. Thus homeopaths noted a dilution of one in ten as IX; one in 1,000 as $3X$; one in 1,000,000 as $6X$; and so forth.[4]

Until 1829, Hahnemann disapproved dynamizing medicines higher than the thirtieth dilution, believing that at some point there was no longer a medicine present in the medium. "There must be some end to the thing," he cautioned, "it cannot go on to infinity."[5] Accordingly, he set bounds to the succussion process to ensure the effectiveness of the potency. He also concerned himself with the most convenient method for transporting dilutions because a medicinal fluid that had already been potentized received additional succussions during transport that likely increased its power beyond safety. To minimize accidental shaking, he proposed that 100 granules of a neutral substance (e.g., sugar of milk) moistened with a single drop of a medicinal substance as the most appropriate medium for transporting medicines.[6] Because of this, homeopaths were often called "sugar doctors," a term that proved decidedly popular among children.[7]

But Hahnemann's most ardent disciples rejected his cautions and continued to test the full potential of their medicines. In 1831, Semen Nikolaievitch Korsakov (1788-1853), a Russian nobleman who practiced homeopathy, remarked in a paper published in the *Archives of Homeopathic Medicine* that he had personally diluted medicines up to the 1,500th attenuation and still found them efficacious. He modified Hahnemann's method of potentization by taking one drop of the *tinctura fortis*, or one grain of a dry substance, mixing it with 100 drops of water, shaking it twice, and then emptied the vial by throwing the mixture out with a jerk of his arm. The amount that remained on the inner surfaces of the glass vial served as the basis for the next attenuation. This he mixed with ninety-nine drops of water, succussed, and again discarded most of the mixture.[8] Korsakov theorized that although the division of the material substance attained its limit at the third or sixth dilution, all subsequent attenuations obtained their medicinal power by some form of "infection or communication of the medicinal power, after the manner of contagious diseases." Thus, the actual force of the material medicine declined with the higher dilutions, but the organism itself remained strongly affected by its immaterial powers. Impressed by Korsakov's remarks,

Hahnemann concluded that the power of medicinal substances was almost unlimited at the higher dynamizations. The greater the "dematerialization" of the substance, the more penetrating and rapid its operation.[9]

Other homeopaths as well aligned themselves behind the medicinal powers of the higher attenuations. German homeopaths Wilhelm Gustav W. Gross (1794-1847) of the original Prover's Union, Johann Ernst Stapf, and Clemens Maria Frans von Bönninghausen favored dilutions from the 200th to the 1,500th potency, while a Dr. Nunez of Madrid, Spain, claimed success with dilutions of the 2,000th potency for both acute and chronic complaints. Law student and horse breeder Julius Caspar Jenichen (1787-1849) of Wismar, Germany, who was introduced to homeopathy by Wilhelm Gross, potentized his medicines by succussion with 60,000 shakes, carrying his dilutions to the 16,000th power.[10] These dilutions, they all vowed, represented the very essence of pure *Hahnemannianism,* a term that would acquire special meaning among conservative homeopaths in the decades to follow.[11]

Hahnemann now began speaking favorably of attenuations of the 60th, 150th, and 300th potency, ascribing them as quicker and more penetrating but also of shorter action. As a rule, however, he continued to prefer the thirtieth dilution.[12] In the 1833 edition of *Organon,* Hahnemann wrote of a *dynamic* capability in a substance when undergoing succussion or trituration. He warned that excessive shaking or rubbing of medicinal substances could sometimes make them too dangerous to use. "One drop of the thirtieth potency of Drosera with twenty concussions of the arm at each dilution, would endanger the life of a child sick with whooping-cough," while a single pellet the size of a poppy seed of the same potency, prepared with two concussions at each dilution, easily cured the disease.[13] It was this spiritlike view of potentization that not only irrevocably separated Hahnemann's New School from Old School medicine but also entangled the movement in endless discussions, differences, and feuds over its increasingly metaphysical direction. In following this path, however, homeopathy articulated a philosophy that not only encouraged a connection between the material and spiritual dimensions of the culture but also seemed to satisfy the public's search for a less invasive therapy.

Hahnemann also contended that the individual who shook the bottles or pulverized the medicine in the mortar could transfer his or her mental power to the medicine. This explains his fascination with Viennese physician Franz Anton Mesmer's (1734-1815) novel healing science known as animal magnetism, the efficacy of which Hahnemann concluded "none but madmen can entertain a doubt." Influencing the body of the patient by means of touch ("gliding the hands slowly over the body from the crown of the head to the soles of the feet"), the mesmerizer distributed vital power to the part affected and uniformly through the body. For Hahnemann, the most effective mesmerizers were men in "the full vigor of life" who were able to "suppress all their desires," including their "inclination for sexual intercourse." Such men contained "an abundance of the subtle vital energy" and, rather than employing it in the production and secretion of semen, used it to communicate homeopathically with patients through the "medium" of touch and "a strong intention of the mind."[14]

Although not directly making a connection between the vital energy imparted by the mesmerizer and his principle of potentization, Hahnemann clearly saw a relationship between his nonmaterialistic ideas and the remarkable energy field discovered by Mesmer. Thus he recognized the necessity of limiting succussion and trituration for fear that the spiritual or dynamic power of the medicine would be too dangerous to the patient. Here Hahnemann and many of his followers diverged, some choosing the lower potencies (third to twelfth) while others preferring the more rarified dilutions. Though Hahnemann cautioned that more than two shakes would make his medicines dangerously potentized, high dilutionists such as Dr. Benoit-Jules Mure prepared their potencies with as many as 300 shakes.[15]

The storm that raged within the ranks of homeopathy over the subject of proper dosage also affected relationships within the entire medical community. Not surprisingly, potentization became the focus of continual derision by Old School doctors who pointed to the high dilutionists as reason alone to discount the entire system. Opponents referred to Hahnemann's homeland as "the land most congenial to ghosts, goblins and devils," and the "region of romance and fiction, of science and folly." Only fiction or folly could explain the infinitesimal doses or how a quadrillionth part of a grain of charcoal, flint stone, table salt, or marble could have powerful medicinal capabilities when administered every six weeks. Hahnemann's declarations on the "itch" were equally derided.[16]

One of the impediments to the effectiveness of the high dilutions was the lifestyle of the patient. Writing in the *North American Journal of Homeopathy* in 1856, J. T. Houghton explained that high dilutions had little effect on patients who were users and abusers of alcohol, tobacco, coffee, and patent medicines; those who garnished their foods with pickles and hot sauces; and those who washed little and lived in badly ventilated apartments. For these patients, he prescribed low dilutions, tinctures, first triturations, and even crude drugs, "repeated . . . oftener than the strict homeopathic rules permit."[17]

Critics were quick to conclude that the extraordinary medicinal powers attributed to infinitesimal doses defied sound reasoning. That the number and forcefulness of rubbings or energetic shakings could affect the inherent virtues of a medicine caused regulars to question the effects on homeopathic medicines carried long distances by buggy or horseback; of instructions which doctors gave for medicines "to be well-shaken before taken"; and of the utterly confounding power of an octillionth part of a ten-millionth of a grain of medicine. Regulars scoffed that a patient would need to consume 7,874 gallons of water to acquire a single molecule of medicine at the 30X power. To admit to the credibility of such "Lilliputian doses" became a matter of faith because there was no satisfactory way to prove their medicinal virtues. Medicines attenuated to the thirtieth power, they explained, had as much influence over disease as the fluttering of butterfly wings had on weather.[18]

EARLY INTERPRETERS

In 1836, the first American edition of Hahnemann's *Organon* was published from the 1833 British translation of the fourth German edition by individuals associated with the North American Academy of the Homeopathic Healing Art at Allentown, Pennsylvania.[19] In the preface, Constantine Hering (1800-1880), professor of materia medica at the academy, explained that homeopathy was a method of cure based upon new discoveries in natural philosophy, physiology, and biology. The particular method of preparing remedies made the New School a part of natural philosophy, having elements common to the principles of magnetism, electricity, and galvanism. Its peculiar effects upon the human organism made it also a part of the natural sciences. Hering went on to write, however, that since his first acquaintance with homeopathy in 1821 he had "never yet accepted a single theory in the *Organon* as it is there promulgated." Rather, he found himself enamored with the "genuine Hahnemannian spirit" which urged opposition to all theories that conflicted with the results of "pure experience." In this regard, Hering rejected Hahnemann's "polemical matter" as superfluous to the singular doctrine of *similia similibus curantur.* This remark represents a clear and unambiguous statement, as early as 1836, that individuals within American homeopathy considered the principle of similars the only legitimate doctrine of homeopathic medicine.[20]

Not surprisingly, then, American homeopaths decried attempts to define their beliefs simply on the basis of infinitesimals. "If our claims depend on that, and that only, I for one am ready and willing to discard her [homeopathy] instantly," wrote Storm Rosa, a teacher of homeopathy at the Eclectic Medical Institute in Cincinnati.[21] But the facts were different: Small doses had nothing to do with the "science" of homeopathy. "I, as a Homeopath, have the right, and shall exercise it if I think proper, of using any amount of a medicament that is appropriate, and well-selected under the principle of similarities," Rosa explained. Homeopathy had but one infallible law—the law of similars. On that law alone the system should stand or fall.[22]

Erastus E. Marcy (1822-1901), editor for fifteen years of the *North American Homeopathic Journal* and a self-proclaimed conservative homeopath, reminded readers in 1853 that the true spirit of homeopathy was in its reformation of antipathy and allopathy by replacing the law of contraries with the law of similars. He noted how opponents of homeopathy had taken great sport in discussing the subject of dosage, mocking the system as little more than the administration of infinitesimal quantities of drug. The high dilutionists had made it an easy target for derision. Nonetheless, he admitted that smaller quantities, reduced by Hahnemann until the atoms of the drug had become "imponderable," were sometimes capable of affecting a diseased structure in a manner as to cure *tuto, cito, et jucunde.* Recognizing that proper dosage was governed by a host of variables, including age, sex, temperament, and susceptibility, Marcy concluded that it could not be regulated "by any fixed rules" but depended ultimately on the judgment of the individual practitioner, thus making homeopathy a real medical art.[23]

French homeopath and author F. A. Espanet (1811-1886) added to Marcy's comments, noting that the novel pharmacodynamics introduced belatedly by Hahnemann had caused "grave and studious men" to mock the system in its entirety. He modestly suggested that homeopathy's essential law of similars ought not suffer the consequences of eccentricity simply because of this one aspect. Although fond of infinitesimals as both benign and easy to use, he insisted they did not represent a law or even an essential principle; more to the point, they were "not a necessary condition of cure." The higher dilutions were assuredly superior in their efficacy to massive dosing, but the nuances of Hahnemann's theory of dynamization should be left to those "who have deeply investigated the science." Most homeopaths were content to reduce treatment and the science of drug dosage to their "simplest expression" and insisted upon the law of similars alone as fundamental to the art and science of homeopathic medicine. Perhaps the experts in pathogenetics could demonstrate the medicinal power of their globules and high dilutions. "But let them suffer the little ones who are just beginning, to reach their position by gradual steps, commencing by ponderable doses," Espanet cautioned.[24]

Yet homeopaths could agree neither on the proper dilution level nor on its modus operandi. Taking a position similar to Marcy's, associate editor John F. Geary of the *Philadelphia Journal of Homeopathy* made a pointed effort in 1858 to explain that Hahnemann's theory of dynamization and the practice of using high and low dilutions or potencies did not constitute a scientific law, only variations of individual experience: "We have ourselves used what are called 'low' potencies, and as far as we have been able to ascertain, they have done us all the good service we could expect from them," Geary wrote.[25]

Homeopath S. Remington, MD, urged colleagues to test the full therapeutic virtues of the high attenuations. Any medicines taken homeopathically, even at the higher dilutions, produced "slight aggravations" of the symptoms. True, some potencies were not always felt, but instead of concluding that a particular medicine was of little or no value to the patient, or that another medicine should be substituted, Remington proposed continuing with the original medicine until convinced it produced no desired effect. To the question whether nature alone brought the case to a successful conclusion or whether it was nature aided by the medicine, Remington answered the latter. "If the high potencies have produced aggravation in one single case," he rea-

Lodge's Homœopathic Pharmacy,

Nos. 57 and 59 Wayne Street.

DETROIT, MICH.

As some have understood, because this Pharmacy was offered for sale, that its business has been falling off, I think it necessary to state that there was A LARGE INCREASE FOR THE YEAR 1872. It is still offered for sale on very liberal terms, but customers may feel assured that it will not be disposed of to any incompetent person. To one properly qualified, who can come with undoubted recommendations, good terms will be offered. I have conducted this business for about fourteen years, and it has now a trade of regular customers who purchase their supplies for cash.

The "American Observer" is NOT offered for sale. We expect to conduct it as heretofore, and in selling out the Pharmacy hope to be able to give it more undivided attention.

Letters of enquiry should be addressed: E. A. LODGE, 57 Wayne St., Detroit, Mich.

Preparatory to selling out my Pharmacy, I wish to reduce the present stock, and make the following offers to the profession to purchase now FOR CASH:

1. PURE MOTHER TINCTURES at twenty cents per ounce.
2. FIRST DECIMAL TRITURATIONS at 20 cents per ounce.
3. LOW DILUTIONS at 15 cents, and HIGH DILUTIONS, 30 cents per ounce.
4. PAGE'S BEST GLOBULES (pure Sugar of Milk) at 50 cents per pound.
5. ALL SUGAR GLOBULES at 45 cents per pound. (10 lbs., $4.00.)
6. REFINED SUGAR OF MILK of best quality, at 30 cents per pound.
7. PURIFIED AND RE-DISTILLED ALCOHOL one dollar per quart. (Bottles free.)
8. MEDICAL TEXT BOOKS at Ten per cent. discount.
9. DOMESTIC WORKS at Fifteen per cent. discount.
10. SURGICAL INSTRUMENTS at Ten per cent. discount.
11. ON CORKS AND OTHER PHYSICIAN'S SUPPLIES Ten per cent. discount.
12. MEDICINE CASES AND MEDICINE CHESTS Fifteen per cent. discount.
13. Best Vials, per gross, drams, $3.25. Half-drams, $1, 2 drams, $1.50. Half-ounce, $2.00. One Ounce, $4.00.
14. Best Corks, per gross... No. 1, at 30 cents. No. 2, at 40 cents. No. 3, at 60 cents. No. 4, at 80 cents. No. 5, at 70 cents. No. 6, at 80 cents. No. 7, at 90 cents.
15. On all Goods now in Stock, 10 to 20 per cent. discount.

* The above rates are STRICTLY FOR CASH. If the order is not accompanied by a remittance, Goods will be sent C. O. D. Charges for collection of money will be paid by me on all orders exceeding ($5), five dollars.

Remittances to be made by Banker's Drafts on Eastern Cities, to my order, Postal Money Order, or by Express, receipted for as money packages. Bank notes sent by mail in unregistered letters, NOT AT MY RISK.

Address orders,

E. A. LODGE,

59 Wayne Street, Detroit, Mich.

Complete Price-List of Physicians' Supplies mailed free to any address desired.

** Above reduced rates are only to Physicians.

Advertisement for E. A. Lodge's Homeopathic Pharmacy, Detroit, 1873. (*Source:* Courtesy of the Lloyd Library and Museum, Cincinnati.)

soned, "it proves that they are capable of affecting the human organism, and that alone establishes their utility." He pointed to numerous instances in which attenuations had been effectively administered at the 200th and some at the 700th power.[26]

Curt Pretsch, MD, complained bitterly that the belief in dynamization had caused homeopathic physicians to be looked upon with distrust and scorn, if not outright ridicule. In fact, the effort to make it into one of nature's laws threatened "to tear up our ranks, much to the satisfaction of our opponents." To prevent this from becoming a self-fulfilling prophecy, he encouraged homeopaths to look upon dynamization as a form of electricity. In preparing medicines through shaking and trituration, he hypothesized, homeopaths increased the drug's power in the same manner that one created an electrical charge by rubbing different substances on a cushion. His explanation, although seeming to restore harmony with unseen material forces, failed to convince those who preferred a more spiritual or metaphysical view of healing.[27]

Other explanations were similarly met with hostility by mainstream homeopaths. It was wrong, reasoned Hamilton Ring of Ann Arbor, Michigan, to expect that homeopathic law applied in every case. "Let us not underrate or overrate the infinitesimals," he cautioned, "neither let us underrate or overrate appreciable doses of medicine."[28] Ring divided the human body into higher and lower planes of importance, i.e., those requiring high dilutions and others more responsive to the lower potencies. Observing that Ring was trying to make homeopathy rational in some cases and irrational in others, E. W. Jones of Taunton, Massachusetts, suggested that Ring's opinions be taken *cum grano salis* and that homeopaths should "give him a fraternal shake of the hand and bid him good-buy."[29]

By the late 1850s, a decided opposition to the so-called high potency advocates had emerged among Hahnemann's followers. In 1857, Dr. Carl F. G. Trinks (1800-1865), a veteran homeopath and author of *Handbuck der Homoopathischen* (1848), wrote to the president of the Central Society in Germany complaining that high potency homeopathy was inflicting "great injury" upon rational homeopathic science. It had become a "pernicious" dogmatism full of contradictions and inconsistencies. He wrote:

> I confess openly that the action of many homeopathic physicians filled me with disgust, and would long ago have estranged

me from homeopathic practice, had not an experience of nearly thirty-five years convinced me of the undeniable superiority of this system. (pp. 250-251)

In studying experiments on patients under the care of "high homeopathists," he observed that acute diseases took "as slow a course as if no remedy had been used," and it became "a matter of conscience" for him to refrain from this form of treatment. He like-wise found chronic diseases little affected by the high dilutions, forc-ing him to resort to larger, stronger, and more frequently repeated doses. He concluded that high potency homeopathy was "erroneous in theory and practice . . . injurious to the sick, and to medicine as a science and as an art." Worse still, it opened the door to "charlatanry, delusion and deception."[30]

Homeopaths struggled to find a rationale that would justify their belief in high dilutions. Some, for example, continued to look to ma-terialistic explanations in forms that were thinly veiled behind spiri-tualistic rhetoric. Dr. I. G. Rosenstein of Louisville remarked in 1840 that the progress in mechanics and the newer discoveries in electro-galvanism had brought "miraculous changes" to the scientific world.[31] The same was true of the medical arts where the rude inven-tions of prior ages paled in comparison with the astonishing achieve-ments of Hahnemann in etiology, materia medica, and therapeutics. Like Marcy and others before him, Rosenstein believed that the ques-tion of dosage was independent of the principle of similars. He recog-nized that strong doses aggravated symptoms and that Hahnemann had gradually reduced his doses until the aggravations diminished. He also accepted, as did Hahnemann, that substances previously con-sidered inert (e.g., charcoal, lycopodium, silex, and graphites) be-came active agents under continued trituration in a mortar or shakings in a vial. Thus the most basic elements of "brute matter" could be "spiritualized" by friction and succussion.[32]

Having stated a case for smaller doses, Rosenstein dismissed the critics of infinitesimal dosages as ignorant of modern physics. "Is the activity of medicinal substances, or the doses which homeopathy prescribes, more repugnant to reason than the velocity with which light traverses space?" he asked rhetorically. Certainly not. Homeo-pathic remedies were merely "stripped of their bodies" so that their spirit could be more palatable to the organism. He challenged those who refused to admit their efficacy to explain how cholera, smallpox, scarlet fever, or the plague had become such fearful scourges without any visible or perceptible cause. Why should medical skepticism be reserved for the doctrine of infinitesimals when other forces with invisible causes were admitted? Clearly nature's greatest powers were "concentrated in atoms."[33]

Although differences existed among homeopathic physicians as to the selection of high or low dilutions of medicines, cures were effected with "all kinds of dilutions"—from undiluted tinctures to decillionths. Rosenstein divided symptoms into three classes: those affecting moral tendencies; those influencing the intellectual faculties; and those connected to the organic economy. Because of these distinctive classes, it was important to carry out a full examination of the patient and to recognize that each class of symptoms could be affected by different attenuations of a particular medicine.[34]

For homeopath Harris Dunsford, MD, chalk, charcoal, common salt, and sulfur ranked among "the most active substances, capable of producing, and consequently of curing, the most frightful diseases." In explaining this, Dunsford observed that remedies were directed not merely to the disease but to the patient's state of mind, and this latter characteristic distinguished homeopathy from all other medical systems. Believing that their medicines could directly influence the "moral" aspect of the individual, homeopaths were constantly challenged to select their drugs with knowledge of the "specific influence upon the mental state and feelings." This allowed the practitioner to reach into the innermost recesses of the patient and exert an influence over the mind as well as the body. In this manner, homeopathy was considered particularly effective in the treatment of women, "for in these patients, the moral feelings are in the highest degree sensitive and influential."[35] Whether cures were achieved by some form of electricity or analogous power remained a question. Dunsford felt, however, that whatever the source of power, it was "quite sufficient to account for the energy of the homeopathic globules."[36]

Benjamin F. Joslin, fellow of the Albany Medical College, found refuge in a simple mechanical explanation to describe the modus operandi of high dilutions. In 1846, and later in 1850, he wrote that Hahnemann had increased the power of his medicines by effecting a comminution, meaning "subjecting every particle of the medicinal substance to [a] mechanical, tearing asunder operation."[37] The power of the drug spread through the inert material by increasing its surface area when the medicine broke into fragments. Each attenuation exposed more surface area, and this increased surface area acted on the body. The intrinsic properties of the substance increased with the continued separation of the particles, giving physicians the ability to send their comminuted medicines into the body's narrowest recesses where coarser medicines failed to travel. This explanation seemed to satisfy skeptics within academic homeopathy who could more easily visualize how the grinding of a grain of medicine increased its surface with every fracture and thus increased its potential distribution and effectiveness in the organism. [38]

Fincke's Fluxion Potencies

Those American homeopaths who favored the higher potencies were heartened by news that the 1853 Congress of German Homeopathic Physicians supported dilution levels to the 2,000th power and even higher.[39] As a consequence, American medical literature in the 1860s was filled with notices of highly potentized homeopathic remedies, the rationale of which was little understood except to say that they seemed to catch the imagination of many who were at home in a more immaterial encounter with healing. Along with the remedies, several theories emerged to explain or redefine Hahnemann's high dilutionism, including Bernhardt Fincke's fluxion potencies and Charles J. Hempel's theory of specific homeopathy.

Bernhardt Maximillian Fincke, MD (1821-1906), was born in Saxony, Germany; became a homeopath in 1851; immigrated to America a year later; received his medical degree in 1854 from the University Medical College of the City of New York; and settled in Brooklyn where he manufactured high potency remedies. Author of *On High Potencies and Homeopathics* (1865), he explained that the higher dynamizations and dilutions had always been part of the doctrines taught by Hahnemann and, therefore, it was "logically impossible to separate *quantity* from *quality, infinitesimality* from *simility.*" The scientific study of dosage, he argued, was at the heart of homeopathy.[40] To support his position, Fincke reported on a series of clinical cases treated with the higher potencies, pointing out that each homeopathic remedy exhibited its own pathognomic character. True pathognosis required finer microscopical and microchemical observations than had been achieved by contemporary physicists, chemists, and physiologists. An avowed transcendentalist, Fincke referred obliquely to German metaphysician Immanuel Kant (1724-1804) and his conception of "chemical interpenetration," and recounted clinical cases using a variety of levels of potencies up to the 71,000th potency.[41]

When challenged by the more cautious American Institute of Homeopathy to explain his preparations, Fincke responded that he would do so only when he could find a publisher. Until then, he continued to assert that his medicines not only cured but produced provings.[42] Fincke packaged his Fluxion Potencies in vials of 1,000 pellets that sold for eight dollars.[43] Odo-Magnetic Sugar of Milk was one of his favorite potencies, used for nervous disorders and debility. Its modus operandi, however, puzzled inquiring homeopaths. What was its intrinsic merit? How was it prepared? What was the evidence of its pathogenesis? Fincke refused to say.[44]

The editors of the *North American Journal of Homeopathy* were polite to Fincke but skeptical of his claims of "astonishing cures." They asked, by what processes were these high dynamizations reached?[45] Again, Fincke remained silent. The editors of the British *Monthly Homeopathic Review* were less reticent in their remarks. On reading a description of Fincke's method of attenuation at the U.S. Patent Office, they judged it "impossible for practitioners to place any reliance on the preparations."[46] The editors of the *American Homeopathic Observer* in Detroit promised not to write so sarcastically about Fincke's high potency nostrums provided he divulge the process used for their preparation. Until then, they considered his claims to be "Nux absurda 100,000."[47] Eventually the editors procured a copy of Fincke's patent (No. 93,980, August 24, 1869) and discovered that the language describing the process was as obscure as Fincke's public announcements. According to the inventor, the process of "fluxion" consisted of "gradually lessening, comminuting, attenuating, refining, rarefying, and infinitesimalizing substances" by dilution.[48] Fincke claimed to have improved on the Hahnemannian and Korsakoffian techniques by directing a "regulated flow of water . . . upon the substance to be potentiated or diluted." In other words, his patented process involved running a premeasured amount of water through a vial of a calculated potency. In 1896, Fincke was elected president of the International Hahnemannian Association, formed in

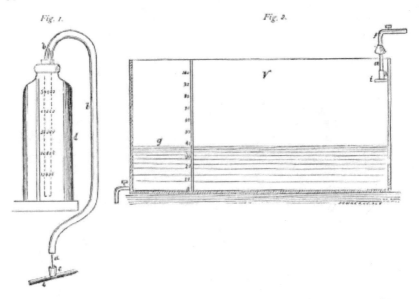

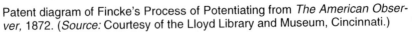

Patent diagram of Fincke's Process of Potentiating from *The American Observer*, 1872. (*Source:* Courtesy of the Lloyd Library and Museum, Cincinnati.)

reaction to the low potency tendencies of the American Institute of Homeopathy.[49]

Charles Hempel

Author, translator, compiler, and critic Charles Julius Hempel (1811-1879) exercised a wide influence over American homeopathy in the nineteenth century. Born in 1811 in Solingen, Prussia, he received his university training in both Germany and France before immigrating to America, arriving in New York in 1835 at the age of twenty-four. Already a convert to homeopathy, he received his medical training at the New York Medical College. Hempel made homeopathy better known among English-speaking audiences. His more noted translations included Hahnemann's *Chronic Diseases* (1845) and *Materia Medica Pura* (1846); G. H. G. Jahr's *New Manual* (1848); Franz Hartman's *Diseases of Children and Their Homeopathic Treatment* (1853); Alphonse Teste's *The Homeopathic Materia Medica* (1854); and Jean Paul Tessier's *Clinical Researches Con-*

cerning the Homeopathic Treatment of Asiatic Cholera (1855). He also authored *The Homeopathic Domestic Physician* (1846); *Organon of Specific Homeopathy* (1854); and *System of Materia Medica and Therapeutics* (1858), among others. Hempel was co-editor of the *Homeopathic Examiner* (1843-1845) and, for three years, chair of materia medica and therapeutics at the Homeopathic Medical College of Philadelphia.[50]

Like Hahnemann, Hempel considered himself a vitalist, believing that the material substances composing the living organism followed the spiritually dynamic law of vital force. Disease, a "dynamic derangement" of organic vitality, represented an abnormal condition in the true character of the organism. But the physician who availed himself of all resources, including the stethoscope, could arrive at a correct diagnosis of disease symptoms. Any disease without symptoms was beyond the reach of treatment. As for the actual removal of the morbid symptoms, Hempel held with Hahnemann that disease was cured by the active substance in medicine, producing a dynamic change in the vital condition of the organism. Every true drug contained a dynamic principle, force, or "pharmaco-dynamic property" that removed the symptoms of disease.[51] While Old School doctors chose medicinal agents such as mercury to modify the physiological functions of the organism, Hempel chose a drug effect ("cosmic principle") of the same order and magnitude as that which developed disease.[52]

Each true medicine, whether animal, vegetable, or mineral, presented a triune set of principles: "the cosmic or creating factor; the germinal principle . . . in the soil of the planet; and the material product resulting from the action of the cosmic factor upon the germ in suitable conditions of atmosphere, heat, light and moisture." Every true drug, regardless of dilution or attenuation, acted by virtue of this "trinity of principles." Hempel denied the claims of both the high dilutionists and the low potency advocates, arguing that the division between the highs and lows was artificial and founded in misunderstanding. Yet natural limitations did occur. Although some drugs were efficacious in attenuations as high as the 200th, he rejected the higher potencies as beyond the pale of the fundamental principles of homeopathic science.[53]

Hempel understood that certain diseases could not be reproduced in humans by artificial means. These included cutaneous eruptions, fevers, enlargements of organs, arthritic conditions, and diseases of the brain, chest, and abdomen. In other words, no drug ever succeeded in developing an exactly similar condition in a healthy individual. This meant a strictly literal interpretation of Hahnemann's law was impossible. Physicians had to be satisfied with simply noting the external manifestations that accompanied pathological conditions. It had never been Hahnemann's intention "to degrade the Science of Therapeutics to the mechanical business of taking a record of symptoms, and of adapting to them a parallel record of drug-effects."[54] By itself, knowledge of the pathogenetic effects of drugs was insufficient in selecting a specific remedial agent. In truth, drug effects derived their quality from the tissues involved, from the nervous centers upon which the drug acted, and from the relation of the drug effects on the natural disease. "This doctrine may not have been that of Hahnemann's original disciples," Hempel reasoned, "but it is in accordance with Science, and professional minds must sooner or later adopt it as the basis of a true system of Therapeutics."[55] In this manner, Hempel urged fellow homeopaths to go beyond the strict symptomatology of Hahnemann by seeking out the more recent achievements of French and German clinicians.

Hempel explained that Hahnemann had introduced the processes of trituration and succussion as a mechanism for detaching the drug force from its material foundations, thereby permitting it to act with greater freedom and power on the organism. However, to believe that the whole structure of homeopathy rested on the theory of potentization defied common sense, particularly when most homeopathic practitioners relied on much larger doses of medicine. The public needed to realize that there was no uniform homeopathic rule on doses except to say that "a large margin must be left to the discretion and judgment of the physician." Each physician was entitled to use any level of potency—from a fifth of a grain to a two-hundredth attenuation—provided it not be used inappropriately or mischievously.[56]

Although Hempel praised the four volumes of provings in Hahnemann's *Materia Medica Pura,* he considered the writings that came afterward to be "utterly worthless." The only other provings he considered reputable were those of the Prover's Union (formed around 1815 by several of Hahnemann's followers who took small doses of remedies and recorded their drug symptoms in minute detail) and isolated provings of certain German, English, French, and American homeopaths.[57] In a speech before the Michigan Homeopathic Institute in 1866, Hempel explained that Hahnemann had been a "fallible mortal" who regarded dosage as a subject of "minor importance" in his early years but who had gradually moved to the smaller doses because "the spook of medicinal aggravation haunted him with unrelenting tenacity." Hempel called this an "infatuation" and criticized ultra dilutionists such as Bernhardt Fincke and Philadelphian Adolphus Lippe for foisting "hyper-metaphysical . . . nonsense" upon those with "highly-wrought" minds and a "morbidly excited imagination." Hempel regretted the claims of these "enthusiasts" whose works of fancy had introduced into the homeopathic materia medica a number of "puerile and unreliable observations." Most homeopaths, he asserted, were earnest practitioners who met the needs of their patients with lower potencies.[58]

At one end of the spectrum, explained Hempel, were those physicians who preferred crude drugs and the lower triturations and attenuations. At the other end were those such as Fincke and Lippe who continued the process of attenuation "up to the point where the boldest imagination can no longer conceive of the possibility of curative action." The advocates of these incredible high potencies did so with a "dogmatic tenacity" and a "poetic arrogance" that defied rational discourse.[59] As for himself, Hempel refused to accept any theory that explained the effectiveness of the drug on the breaking up of its molecules to the point of "disengaging the spirit and securing its perfect activity." The absolute disintegration of the drug molecule was impossible. "If the high-potentialists mean to advocate the doctrine that an indefinite division of matter spiritualizes matter itself," this was no more than a "new-fangled system of transcendental materialism" grafted onto homeopathic science. He blamed this "insulting arrogance" on the faculty of the "Philadelphia Synagogue," a term he used to describe the Homeopathic Medical College of Pennsylvania after it turned ultraconservative in the 1860s.[60]

Hempel insisted that the virtue of a drug remained a "fruitless abstraction" unless presented in material form. "Spirit without a material form," he explained, was vague and indefinable. Similarly, matter without an "indwelling spirit" remained "a shapeless, mechanical juxtaposition of molecules, utterly destitute of power, either for good or evil." No drug could be divided or subdivided, shaken or triturated to the point of losing its material basis. Only Lippe, Fincke, and the

Philadelphia professors of "high Homeopathy" believed in such absurdities, Hempel explained. But then, these same individuals were "inflated with all the pompous pride which a solid dogmatism is so apt to beget in the hearts of young doctors."[61]

Although open to thoughtful dialogue on the matter and willing to examine every case showing the efficacy of high potencies, Hempel urged physicians to be guided by the nature of the malady, along with the duration, habits, constitution, and idiosyncrasies of the patient, in determining the size of dosages. Between the "ideal truth" of homeopathy and its application there existed a "vast gulf . . . which cannot be bridged over by human cunning and dogmatic assertions."[62] For beginners, he recommended the lower attenuations (second or third) or triturations during the first stages of all acute and even most chronic diseases.[63]

Equally significant, Hempel urged homeopaths to quit their opposition to the use of palliatives. A mustard plaster, a gentle laxative, and even morphine could be used humanely and effectively. The "exclusivists" within the homeopathic family should never subordinate the needs of the patient to the "technical letter of a formula." Hempel hoped that "prejudice, pride, and sordid interest" would not prevent the two schools of allopathy and homeopathy from eventual unification. "Let them but listen to each other with respectful forbearance, and they will soon find that they may impart an immense fund of knowledge to each other."[64]

In 1870, Hempel urged fellow homeopaths to read the works of Eduard von Grauvogl (1811-1877), particularly his *Lehrbuch der Homeopathie* (1870). A determined opponent of dogmatism, Grauvogl had dedicated himself to presenting homeopathy as a "liberal and progressive science." Hempel praised Grauvogl for opposing the concept of dynamization in medicines; attacking orthodox homeopathy; defending the alternation of drugs; and suggesting that the law of similars and the principle of *contraria contrariis* were complementary of each other. In other words, the law of similars had limits and could not be depended upon as a guide in all cases. Neither was it superior or inferior to the principle of *contraria contrariis;* instead, the two principles "reciprocally complete each other."[65]

SORTING IT OUT

Ultimately, clinical judgment became the common ground between the highs and lows of homeopathic practice. Those who preferred medicines as low as the first and third decimal or as high as several hundred were not embarrassed to admit they had also experienced situations where they prescribed the opposite.[66] In responding to the question of dilution, H. C. Allen, MD, wrote: "I can neither treat successfully nor satisfactorily all the cases that come under my care with either low or high dilutions exclusively."[67] For J. S. Douglas, MD, of Milwaukee, high dilutions made the needed impression on those with "highly exalted" sensibilities. On the other hand, where the sensibility was depressed, low dilutions readily roused the organism to action.[68] In effect, the options available in the different attenuations corresponded to the degrees of vitality found in the organism.

Charles Cropper, MD, of Cincinnati, viewed each attenuation or potency as a "different remedy" and, therefore, kept the provings entirely distinct. This was because potencies developed drug symptoms peculiar to the particular attenuation. A dilution of a 3rd or 12th potency differed in action from a 132th, 200th, or 2,000th potency. Since medicines gained in their intensity by the process of potentization, and since acute diseases were more intense in their manifestations than those of a chronic nature, it followed that the higher potencies were more applicable to acute than to chronic diseases.[69]

However, Cropper's views were not widely accepted. To the question whether succussion and trituration increased the power of a medicine, I. S. P. Lord, MD, of Chicago, explained that certain substances were at the maximum of their dynamic power and no manipulation could increase their force. This group of substances included air, alcohol, ammonia, bromine, carbonic acid, chloroform, ether, sugar, and water. Some substances represented the medium level of dynamization, and doctors could increase their dynamic power more or less by manipulation. These included belladonna, bryonia, camphor, cannabis, cantharis, cimex, cina, fluoric and hydrocyanic acid, hellebore, hyoscyamus, ignatia, ipecac, nux vomica, opium, pulsatilla, sambucus, secale, senega, tartar emetic, and veratrum. Finally there were substances whose dynamic powers could be increased indefinitely. These included alumina, antimony, argentum, arium, arsenium, carbon, causticum, cuprum, ferrum, graphites, mercury, plumbum, silex, stannum, and sulphur.[70]

Carl Müller, editor of the *American Homeopathic Observer,* walked a middle ground between the low and high dilutionists. He had no trouble criticizing the fanciful claims of Fincke's potencies. "Our greatest objection . . . is purely ethical," wrote the editor. "We don't believe any one can combine the physician and apothecary without producing a hybrid which consists of the worst features of both—a creature which is named like the cry of a duck."[71] Nevertheless, to those who poked fun at the efficacy of high dilutions, he suggested that the fault lay more often in the prescription than in the dilution itself. Being bound to no set or range of potencies, Müller urged students of homeopathy to rely on the clinical test itself to steer them on the right course.[72]

The debate over the low and high potencies consumed much of the rhetoric within homeopathy. Eventually, most were willing to subscribe to the following two propositions: *First,* certain classes of remedies were more effective when given in low attenuations. *Second,* some remedies showed no effect when given in a crude state and "an unloosing and separation of the molecules [was] necessary to furnish to the organism . . . a great number of points of contact." The effect of these two propositions was to place no limits other than the susceptibility of the organism to the stimulant. This meant "every physician may use the entire scale of potencies according to his own discretion."[73]

In the last analysis, however, the two propositions left unresolved the division within homeopathy between the "highs and lows" and between the vitalists and materialists. In an age about to be overwhelmed by an increasingly scientific culture, the stubborn and inelegant nature of this standoff tended to alienate New School reformers from mainstream medicine and, in time, created an internal disenchantment that would result in a rupture within homeopathic ranks. Dynamization, however defined, became a devilish tormentor of homeopathy's public face. Clearly, it appealed to the oracular and mystical elements within homeopathy, particularly those whose kinship was closer to liberal Christianity and the transcendental and Swedenborgian spirits that both animated and inspired lay practice. But for an increasing number of academically educated practitioners, the spiritual interrelatedness between humans and nature was secondary to the forcefulness of scientific rigor. Given the infusion of clinical and laboratory science into the discourse over matter and spirit, homeopathy was left with an inner uneasiness that soon translated into a tangled web of confusion and ultimate conflict over the metaphysical rationale for the efficacy of its healing practices.

Chapter 4

Lies, Damn Lies, and Statistics

Spurred by the establishment of the Société Royale de Médecine (1776) and the later Bureau de Statistiques (1800), and encouraged by the secular and humanitarian spirit of the Enlightenment, individuals such as Jakob Bernoulli (1758-1789), Marie Jean De Condorcet (1743-1794), and Pierre-Simon de Laplace (1749-1827) sought to illuminate knowledge with the more exacting methods of mathematics.[1] Enhanced by the Napoleonic legacy of data collection to support the administrative fabric of the First Empire, Europe's savants sought through quantification a more reassuring basis for their political, scientific, and philosophical thinking. Beginning with classifications in botany and mineralogy, and moving into other fields of natural history, they introduced a whole new way of looking at the world. Opinions, however extreme or inarticulate, rested more comfortably behind the surety of numerical expression.

Before long, such medical men as Philippe Pinel (1745-1826), Étienne Pariset (1770-1847), August François Chomel (1788-1858), Gabriel Andral (1777-1876), Jean Baptiste Bouillaud (1796-1881), and Pierre Charles Alexandre Louis (1787-1872) were bringing these same mathematical techniques into the nosography of diseases, the beneficial effects of particular forms of treatment, and, ultimately, calculations of life and death.[2] To be sure, the value and utility of the calculus of probabilities, statistical analysis, and more basic numerical methods did not enter medicine without challenge, but worked their way into acceptance by first demonstrating their importance to public health officers on matters such as bills of mortality, tracing the course of yellow fever, and accounting for the control of smallpox through vaccination. The initial applications of quantitative methods to issues of public health were often carelessly recorded, highly selective, and used uncritically, evoking at times a storm of criticism and misunderstanding; but advocates eventually overcame the arguments of opponents by demonstrating a clearer and more dramatic understanding of evidentiary materials than heretofore possible.[3]

As James Cassedy explained in his *American Medicine and Statistical Thinking, 1800-1860,* Louis's numerical method became an engine of authority for regular medicine in the nineteenth century and attracted numerous American students, including John Y. Basset, Josiah Nott, and Peter C. Gaillard from the South; William W. Gerhard and Alfred Stille from Philadelphia; Alonzon Clark and Valentine Mott from New York; and James Jackson Jr., Oliver W. Holmes, and George C. Shattock from Boston—all of whom acquired a lasting appreciation for numerical analysis and systematic methods of investigation. Nevertheless, orthodox physicians and state and local medical societies struggled to reach consensus on the uses of statistical information, often stumbling in their observations, experiments, deductions, inductions, and calculations. Daunted in the absence of European-type hospitals and organized record keeping, American doctors were nevertheless able to endorse the Baconian ideal. By the second half of the nineteenth century, American hospitals had progressed to more careful record-keeping habits, and their early calculations contributed significantly to the quest for greater certainty in their medicines and procedures. Leading regulars such as Holmes, Austin Flint (the "American Louis"), and Jacob Bigelow utilized an assemblage of data to question traditional methods of bleeding, purging, and other heroic therapies and, over time, moved inexorably toward a more "expectant" regimen of healing.[4]

Medical orthodoxy was by no means in agreement on either the efficacy or on the appropriate "system" for treatment. The best that could be said was that past methods were uncertain and many diseases, as explained by Jacob Bigelow of Harvard, were self-limited in the degree that they were controllable by any treatment. [5]At the same time that regulars were turning inward as they tested and eventually challenged the conclusions of Cullen, Rush, Broussais, and other authoritative figures with the techniques of numerical analysis (and in the process developed a whole new consensus as to what constituted rational or orthodox medicine), Louis's numerical analysis also became the method of choice among the century's sectarians. Seeking to garner greater respectability for themselves and their movements,

Thomsonians, eclectics, homeopaths, and other irregular medical groups embraced the new methodology to justify their own particular theory and advance their claim to superior medicines. For those enamored with the prospect of giving each individual responsibility for his or her own health and welfare, statistical calculations were given equal billing with spiritual and intellectual authority.

In the war of words between regulars and their homeopathic rivals, early indications suggested that mortality from homeopathic treatment was appreciably lower. Having graduated from the same schools as regulars, many homeopaths were appreciative of Louis's emphasis upon observation and exactness in data gathering. Homeopaths had long benefited from an emphasis on symptomatology, a procedure that encouraged observation, classification, and numerical analysis. As the combatants came head to head over numbers, homeopaths paid careful attention to bills of mortality and applauded the role statistics played among members of the Paris clinical school who so strongly influenced changes in medical treatment in the early decades of the nineteenth century. Feeling increasingly secure in the meticulousness of their data and in the effectiveness of their medicines, they chose to downplay Hahnemann's initial opposition to clinical science and decided instead to claim the high ground by announcing that homeopathy offered the only rational alternative to the chaos of orthodoxy's many systems. Moreover, in addition to lower mortality, the mean duration of their treatment was significantly less, and at a fraction of the cost of allopathic treatment.[6]

CHOLERA

In its battle with regulars, no disease served as a greater catalyst to homeopathy's success than the worldwide pandemic of waterborne cholera that emanated from the Ganges Delta in March 1817. Within a year, it had moved through India, and by 1819 had spread to Samatra, Singapore, Siam, and Ceylon. A year later, cholera visited southern China and the Philippines, and the following year, the Indian Archipelago, Arabia, and Persia. During succeeding years, it spread into central and northern China. It then receded, only to break out once more from the Ganges Delta in 1827; and by 1829 it had penetrated Russia, Poland, Austria, and Moldavia. A year later, it traveled with caravans from Mecca to Cairo, reaching Constantinople in August 1831. That same month, it also appeared in Berlin and Hamburg. The new year brought the disease to Newcastle and London, from where it spread to Scotland. On June 8, 1832, when the *Carrick* arrived in Quebec from Dublin, forty-two of the passengers and crew were already dead from the disease that promptly spread into the city. Within days, it had traveled up the St. Lawrence River to Montreal. On June 26, the ship *Henry IV* arrived in New York harbor with sick passengers and the disease broke out shortly afterward in the city. From there it moved up the Hudson River and also to Philadelphia before traveling westward. Within weeks, it had spread to Charleston, St. Louis, and New Orleans.

In 1847, another pandemic broke out of India, and by the spring of 1848 had spread through Europe, reaching London and Edinburgh by late summer. In December the disease arrived in North America in two vessels that sailed from Le Havre: one docked at Staten Island and the other at New Orleans. By spring, cholera had traveled up the Mississippi and Ohio Rivers, surfacing in Cincinnati and St. Louis, and eventually engulfing the whole Mississippi Valley. From there it moved north to the Great Lakes and Canada and west to Sacramento and San Francisco.[7] Former President James Polk (1795-1849) reputedly died of cholera in Nashville, Tennessee, in June 1849, as did Congressman Joshua Mathiot (1800-1849) of Ohio, Senator Thomas H. Blake (1792-1849) of Indiana, President Zachary Taylor (1784-1850), and former Governor James Clarke (1812-1850) of the Iowa Territory.

In October 1853, cholera once again visited the United States when twenty-eight ships were quarantined at Staten Island with 1,041 cases of the disease. Although cholera seemed to run its course during the winter, it returned in the spring as arriving vessels brought new cases to New York. By May and June, the disease had spread to cities along the post, rail, and water routes of transportation.[8] Other visitations came and went, each originating in India and sweeping across the trade routes of the world. On May 29, 1866, cholera returned to the United States, arriving in New York on the steamer *Union* from Liverpool. A day later, another steamer from Liverpool, the *Peruvian,* docked with thirty-five of its passengers and crew dead from the disease.[9] Within days, the steamships *Atlanta, Helvetia,* and *Virginia* arrived in New York with similar numbers of victims.[10]

Medical journals of all stripes tracked the cholera pandemics, making note of deaths and comparing the results of different treatments. The many published reports, some arranged by country and others by region, city, or simply by hospital, recounted the different types of treatment; in others, the information was less clear.[11] The suspected causes of cholera were many and varied. Theories ranged from a specific poison in the alimentary canal to microscopic insects; changes in the atmosphere (including a deficiency of ozone); calcium or magnesium salts in the drinking water; spontaneous productions from masses of people in motion; immorality; and specific viruses or poisons generated by a mode not yet known or understood and received into the body by inhalation, fear, intemperance, or improper diet.[12] Directions on avoidance generally followed a blind empiricism that knew few bounds. These included avoiding crowds (dwellings, ships, prisons, camps); observing physical and moral cleanliness; maintaining good ventilation of air and sun; abstaining from such foods as beans, broccoli, cabbage, carrots, green corn, cucumbers, unripe fruits, mushrooms, peas, new potatoes, rhubarb, shellfish, spinach, tomatoes, and turnips; avoiding alcoholic and acidic drinks as well as mineral water; and prohibiting cathartics and all forms of moral and physical excess.[13]

Among regulars, treatment for cholera oscillated between contagionists and miasmatists as well as between those who favored more active intervention versus those who preferred waiting on the power of nature. Therapies included the imbibing of alcoholic drinks as a preventive; prescriptions of cajeput oil, creosote, croton oil, mustard emetics, and quinine; large and small quantities of morphine, opium, and tartar emetic; teaspoon doses of calomel in brandy; bleeding and leeches to the epigastrium; plugging the anus; pills of acetate of lead and combinations of opium and camphor; inhalation of oxygen; and galvanism. In addition, physicians urged families and public health officials to use disinfectants such as sulfate of iron, quicklime, chloride of zinc, carbolic acid, and vinegar to clean private and public rooms.[14] The results of these regimens were not often pleasant. In one French army regiment, 700 men reportedly died within six days under heroic doses of tartar emetic.[15]

Sectarians welcomed the opportunity to test the efficacy of their regimens against orthodox practices and were confident in the outcome. In New York City alone, where regulars were accused of losing one out of every two patients to cholera, the Thomsonians claimed to have saved 4,978 of the 5,000 they treated for the same disease.[16] Similar claims were made by sectarians up and down the Atlantic seaboard and inland through the waterways to the Midwest.

Assisted by the fact that traditional mainstays such as bleeding, calomel, antimony, and opium had done little to merit any confidence, it was not unusual for individuals and families to reach out to all manner of claims, including the infinitesimal therapies espoused by Hahnemann's followers. Indeed, regular medicine lost its largest single number of adherents during the cholera pandemics of 1832 and 1849. Having despaired of measures to contain the disease, significant numbers of worried patients migrated to the ranks of the botanics, eclectics, hydropaths, and especially the homeopaths. Unlike regulars, homeopaths tended to underprescribe for their cholera patients, a factor that had a surprisingly positive effect. During the 1831-1832 epidemic, Samuel Hahnemann had recommended the use of camphor, cuprum, and veratrum as individual remedies. Compared to the harsh regimens of regular medicine, these medicines were relatively benign and Hahnemann's disciples were similarly inclined to prescribe in a minimalist manner. Believing the cause of cholera to be "some poisonous modification of the atmosphere, acting directly on the blood through the lungs," some prescribed only camphor, giving five drops of the tincture every five minutes until improvement set in, and then gradually reducing the amount. In New York, this was known as the "German treatment." Other regimens included aconite, arsenicum, carbo vegetabilis, colocynth, ipecacuanha, laurocerasus, mercurius solubilis, phosphorus, sulfur, and secale cornutum.[17] In addition, homeopaths recommended removal to high land, and exposure to pure air and water.[18] In all, they employed some thirty-five different remedies for cholera.[19] The relative success of these agents played an important role in winning additional friends and supporters for the movement.[20]

Homeopaths turned the 1832 and 1849 cholera epidemics into major public relations campaigns, claiming significant savings in lives and utilizing statistical information to buttress their claims. Although not always consistent, their treatment was usually defined as the use of the principle of similars; the use of minute doses given in the form of one medicine at a time; the perseverance of the same medicine so long as there was improvement; and treating each case in accordance with the totality of the symptoms. Prophylactic treatment involved the use of camphor in the first stages of cholera; ipecacuanha when there was vomiting and watery evacuation, with slight cramps; veratrum when the cholera showed signs of permanent cramps, great thirst, and excessive coldness; and cuprum in cases of convulsions, bloody stools, watery diarrhea, and vomiting.[21]

In an unusual paper published in the *North American Homeopathic Journal,* several New School reformers recommended the "teclectic" and "magnetic" properties of copper, brass, and bronze applied homeopathically to the body. It seems that during the cholera epidemics of 1832 and 1849 in Europe, mines and industries where these metals were either extracted or processed reported significantly fewer incidences of the disease. Suspecting that copper possessed anticholera properties, the authors theorized that minute amounts of the metals had a prophylactic power and pointed out that Hahnemann himself had recommended the use of copper (one pellet in the morning) combined with a regular regimen of cleanliness to act as a "certain and efficacious preservative." The authors recommended prophylactic belts consisting of alternate links of copper and brass, separated by rivets of steel and worn around the waist.[22]

Regulars chose the path of ridicule as the best method for attacking homeopathy's appeal. Explaining the arithmetic implications of the dynamization theory in terms of lakes and oceans needed to contain a single grain of cure, they warned the public of the preposterous nature of homeopathy's claims and challenged as well its statistical evidence as deceptive, if not outright dishonest.

Homeopaths were understandably righteous in their indignation against claims that their statistics were misleading and that they practiced "expectant" medicine (i.e., careful adherence to hygienic rules but without medicine) on their cholera patients. They were equally righteous over the posturing attitude of eclectics who often took the side of Old School practice against them. If eclectics were truly what they represented, argued one homeopathic critic, they had better be open to "free discussion, thorough examination, and candid tests" before adopting the best of each system.[23]

Because deaths from cholera proved fearfully high, comparisons were made of allopathic and homeopathic treatments at hospitals in Austria, Hungary, Russia, and in Bordeaux. In Vienna, the Hospital of the Sisters of Charity opened in 1832 during the cholera epidemic and treated patients until January 1835, offering both homeopathic and allopathic systems of treatment. In 1835, the hospital's director, a Dr. Fleishmann, decided to treat patients exclusively by homeopathic methods.[24] As a result of his success, the emperor of Austria rescinded the statute forbidding the practice of homeopathy and established an institution in Vienna for teaching it.[25] In England, fourteen allopathic hospitals between 1849 and 1854 reported an average mortality rate from cholera of 43 percent; and one American and eight European hospitals in the years 1831, 1849, and 1854, reported an average mortality rate of 54 percent. By contrast, six European homeopathic hospitals for the years 1834, 1849, and 1854 posted a mortality rate from cholera of 27 percent.[26] Between October 1848 and February 1849, the General Board of Health of Edinburgh and Leith reported 66.45 percent mortality for patients treated allopathically and 24.25 percent for those treated homeopathically. The statistics were so compelling that the physician who had presided over a meeting of medical men at Brighton to pass resolutions attacking homeopathy in 1851 announced later his conversion to New School reform.[27]

In 1855, the House of Commons in England requested a report on the management of cholera under the rival systems of homeopathy and allopathy. Dr. John McLoughlin, medical inspector to the General Board of Health, visited all hospitals in 1854 and reported that the number of deaths occurring under homeopathic treatment amounted to only 16.4 percent, while deaths under allopathic treatment had reached 59.2 percent.[28] In the report, McLoughlin reputedly made the astounding admission that had he been afflicted with cholera, he would have preferred the care of a homeopath rather than an allopathic physician. Lord Robert Grosvenor, a member of parliament, forced the government to publish the report.[29]

In October 1866, following an outbreak of cholera in Chicago, the students of Rush Medical College voted to return to their homes to avoid the epidemic. Only a week previously, they had sat through several lectures on the disease and its treatment. Out of 100 students, only twenty chose to remain in the city. "What a commentary in the vaunted confidence of the allopaths in their own medicines!" remarked a cynic in the *American Homeopathic Observer*.[30]

More than any other disease, cholera played a disproportionate role in the claims and counterclaims of regulars and sectarians and precipitated the significant migration of regulars into the camps of so-called irregulars. Distraught and disillusioned with the age-old regimen of regulating intake and outflow of the body's secretions, many regulars found comfort in using doses of medicine that did not assault the patient's own recuperative powers.

YELLOW FEVER

In 1853, the scourge of yellow fever made its annual pilgrimage to New Orleans, Mobile, Vicksburg, Natchez, and other southern cities, killing thousands and causing a seasonal flight north of individuals and whole families seeking to escape the disease. In New Orleans alone, more than 6,500 died in July and August 1853, out of a total population of 40,000.[31] Noted homeopaths treating yellow fever included doctors William H. Holcombe and F. A. W. Davis of Natchez; doctors Gustavus M. Taft, Alexis Leon, J. Vail, James G. Belden, Richard Angell, Adolphe Cartier, and Alexander Burritt in New Orleans; doctors Joseph R. Brown and Richard L. Bryant in Galveston; and Dr. J. Barton in Charleston.[32]

William H. Holcombe (1825-1893) found himself in the middle of the Natchez epidemic and waited anxiously to test New School therapeutics against the disease. Concluding that homeopathy had been successful in fighting cholera, pneumonia, and other life-threatening illnesses, he showed less concern than others for the advancing epidemic. Natchez, a city of 6,000, was situated on a bluff 150 feet above the Mississippi River. In a matter of weeks, the disease had moved through its neighborhoods, where regular doctors relied on the old standbys of bloodletting, emetics, mercurial purges, and diaphoretics in the first stage; and calomel (pushed to salivation) and quinine (three- or five-grain doses) every one or two hours, with brandy or wine, blisters and rubefacients in the second stage. Some regulars prescribed ten- to forty-grain doses of quinine, placing patients under blankets with their feet in hot water; closing the doors and windows; and giving hot drinks. Victims remained in a condition of filth and stale air for a week or more to sweat out the disease. [33]

Holcombe accused allopaths of impairing the vital powers, disturbing the natural processes of cure, complicating treatment, and retarding recovery. Based on the ancient doctrine of *crases,* allopathy's harsh regimens were little more than a "death-warrant" for patients.

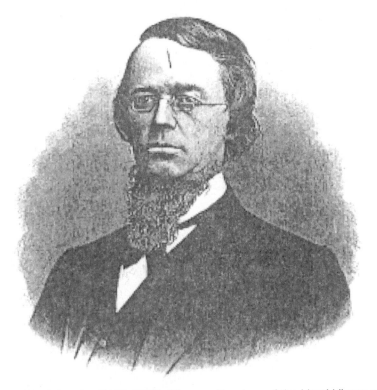

William H. Holcombe (1822-1893). (*Source:* Courtesy of the Lloyd Library and Museum, Cincinnati.)

Although the specific purgative action of mercury operated in a crudely homeopathic manner, its dreary history of abuse negated any slight benefit. There was no more "poignant satire on the medical profession, the meagerness of its knowledge, and the poverty of its resources," wrote Holcombe, than the history of mercury's abuse over the previous half century. He also opposed the expectant treatment of French and Spanish physicians and pointed out the reported 29 percent mortality rate among untreated cases in British Guiana and the equally high mortality among unattended victims in New Orleans. "Nothing but pure blind prejudice or stupidity," he observed, prevented one from seeing the inconsistencies in the expectant form of treatment.[34]

In contrast to either expectant or heroic treatments, Holcombe prescribed aconite and belladonna for the first stages of the disease. In a few cases, he used a drop of pure tincture in half a glass of water; in most instances, however, he prescribed five or six drops of the first centesimal dilution, followed by a similar strength of ipecac, which he administered after each incidence of vomiting. During the second stage, when the patient complained of nausea, prostration, abdominal pain, thirst, and restlessness, Holcombe prescribed a fourth trituration of arsenic or a fifth trituration of lachesis (derived from the bushmaster snake), at one-hour intervals. Although he preferred lower dilutions, repeating them frequently, he admitted to sometimes employing a twelfth or even a thirtieth dilution if the lower dilutions had failed. If the patient continued to sink, he gave a first or second centesimal trituration of nitrate of silver, along with arsenic and lachesis. In addition, he paid strict attention to diet, managing the disease with arrow-root, rice-water, and black tea during the first stage; and ice and teaspoons of cream during the second stage. If no improvement occurred, he considered the case hopeless.[35]

While mortality reports from allopathic doctors ranged from 30 to 42 percent in private home settings, and as high as 66 percent in hospitals, homeopaths reported only a 6 percent loss during the yellow fever epidemics of 1853, 1854, and 1856. During the epidemic of 1853, the Mississippi State Hospital in Natchez reported a 55 percent mortality rate. A year later, under homeopathic control, the hospital reported a rate of only 7.9 percent, and in 1855, a rate of 13.7 percent. On the basis of this surprising evidence, the trustees ended allopathic treatment and adopted homeopathy exclusively.[36]

The patrons of homeopathy understandably grew during the epidemics of cholera and yellow fever when Old School compounds proved so ineffective. To their credit, homeopaths encouraged simple rules: choosing a good diet, avoiding the mixing of medicines, remaining free of anxiety, avoiding any change in accustomed activities, securing fresh air, maintaining cleanliness, and prohibiting the eating of under- or overly ripe fruit.[37]

TESTING THE CLAIMS

In the first half of the nineteenth century, experiments testing the validity of homeopathic practice were undertaken in numerous Western and Eastern European countries. They included the following:

- *1832:* At the Hotel Dieu de Lyon, a thirty-bed ward was placed under the charge of Jacques A. Guerard, one of the most distinguished homeopathic physicians in the city. After selecting fifteen patients suffering from various febrile diseases (pneumonia, erysipelas, catarrh, etc.), he prescribed homeopathic medicines in the presence of sixty students and several physicians. The experiment lasted seventeen days with no perceptible improvement in the patients' conditions. Claiming that the same remedies had been effective in private practice, Guerard attributed his failure to the bodily smells in the ward that neutralized the effects of the infinitesimal doses.[38]
- *1834:* At the Hôpital de la Pitié in Paris, Gabriel Andral experimented over a period of a year on 140 patients diagnosed with various diseases, using aconite, arnica, belladonna, cinchona, and sulphur. He concluded that the homeopathic medicines had produced no visible effect.[39] Even though Andral had taken careful steps to ensure the accuracy of his treatment, homeopaths excoriated him for failing to follow their strict rules. They complained bitterly that he had conducted his trials behind closed doors and only announced his "damnatory verdict" in public. Even though he claimed to be faithful to the principles and ideas of Hahnemann, homeopaths accused him and his intern, Maxime Vernois, of erroneous decisions and procedures. Had they not given wine to patients, deprived them of salt, and shown general indifference to more appropriate medication? Critics also accused the two of not being conversant in the German language and therefore unable to consult Hahnemann's *Materia Medica* in the original. Nor had they made use of the French translation of Hahnemann's *Chronic Diseases.* Ignorant of these important texts, they had prescribed the wrong medicines and stopped treatment far sooner than the rules dictated.[40]

  Other homeopaths weighed in as well. Erastus E. Marcy regarded the experiments as dishonest, and accused Andral of possessing neither the knowledge to employ the remedies properly nor "the moral honesty to administer them fairly if he had possessed this knowledge." Had Andral invited a competent homeopath to carry out the test, perhaps homeopaths would have accepted the results. Instead, Andral found it "more agreeable to his interests and to his preconceived notions that the experiment should fail."[41] Homeopath Abraham Howard Okie accused Andral of being a "leader of a medical clique at Paris," and for attacking homeopathy on the basis of experiments that were decidedly unhomeopathic in nature. Because Andral had "no guide" in the prescription of homeopathic medicines, he reputedly made the wrong applications of the medicines employed, and because no homeopaths witnessed the experiments, Okie dismissed Andral's conclusions as wholly without merit.[42]

Homeopathy's railings against Andral were met with deaf ears by regular doctors. The experiences of American students in Andral's wards at La Pitié were a matter of pride for those who had had the good fortune of attending his clinics, courses, and private lessons. Students the caliber of James Jackson Jr. considered the empirical methods of this French pathologist without equal, and Dr. Oliver Wendell Holmes of Boston found it curious that Andral would receive such harsh criticism when families espousing homeopathy used the very same medicines and drew their instructions from the same texts.[43]

- *1834:* Homeopaths lodged similar criticisms against tests performed at Hôtel Dieu where Victor Baillie invited two homeopathic practitioners, Léon Simon (1798-1867) and Paul Francis Curie (1799-1853), to treat patients over a period of five months. Although Curie chose his medicines from the very pharmacy that supplied Hahnemann, the results proved disappointing. Similar experiments by clinical professor Simon had the same unsatisfactory results. For Dr. Oliver Wendell Holmes, the tests demonstrated "the total worthlessness" of homeopathic medicines that were but a "slippery delusion," nothing more.[44] Once again, homeopaths cried foul, claiming the methods used in the test were not in accord with accepted homeopathic techniques.[45]
- *1835:* The King of Naples ordered a commission formed to test homeopathic remedies. The commission consisted of two professors from the University of the Faculty of Medicine, two

members of the Medico-Chirurgical Academy, two members of Public Instruction, and the directors of the city hospital. All homeopathic remedies were placed under tight security, and control of the twenty-bed clinical ward was placed in the hands of two physicians: one chosen by the attending physician, homeopath Chevalier Cosmi de Hortatus, and the other by the commission. Both maintained separate records on each patient. The choice of patients was left to the attending physicians and commission. Although they admitted both acute and chronic patients, the attending physicians were not obliged to accept patients thought to be incurable. Following a forty-day trial, the commission concluded that homeopathic treatment had been ineffective and, in certain diseases, prevented the employment of remedies that could have cured the patient.[46]

- *1835:* The Prussian government ordered a public test of homeopathy at Charité in Berlin by one of Hahnemann's own disciples. When the results proved negligible, Hahnemann dismissed the disciple as incompetent; a second was put in his place, with the same disappointing results.[47]

- *1853:* In the period up to 1853, the average mortality rate at Vienna General Hospital was 8.5 percent compared with three homeopathic hospitals at 5.3 percent. Astonished with these findings, Josef Dietl, physician to the hospital, initiated tests using four methods of treatment for patients diagnosed with pneumonia: bleeding, tartar emetic, expectant, and homeopathic treatment. As the trials commenced, first upon the doctors themselves and then on patients, disbelief gave way to surprise as long-held theories and revered regimens were found wanting. In comparing patients, Dietl noted an average duration of 35 days for cases treated by venesection; 28.9 days for those treated by tartar emetic; 28 days for those treated by the expectant method; and only 11 days for those treated by homeopathy. Mortality rates were equally surprising. In 85 cases treated by venesection, 17 died, or 20.4 percent; in 106 cases treated by tartar emetic, 22 died, or 20.7 percent; and in 189 cases treated by the expectant plan, 14 died, or 7.4 percent. By contrast, of fifty cases treated homeopathically, only three died, or 6 percent. Similar statistics by Charles H. F. Routh, who had been particularly hostile to homeopathy, revealed that of 783 cases of pneumonia treated in various homeopathic hospitals, 45 died, or 5.7 percent; while in 1,522 cases treated by regular medicine, there were 373 deaths, or 24 percent mortality.[48]

- *1864:* In comparing mortality rates in 1864 from dysentery, typhoid fever, diarrhea, and pneumonia at City Hospital (regular) and Cavalry Depot Hospital (homeopathic) in St. Louis, doctors reported very dissimilar results. Of 169 cases admitted to the regular hospital, 63 died, giving a 37.2 percent mortality rate. By contrast, of 179 cases admitted into the homeopathic hospital, doctors reported only 2 deaths, or a mortality rate of 1.1 percent. In more general areas, the regular hospital treated 990, with a mortality of 120, or 12 percent, while the homeopathic hospital admitted 833 cases, with 5 deaths, or .6 percent, showing a clear gain over its rival of 11.4 percent.[49]

- *1867:* Dr. John Hughes Bennett, a zealous regular and professor at the University of Edinburgh, collected statistics from European hospitals showing the results of regular treatment in pneumonia. The standard calomel and lancet approach to treatment produced mortality rates ranging from 12.5 percent to more than 35 percent, while patients who received no medicine but a careful diet registered a mortality rate of 7 percent. The evidence suggested that regular treatment was "worse than no treatment at all!" Bennett provided the statistics to demonstrate the validity of his own treatment that consisted of small doses of salts to "diminish the viscosity of the blood." This regimen, similar to homeopathy, showed a mortality rate of only 4 percent.[50]

Various longitudinal studies were also noted by both of the competing camps.

- *1794-1856:* Studies of sixty-four European hospitals from 1794 to 1840 indicated an average mortality rate for all diseases ranging from 9 to 10 percent. Similarly, the three largest American hospitals (Massachusetts General Hospital, New York City Hospital, and Bellevue Hospital) reported an average mortality rate of 10 percent from 1792 to 1856. By contrast, fifteen European homeopathic hospitals reported an average mortality rate between 5 and 6 percent in the period from 1834 to 1856.[51]

- *1844-1854:* At the Convent of Refuge in Marseilles, France, under allopathic hands from 1841 to 1848, directors reported a

5.5 percent mortality rate, while the mortality rate under homeopathic supervision from 1850 to 1854 was only 2.9 percent.

- *1848-1853:* At the hospital at Gyöngyös, in Hungary, under allopathic treatment from 1848 to 1853, directors reported a 15.7 percent mortality rate, with homeopathic treatment in the same hospital and during the same period reported at 9.3 percent.[52]
- *1849-1851:* At Hôpital St. Marguérite in Paris, directors allocated 100 beds to homeopathy and 99 to allopathy. The allopathic section accepted 3,724 patients, with an average duration of 29 days of sickness, and 411 deaths, or 11.3 percent mortality. The homeopathic section accepted 4,663 patients, with an average stay of 23 days, and 399 deaths, or 8.55 percent mortality. Treatment in the allopathic section cost 23,522 francs while the homeopathic wards cost a mere 300 francs.[53]
- *1849-1851:* Converted allopath Jean-Paul Tessier (1811-1862) and his assistants claimed success in treating cholera and pneumonia patients at the 100-bed Beaujon hospital in Paris on the basis of homeopathic principles.[54] Having taken into account Tessier's prior tendency to treat his pneumonia patients with successive bleedings, critic Worthington Hooker thought it fortunate for his patients that he had moved to homeopathy, since he had been practicing bad allopathy. Of others who had gone over to homeopathy, they "did not bear the character of judicious practitioners previous to their conversion." These apostates were doing less harm with their "sins of omission" than they would have done with their "undiscriminating overdosing."[55]
- *1850-1852:* During a typhus epidemic in Vienna, doctors at the General Hospital reported a 21 percent mortality, while the city's homeopathic hospital reported less than 11 percent.[56]
- *1850-1856:* At the London Homeopathic Hospital, doctors reported a 4.2 percent mortality rate, compared with 18 percent mortality at St. George's, a regular hospital.

Regular Critics

In response to homeopathy's numerical claims, many regulars explained that homeopathy "only amused the patient, while nature wrought the cure."[57] On the other hand, James Young Simpson, professor of midwifery at the University of Edinburgh, reported that the statistical comparisons did not bear out homeopathy's claims. Indeed, the "infallible evidence" paraded before the public of homeopathy's superiority showed instead the "utter frailty and fallaciousness of the statistical proofs and comparisons." Looking specifically at the comparisons published during the cholera epidemic of 1835, Simpson readily admitted that in the large and crowded metropolitan hospitals of London, Edinburgh, and Glasgow, mortality rates were several percentage points higher than those reported by Fleishmann in the Hospital of the Sisters of Charity. However, the raw statistics failed to explain Fleishmann's choice of patients and diseases.[58] Admissions to general hospitals of pulmonary consumption, organic heart disease, aneurism, kidney disease, and stomach disease far exceeded admissions for similar types of cases at private homeopathic hospitals. The same applied to burn cases and wounds. Here, again, regular hospitals received more serious cases, and from a poorer and less healthy class of patients. Seeing that Fleischmann's data had been significantly skewed by his choice of patients and also by his choice of "very mild and curable affections," Simpson concluded that homeopathy's parade of cures had been a sham. Indeed, he questioned whether Fleischmann's mortality rates should not be viewed as alarming, given the mildness of the cases admitted.[59]

Similar criticisms came from Charles H. F. Routh in his essay "On the Fallacies of Homeopathy, and the Imperfect Statistical Inquiries in Which the Results of That Practice Are Estimated," published in 1852. Routh accused Fleischmann of having excluded from admission any moribund cases (patients admitted several hours before death), as well as the least healthy and poorest class of patients. While public hospitals were open to the most "wretched objects living," Fleischmann had the luxury of restricting admissions to a healthier class of workers. This was particularly evident in cases of consumption where Fleischmann admitted to having no drug that could cure the disease or even retard its progress, yet he claimed a lower mortality rate for patients in his hospital.[60]

Dr. Oliver Wendell Holmes added his voice to the debate, arguing that homeopathy's explanation for lower mortality was an *argumentum ad ignorantiam*. "An honest man should be ashamed" to make such a claim, given that the mortality in hospitals depended not only on the particular treatment but on the class of patients the hospital received, the season, the patient's condition, and many other factors. Patients in the wards attended by Pierre Louis at the hospital of La Pitiè, for example, had sought admission in the last stages of consumption. Not to acknowledge this fact represented "a miserable appeal to the thoughtlessness of the vulgar."[61]

Former homeopath John C. Peters, a practicing physician in New York during the 1849, 1854, and 1866 cholera epidemics, saw himself as both a witness and an authority on the medical practices of his day. In his *Treatise on the Origin, Nature, Prevention, and Treatment of Asiatic Cholera* (1866), Peters took exception to homeopathic claims of statistically safer treatment, arguing that the large public hospitals differed greatly from the smaller homeopathic hospitals in the economic status of patients and in the severity of the diseases treated. Among the poor, cholera mortality reached 70 percent and higher, while cases of cholera among the middle and upper classes were fewer. In their efforts to claim respectability, the eclectics, hydropathists, and homeopaths had made no allowance for these factors.[62]

Crimean War

During the Crimean War of 1854-1856, cholera and other communicative diseases ravaged the camps and hospitals of the contending armies. Accounts of suffering British troops and the acknowledged "insufficiency" of military medical staffs unleashed efforts to provide a homeopathic option for soldiers and sailors. Lord Robert Grosvenor, himself an advocate of homeopathy, brought together a number of influential supporters in February 1855 to discuss the possibility. The result was a committee that drew up a memorial, signed on March 29, 1855, and given to Minister of War Lord Panmure requesting that at least one of the hospitals in the Crimea be placed under the direction of homeopathic physicians.[63] The committee argued that in the United States, Pennsylvania and Ohio had already granted charters of incorporation for homeopathic medical schools to which hospitals were attached; that the German states of Bavaria and Baden had authorized professorships of homeopathy in the public universities; that the imperial government of Austria had instituted professorships and homeopathic hospitals in Vienna, Hungary, and other parts of its dominions; and that homeopathic hospitals were established in Russia at St. Petersburg and Moscow.[64]

This information, along with reports that mortality in homeopathic hospitals was half that of allopathic hospitals, influenced one archbishop, several peers of the realm, officers of all branches in the military, fourteen members of parliament, and other prominent lay and clerical officials to sign the memorial.[65] But Lord Panmure remained unimpressed and, in his reply, explained that he could not justify "lending the authority of government to promote this particular mode of medical treatment in the army." The "great principles" of medicine had been "slowly built" by the labor of "able and learned men," and until these principles were proved "erroneous, and consequently abandoned," the government intended to support them.[66]

Claims and Counterclaims

Homeopaths claimed several small victories in their quest for validation. In Austria, Britain, France, Germany, Italy, Russia, Spain, and Switzerland, professorships of homeopathy had seemingly been authorized in public universities and hospitals. Appointments included Dr. T. Buchner, professor of homeopathy in the University of Munich; Dr. F. Arnold, professor of the theory and practice of medicine in the University of Zurich; Dr. William Henderson, professor of medicine and general pathology, and professor of clinical medicine in the University of Edinburgh; Dr. Edward Martin, professor of the theory and practice of medicine in the University of Jena; Dr. Janer, dean of the faculty and professor of clinical medicine, University of Barcelona; Dr. Chevalier de Horatiis, professor of the theory and practice of medicine in the University of Naples, and president of the Royal Academy of Medicine; Dr. Lambrecht, professor of the theory and practice of medicine in the University of Padua; Dr. J. A. Weber, professor of the theory and practice of medicine in the University of Freyburg; Dr. Quadri, professor of ophthalmic surgery, Naples; Dr. H. Arnith, professor of midwifery in the General Hospital, Vienna; Dr. Bigel, professor of midwifery in the University of St. Petersburg; and Dr. Botto, professor of surgery in the University of Genoa. Other acknowledged homeopaths included Professor Leupoldt at the University of Erlangen; Dr. Reubel at the University of Munich; Profes-

sor Quadranti at the University of Naples; Professor Ribes at Mont-
pelier; and Professor Taglianani at Ascoli.[67]

Although these appointments were highly touted in the homeopathic literature, reports circulated that the claims were in error and
that many European governments had passed legislation prohibiting
the system.[68] In a series of letters sent to foreign governments and
vice consuls and ambassadors at U.S. embassies abroad, regular doctors and their medical societies sought to clarify the claims and counterclaims of the two competing systems. According to a letter from
the Austrian minister of foreign affairs to H. R. Jackson, minister resident of the United States in Vienna, homeopathy was not taught by
publicly appointed professors but by private teachers only. Although
doctors in private practice and in cloister, criminal, and private hospitals (e.g., the private hospital in Vienna belonging to the Catholic
Charitable Society of the Grey Sisters) were permitted to use homeopathic methods, the system was not sanctioned in the public hospitals. In France, Spain, and Prussia, similar rules applied, as homeopathy was neither taught nor practiced in the universities or public
institutions but was allowed in private practice.[69] This implied that
public authorities allowed for homeopathic practice, provided that the
physician who professed such beliefs passed an examination and obtained the degree of MD in a regular medical school.[70] At the University of Munich, Dr. Joseph Buechner was an "honorary professor" of
homeopathy who taught the materia medica, but his appointment had
been authorized by a high government official and not by the medical
faculty. Moreover, he had no rank, no voice in the faculty, and no salary from the university. Nor were students obligated to attend his
course of lectures or take an examination in homeopathy as a prereq-
uisite for their degree.[71]

Even Dr. William Henderson, who embraced the views of homeopathy sometime after his appointment in general pathology at the
University of Edinburgh, admitted to employing the system in his private practice but not teaching the subject in his lectures. Because of
the strong antagonisms between homeopathy and allopathy, Henderson opposed teaching the two systems in the same school and recommended against the establishment of a homeopathic chair within the
allopathic department of medicine at the University of Michigan.[72]

Life Insurance

In the early 1860s, most American and British life insurance companies used the so-called Carlisle table of life expectancy as the basis of their calculations. Within this table were statistics on general mortality of one of the healthiest districts in England from 1777 to 1787, without regard to health or age. Later companies adopted the Combined Experience table, which derived from the experiences of seventeen life insurance companies in England over a later period of years. The new table varied little from the Carlisle table, but it did extend life expectancy and allowed for a reduction in the amount of premium assessed.[73]

Actuaries disregarded differences in medical treatment between and among the different schools of medicine. But claims that individuals using homeopathic treatment were more often cured, and that continued employment of the homeopathic system actually prolonged life, raised questions as to whether life insurance companies would recognize these as factors affecting premiums. In December 1864, the directors of the General Provident Assurance Company of London asked shareholders to consider the potential bearing of homeopathic medical treatment on company policy. The actuaries investigating comparative medical treatment concluded that persons treated homeopathically enjoyed "more robust health," were "less frequently attacked by diseases," and when attacked, recovered "more rapidly than those treated by any other system." In fatal diseases, the mortality rate under homeopathy was lower, and some diseases considered incurable under allopathy were, in fact, "perfectly curable" under homeopathy. Finally, the actuaries determined that the medicines prescribed on the basis of homeopathic theory did less injury to the body. On the basis of the evidence, the company's shareholders accepted the recommendation to establish a "special section" for those treated homeopathically and to charge a lower premium than that assessed on other lives. The stockholders adopted the recommendation without dissent.[74]

The decision taken by General Provident led to the founding in 1866 of an American company that offered a similar discount to those using the homeopathic system of medicine exclusively.[75] The board of directors of Hahnemannian Life Insurance Company of Cleveland, with a capital stock of $200,000 and authority to extend to $1 million, included president Herman M. Chapin, mayor of Cleveland; former U.S. Senator Benjamin F. Wade; S. L. Mather of Cleveland Iron Mining Company; William Hewitt, superintendent of Union Line Express; and Dr. Jabez P. Dake, president of the Dover Bay Grape and Wine Company.[76] Actuary Elizar Wright developed the tables for Hahnemann Life of Cleveland, justifying a 10 percent discount from regular premiums.[77]

At the annual meeting of the Western Institute of Homeopathy in Cleveland in 1865, Chapin and the directors welcomed delegates to the company offices and assured them that the goals of the company and the interests of the profession were the same. Responding on behalf of the delegates, Charles Hempel pledged the institute's support to the company.[78] In 1866, the American Institute of Homeopathy forbade the use of its name in any manner to advertise or promote companies such as the Hahnemannian Insurance Company of Cleveland or the Atlantic Mutual Company at Albany.[79] A year later, however, the Michigan Homeopathic Institute made a similar commitment to that of the Western Institute of Homeopathy, recommending that patrons of the association give their business to any life insurance company willing to reduce premiums for those who employed homeopathic physicians.[80] Later that same year, at the second annual meeting of the Homeopathic Medical Society of Pennsylvania, members passed a resolution expressing their gratitude to those companies that recognized the superiority of homeopathy over other systems. The resolution recognized the companies as "an important coadjutor . . . in medical reform" and urged homeopathic practitioners to acquaint themselves with the special features of these companies so that they might convey that information to their patrons.[81]

By 1869, four additional companies were established in the United States with similar discount policies.[82] In four years, New England Homeopathic Mutual Life issued approximately 2,700 policies on those who followed homeopathic practice, and 500 for those relying exclusively upon allopathic practice. As justification of its discount policy, the company reported that the losses paid to regulars were eight times greater than those paid to homeopaths.[83]

The Atlantic Mutual Life Insurance Company of Albany, New York, proposed not only a 10 percent discount to those using homeopathy exclusively but also promised to make an additional discount from 20 to 25 percent as comparative rates of mortality became more definitely determined.[84] In defending its position, the company referred to statistics showing that, with regard to all diseases, 4.17 persons of every 100 died after being treated by homeopathy while 13.53 died under allopathy. In other words, allopathic mortality was 3.24 times that of homeopathy. In specific diseases, the company reported an allopathic mortality rate 2.94 times that of homeopathy for cholera; 3.95 times for typhus; 5.84 times for pneumonia; and 8.20 times for yellow fever. This resulted in a general average of 8.5 deaths per 100 under homeopathy and 34.39 under allopathy, for a mortality rate of 4.83 times greater from allopathic treatment than from homeopathic.[85] This information, while published frequently in homeopathic journals, was ignored in regular medical journals.

During its first three years, Atlantic Mutual Life was true to its promise and provided a deduction of 10 percent from the usual rates. However, company officials found that the discount tempted persons to misrepresent themselves in their applications.[86] As a result, the company eliminated the discount in 1869 and set the same rate for all insured persons. It did, however, keep separate accounts for regular and homeopathic insured and, in 1872, reconsidered its decision and not only reinstituted the 10 percent deduction but increased it to nearly 19 percent.[87] The prosperity of Atlantic Mutual remained a continual matter of discussion among homeopaths since three-fourths of the company's policies were issued at a reduced premium. The company's published tables showing the superiority of homeopathic over allopathic treatment and its directors hoped that the profession would communicate that information to patients.[88]

A third company, the Homeopathic Mutual Life Insurance Company, obtained a charter in 1868 to operate in the city of New York.[89] By 1870, the company was writing 130 policies a month, and paying dividends averaging 18 to 35 percent.[90] From tables prepared by the company's actuaries, homeopathy lost ten patients to every seventeen lost by allopathy. These were statistics of private practice, compiled from official records, and used by the company in its justification for insuring homeopaths at less than the usual rate.[91] By 1880, the company had written 11,293 policies and its president, Dr. E. M. Kellogg, sent leaflets documenting the company's statistics to many parts of the world, including India.[92] In comparing mortality rates for the cities of New York, Boston, and Philadelphia, Kellogg provided the results shown in Tables 4.1 and 4.2.[93]

Advertisement for the Homeopathic Mutual Life Insurance Company, New York, 1873. (*Source:* Courtesy of the Lloyd Library and Museum, Cincinnati.)

Kellogg's tracts also included medical statistics comparing mortality rates of homeopathic and regular doctors in the cities of Brooklyn and Philadelphia. For every 100 deaths by regular doctors, Kellogg provided a corresponding ratio for homeopathy. The results (see Table 4.3) showed that the death rate among those treated homeopathically was almost half that of patients treated allopathically.[94]

Of the approximately ten insurance companies that offered discounts to persons adhering to the homeopathic system, only one survived to 1880. The rest merged, were bought out, or went out of business. Nevertheless, homeopathy had made its mark in the commercial world of annuities and life insurance by being singled out among the schools of medicine for special treatment.[95]

SUMMARY

With rational or orthodox medicine under siege, it was understandable that homeopaths saw themselves as "honest laborers after truth" who sought to "clear away the rubbish of former theories" that included the humoral beliefs of Hermann Boerhaave, the nervous doctrine of William Cullen, and the gastroenteric ideas of François J. V. Broussais. Although homeopaths claimed vindication with information derived from medical statistics, surprisingly they paid little attention to the early achievements in pathological anatomy. The Paris clinical school had taught physicians to compare abnormal tissues

TABLE 4.1. Mortality rates: Allopathic treatment.

City	Year	Physicians	Deaths	Ratio
New York	1870	944	14,869	15.75
	1871	984	15,526	15.78
Boston	1870	218	3,872	17.76
	1871	233	3,369	14.46
	1872	233	4,575	19.63
Philadelphia	1872	655	12,468	19.03
Average				16.73

TABLE 4.2. Mortality rates: Homeopathic treatment.

City	Year	Physicians	Deaths	Ratio
New York	1870	143	1,287	9.00
	1871	156	1,243	7.97
Boston	1870	40	402	10.05
	1871	44	363	8.25
	1872	54	446	8.26
Philadelphia	1872	168	2,162	12.87
Average				9.75

TABLE 4.3. Comparative mortality rates by disease.

Disease	Homeopathic	Allopathic
Bronchitis	48	100
Cerebrospinal meningitis	44	100
Cholera infantum	64	100
Croup	87	100
Diarrhea	85	100
Diphtheria	63	100
Dysentery	39	100
Erysipelas	33	100
Inflammation of brain	69	100
Inflammation of bowels	33	100
Inflammation of lungs	39	100
Scarlet fever	69	100
Small pox	61	100
Typhoid fever	88	100
Total	722	1400

with healthy ones and give a scientific estimate of those changes, but according to homeopath I. G. Rosenstein pathological anatomy could "accomplish nothing beyond this" since autopsies yielded "very imperfect information."[96] Stung in part by the harsh criticisms of Gabriel Andral, the earliest homeopaths chose not to look at the lessons drawn from postmortem examinations but, instead, turned to ancient theories (e.g., no two similar diseases can exist in the body at the same time) and so-called natural laws. Eventually, they would lay claim to the findings of the Paris clinical school and its emphasis upon empirical observation, but not until they had moved beyond the metaphysical constraints imposed by their founder.

In due time, academic homeopaths discovered that the findings of morbid anatomy offset Hahnemann's indifference to specific diseases and the internal changes produced by them. From the Paris clinical school and the opening forays of statistical medicine, trained homeopaths learned to appreciate the similarities rather than the uniqueness of patient cases, a change in thinking that required a true mental leap of faith for New Schoolers who had cut their teeth on the uniqueness of each patient. This also required experienced practitioners to make use of solid scientific research, not just a simple belief in nature and God. One unanticipated outcome of this change in doctrine was to reverse homeopathy's opposition to the objectification of therapeutic knowledge while retaining its rhetorical emphasis on symptomatology and the distinctiveness of the individual patient. Another unanticipated outcome was for academic homeopaths to minimize the centrality of the doctrine of similars while stressing instead the lower dilutions and supporting regimens common within regular medicine.[97]

As explained by James Cassedy in his *American Medicine and Statistical Thinking,* the data collected in antebellum medicine "were crude and faulty, often scant and incomplete in quantity and suspect in quality." Carelessly collected and often using only selected information, the data were all too often used uncritically to serve personal wants and needs. Misuses, misapplications, and wild claims abounded during this period of emerging statistical science. Nevertheless, they were a "symbol of medical progress," an initial step toward attaining some degree of medical certainty, and one of the more productive sources of the century's new knowledge.[98]

Overall, the rank and file of both allopathy and homeopathy were conspicuously overbearing in their public pronouncements of statistical superiority. Their denominational rivalry left each with undoubting confidence in their own numbers and a determination to discredit the claims and reputation of the other. As no standards existed to settle their differences, the public was left with a statistical stalemate. At best, the two schools had become victims of their own propaganda. This was one area where regular medicine met its match. Here, homeopathy wrestled with the arrogance of ill-tempered regulars and came away with a sense of righteousness and self-sufficiency.

Chapter 5

The Passing of Knowledge

For more than a century, American homeopaths benefited from professional options available to few other sectarians or their European counterparts. In effect, they could obtain their degrees from a regular medical school and supplement their education with a homeopathic apprenticeship or postgraduate instruction on homeopathic principles and therapeutics. Those who took their education at a regular school before turning to homeopathy, however, were sometimes faced with revocation of their diplomas. This hostile act proved to be an exception rather than the rule, because regular medical schools and their faculty tended to turn a blind eye to the practice. Over time, however, the practice of obtaining a regular medical education first and then taking postgraduate work in homeopathy worried homeopathic educators, who feared the loss of potential New School doctors to regular medicine. Too much importance was attached to the mere possession of a diploma, wrote homeopath L. M'Farland in 1854 (p. 145), "as if the exhibition of that was sufficient to settle the question of professional competency."[1]

Homeopaths generally applauded the establishment of their own colleges, but the sentiment was not unanimous. One critic, writing anonymously in 1859 in the *North American Journal of Homeopathy,* complained that most homeopathic colleges were not in a "ripe state of learning," and lacked the necessary clinical appliances to warrant a broad educational environment. He found the lectures inadequate and the professors lacking the most elementary scientific knowledge and practical sense.[2] Reflective of efforts initiated by the early Thomsonians and eclectics, the author of the article urged the creation of one "noble school," a national college, that would teach the science of medicine while a "well conducted" hospital would illustrate homeopathy's practical applicability at the bedside of the sick. True medical education required both the clinical advantages of a good hospital and the scientific foundations that were taught in the classroom. "Books may take the place of the professor's lectures, but they can never bring the student into actual contact with the various forms of disease that fill the wards of an infirmary in a populous city," the critic wrote. No longer should diplomas be easily obtainable from medical colleges. This deplorable practice had "sunk the profession in the eyes of the people." Men unable to read, spell, or write, but who had obtained medical degrees, brought the social position and the income level of the physician to the lowest level. "Make it impossible for the butcher in 1858 to be the 'MD' of 1859!" he concluded. Abraham Flexner used nearly the same language fifty-two years later.[3]

The call for a single national homeopathic university, preferably located in the east, did not resonate well with the majority of New School reformers. Reflecting the interests of a broader and less regionally dominated reform movement, editor Edwin M. Hale of the *North American Journal of Homeopathy* hoped instead to see a college in New Orleans, another on the shores of the Pacific, and others in the emerging cities east and west.[4] He viewed competition between and among the institutions in Philadelphia, Chicago, St. Louis, and Cleveland as healthy, honorable, and high-minded in that it elevated the standard of medical education. Only when rivalry turned nasty and cliquish did it become self-serving and destructive. For this reason, he urged the avoidance of "slanderous and cowardly attacks" on competing schools as detrimental to the future of homeopathy.[5]

Over the course of the late nineteenth century, Hale's opinion predominated as growing numbers of homeopaths saw the wisdom of establishing a collective identity via their own schools. As a result, dozens of departments and freestanding schools opened. Many were proprietary in nature and not unlike regular medical colleges in the first decades of the century. Others were affiliated with state-funded or private universities. Approximately one-third of the colleges were established in Pennsylvania, New York, Massachusetts, the District of Columbia, and Maryland, and the remaining two-thirds in Ohio, Kentucky, Illinois, Missouri, Michigan, Minnesota, Iowa, Colorado, and California (see Appendix B).[6] By the turn of the century, twenty-one of these schools still operated, with a combined enrollment of approximately 2,000 students and a graduation rate of about 400 doctors annually. Ten years later, following the publication of Abraham Flexner's *Medical Education in the United States and Canada* (1910) and the increased regulation by the American Association of Medical Colleges and the Council on Education of the American Medical Association, the number of schools declined to fifteen, with a student enrollment and an annual graduation rate cut almost in half. By 1923, only two schools remained (Hahnemann Medical College and Hospital of Philadelphia and New York Homeopathic Medical College and Flower Hospital), leaving homeopaths to ponder the future of their system.

PENNSYLVANIA'S DISCORDANCE

In August 1834, doctors Henry Detwiller, William Wesselhoeft, John Eberhard Freitag, John Romig, Joseph H. Pulte, Adolph Bauer, J. C. Gosewitch, and Gustav Reichhelm, along with four ministers, formed the Homeopathic Society of Northampton and Counties Ad-

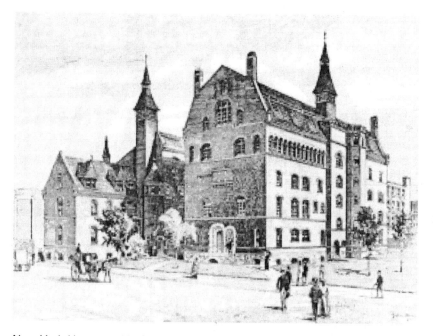

New York Homeopathic College and Hospital, 1889. (*Source:* Courtesy of the National Library of Medicine.)

jacent.[7] Out of their meetings, America's first homeopathic college was founded on April 10, 1835, the eightieth anniversary of the birth of Samuel Hahnemann. The society invited Dr. Constantine Hering (1800-1880) of Philadelphia to become president of the college.[8] Hering, an enthusiast of German democracy, had received his medical degree from the University of Würzburg in 1826 before joining a botanical and zoological expedition to Surinam in South America during which time he lived in a German Moravian colony and became a convert to homeopathy. On learning that his newfound medical interests were unappreciated by the king of Saxony, Hering migrated to Philadelphia where he joined a small group of homeopaths seeking charter for an academy. Hering agreed to assume the school's leadership provided the society could guarantee him a salary equivalent to a "first-class Allentown clergyman."[9]

The curriculum devised by Hering and the society consisted of a course of lectures during the summer months (when regular medical schools were not in session). On June 17, 1836, the Pennsylvania legislature incorporated the college as the *Nordamerikanische Akademie der homöopathischen Heilkunst* (North American Academy of the Homeopathic Art).[10] Like most other proprietary medical schools of the day, the academy formed as a stock company with subscribers from Allentown, Bethlehem, Philadelphia, and New York. The company purchased land in the center of Allentown and constructed two red brick buildings housing classrooms, faculty offices, and chemical, anatomical, and dissecting rooms. A botanical garden also occupied the grounds. Lectures, given in German, were intended to supplement regular medical college curricula. Subjects included clinical instruction, pharmacodynamics and materia medica, medical botany, dietetics, surgery and obstetrics, medical jurisprudence, general therapeutics, symptomatology, anatomy and physiology, chemistry, zoology, astronomy, mathematics, history of medicine, and history of the natural sciences. Those completing the course of studies were required to pass an examination, present a résumé, and prepare a dissertation.[11]

The academy was short-lived, undermined by the failure of the Allentown Bank where its funds were deposited. Instruction ended in 1839, and in 1842, following several false starts, the academy closed and its buildings were sold to pay the school's mortgage. During Hering's tenure as president, he organized an archive for case histories of provings and edited the *Correspondenzblatt der Homoopatis-chen Aerzte* (1835-1837), which provided the principal source of communication between American and German homeopaths. The academy also provided Hahnemann's wife, Mélanie, with a diploma in 1840.[12] After the academy closed, Hering returned to Philadelphia where he once again opened a general practice and continued his research and writing, contributing to the materia medica, publishing books on domestic medicine, and playing a decisive role in the founding of the Homeopathic Medical College of Pennsylvania and its successor, the Hahnemann Medical College of Philadelphia.[13]

In February 1848, doctors Hering, Jacob Jeanes (1800-1877), and Walter Williamson (1811-1870) petitioned the legislature to charter a homeopathic school in Philadelphia. Two months later, the Homeopathic Medical College of Pennsylvania was established. The school's board of trustees then formed a committee to develop curricula in anatomy, physiology, pathology, surgery, materia medica, chemistry, toxicology, botany, medical jurisprudence, and obstetrics—as well as in homeopathic subjects.[14] Original faculty and staff included Williamson, dean and professor of midwifery and diseases of women and children; Jeanes, in principles and practice; Caleb B. Matthews (1801-1851), in materia medica; Francis Sims, in surgery; Samuel Freedley, in botany; Matthew Semple (1813-1867), in chemistry; William A. Gardiner (1823-1863), in anatomy; Alvan E. Small (1811-1886), in physiology and pathology; and John S. Foley, as janitor.[15] The faculty pledged to adhere firmly to the principles of Hahnemann and never to compromise with allopathy, hydropathy, or eclecticism.[16]

Mention of the janitor in the college's publications was typical of medical schools of the day, since the janitor's role was critical to both faculty and students. Not only did he maintain the cleanliness of the premises, he also arranged for the acquisition of anatomical material and, like a French concierge, served as broker between students and local tradespeople for food, lodging, laundry, and other necessities. Good janitors were cherished as beloved and essential fixtures in nineteenth-century medical schools.

In 1850, the college moved to Filbert Street, near Eleventh, in the central part of the city, in a building previously occupied by the Pennsylvania Medical College. The basement was used for practical surgery and to store anatomical material; the first floor held a lecture room with laboratory; the second floor housed the school's museum;

the third floor contained an amphitheater and dispensary; and the top floor, typical of most medical schools, was reserved for dissection so that the smells of the dead bodies exited the windows and did not linger in the corridors of the building.[17] In 1855 the trustees purchased the building on Filbert Street, which they had previously rented, as well as two adjoining buildings, which allowed for expanded clinical instruction. The college remained on Filbert Street for thirty-six years and then moved in 1886 to larger and more accommodating facilities on Broad Street.[18]

Among the medical colleges of Philadelphia for the 1852-1853 school year, the Homeopathic Medical College of Pennsylvania ranked fourth in the production of doctors.[19]

School	Graduates
Jefferson Medical College	223
University of Pennsylvania	160
Pennsylvania Medical College	56
Homeopathic Medical College	55
Philadelphia Medical College	25
Female Medical College	7
Total	526

As in most medical schools of the day, financial problems and dissension among faculty and between faculty and trustees were part of the everyday landscape. At the Homeopathic Medical College of Pennsylvania, power resided in the hands of a twelve-member lay board of trustees that viewed New School reform differently than did the faculty. While faculty focused on preparing professional doctors, lay board members often advocated domestic kits and proprietary medicines. Thus, the college's first internal controversy came when Frederick Humphreys (1816-1900), hired by the board to teach institutes of medicine, was accused by the faculty of promoting and selling his own patent medicines. Rather than permit the disagreement to become public, Humphreys resigned his position, preferring the life of a wealthy pharmaceutical manufacturer to that of a struggling teacher.[20]

Other matters were not so easily resolved, such as the growing debate between the school's liberal and conservative factions. Preeminent among the college's conservative proponents was Adolphus

Lippe (1812-1888) who immigrated to the United States in 1837 and graduated from the North American Academy of the Homeopathic Art in 1841. As one of the original supporters of the Philadelphia college, he sought to influence the institution to be more conservative by aggressively attacking its more liberal faculty, especially Charles Julius Hempel (1811-1879) who had emigrated from Prussia to the United States in 1835. Hempel had received his medical degree from New York University Medical College before discovering homeopathy through pharmacist and publisher William Radde (1800-1884). Over the years, Hempel supported New School reform and established his reputation by translating many of the early homeopathic works into English.[21]

Hempel did not forgive or forget the treatment he received from Lippe, viewing his attacks as an assault on the true principles of homeopathy. In a communication to the editor of the *Philadelphia Journal of Homeopathy* in 1854, he identified Lippe as a "former gentleman and . . . the greatest ignoramus living."[22] In subsequent years,

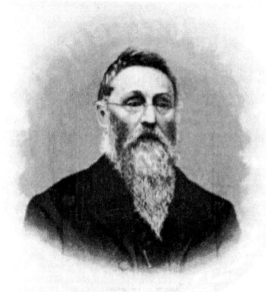

Adolphus Lippe (1812-1888), founder of the International Hahnemannian Association. (*Source:* Courtesy of National Library of Medicine.)

Hempel accused Lippe and his "clique" of high dilutionists of having undermined the reputation of the college.[23] Lippe and his supporters had endorsed provings of the 1,000th potency, substituted "sophistical reasonings" and "high-potency hocus-pocus" for common physiology and pathology, and had recklessly permitted their own scholastic thinking to replace the significant findings of Rudolf Virchow's cellular pathology.[24] In a letter to the editor of the *American Homeopathic Observer*, Hempel claimed that Lippe's teachings were "utterly destructive" of the truths of homeopathy, and anyone who endorsed his doctrines was similarly guilty of disgracing the homeopathic school with "silly assumptions [and] perversions."[25]

From 1854 to 1857, Hempel held the chair of materia medica and therapeutics at the college. Two days before commencement exercises in 1857, for which he had been invited to give the valedictory address, he was fired by the board of managers for not adhering to the teachings of pure homeopathy. Hempel questioned the board's power to remove professors at its pleasure, believing that faculty should be removed only for "grossly immoral conduct" or for "evident incapacity to discharge the duties of their office." Any other reason simply was not justified.[26] Observing that the college had become a battleground between the "great principles of philosophical organization, of scientific truth and moral integrity," and a "clique of secret mischief-workers [in] the black arts of intrigue and slander," Hempel concluded that his dismissal was inevitable.[27] The era of homeopathic science had begun, but the ideal it sought to attain was impossible until the college removed from its ranks those dogmatists who "planted the iron hoof of an unmeaning and frivolous conservatism upon the neck of Homeopathy." Entrenched in their ways, they had transformed the school into a "Synagogue of Satan."[28]

Hempel accused Lippe of having distorted Hahnemann's ideas with "childish extravagances" and of moving away from the principles of true reform medicine. While Hahnemann had repudiated pathological speculations, those at the college denied the entire pathology of disease. Similarly, while Hahnemann had taught that symptoms were the only *reliable* guides, Lippe and his colleagues taught that symptoms constituted "the alpha and omega of disease."[29] Hempel regarded symptom mania as the first obstacle on the road to a "new medical Gospel." This mania had elicited "smiles of incredulity" from friends and opponents alike and had enticed homeopathic

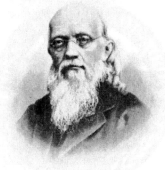

Charles J. Hempel (1811-1879). (*Source:* Courtesy of the National Library of Medicine.)

physicians to lose confidence in the healing power of nature. This attitude had arisen partly from Hahnemann's position on the expectant method in vogue among certain members of Old School medicine. Nevertheless, nature's own restorative energy constituted one of the pillars of Hahnemann's system, evident in his early emphasis upon diet and his practice of giving single infinitesimal doses of sugar of milk to his patients.[30]

Hempel's experiences at the hands of Lippe and the board represented the beginning salvo of the school's ideological feuds. At the close of the 1859-1860 session, with open dissension among the faculty due to the board's decision to substitute corporate script for salaries, the trustees vacated the chairs and filled them with new faculty.[31] The thirteenth annual announcement (1860-1861) of the college gave notice of this change.[32]

During the 1863-1864 session, trouble again arose between the faculty and trustees and, at the end of the session, the trustees once again replaced the chairs. Insisting that the college remain true to Hahnemann's principles, Lippe tried to acquire controlling interest (thereby dictating the school's medical theory) or, alternatively, organize a competing school. From his position as chair in materia medica at the college (1864-1869), Lippe gained both managerial and political control of the college. In 1865, the trustees obtained a new charter, forming a stock company with capital of $60,000 (3,000 shares valued at $20 per share). Unlike the former charter, under which the stockholders chose the trustees to govern the college on a continuing basis, the new charter authorized the stockholders to elect a board of trustees to serve single-year appointments. These trustees, in turn, appointed faculty on year-to-year contracts. Power resided in the stockholders, which in this case reverted to a single individual, Lippe, who controlled the majority of stock.

One immediate issue was the appointment of Charles G. Raue (1820-1896) to the new chair of special pathology and diagnostics. This position had been pushed by liberals seeking to align homeopathic science with the newer findings of the Paris and German clinical schools. Unfortunately for the liberals, the appointment of Raue came at a difficult moment in the school's financial state. As majority stockholder, Lippe's first order of business was to remove the chair of special pathology. Numerous faculty members, including Hering, John C. Morgan, and Lemuel Stephens, resigned in protest. Unable to weather the storm, the college closed after twenty-one years.[33]

Several faculty who left the Homeopathic Medical College of Pennsylvania to protest its peculiar form of governance and Lippe's managerial dominance acquired the charter of Washington Medical College of Philadelphia and, by an act of the court in 1867, changed its name to the Hahnemann Medical College of Philadelphia. Faculty and staff included Hering as dean and chair of institutes and materia medica; Charles G. Raue (1820-1896) in practice of medicine, special pathology and diagnosis; John C. Morgan (1830-1903) in surgery; Henry Noah Martin (1829-1889) in midwifery, diseases of women and children, and lecturer on clinical medicine; Richard Koch (1838-?) in physiology, general pathology, and microscopic anatomy; Amos R. Thomas (1826-1895) in anatomy; Lemuel Stephens (1817-1892) in natural philosophy, chemistry, and toxicology; H. Ryland Warriner in forensic medicine; C. H. Von Tagen as demonstrator and lecturer in surgical anatomy; and William Ware as janitor.[34] Professors Hering, Raue, Morgan, Koch, and Stephens had formerly held chairs in the Homeopathic Medical College of Pennsylvania, and Warriner had been a trustee.[35]

After a faltering beginning, the trustees acquired the charter and physical facilities of the former Homeopathic Medical College of Pennsylvania in 1869 and the two colleges merged as one corporation, the Hahnemann Medical College of Philadelphia. The merger was arranged by Henry N. Guernsey (1817-1885) who, disappointed with the ideological destructiveness of Lippe and his colleagues, managed to acquire Lippe's shares and sell them to Hering, thus ending Lippe's hold on the school. Guernsey, a devout Swedenborgian, became professor of obstetrics at the college, author of *The Application of the Principles and Practice of Homeopathy to Obstetrics and the Disorders Peculiar to Women and Young Children* (1873) and an early advocate of high potencies.[36]

To its credit, the newly consolidated college avoided the dissension of earlier years by offering tenure to the faculty instead of annual appointments. This settled, the college embarked on a period of stability and the faculty focused on expanding the curriculum, tightening standards, and taking a more progressive approach to homeopathic theory and practice, particularly regarding dosage.[37] The school announced in 1869 an optional track that offered students more specialized training during a third year in special pathology and diseases, materia medica, surgery, clinical surgery, clinical medicine, midwifery, diseases of women and children, toxicology, and medical jurisprudence.[38]

As successor to the Homeopathic Medical College of Pennsylvania, the Hahnemann Medical College of Philadelphia boasted of being the oldest homeopathic college in the world, with 800 alumni, a renowned anatomical museum, clinical privileges in both homeopathic and allopathic hospitals in the city, and a permanent and experienced faculty.[39] In 1885 the trustees changed the name to the Hahnemann Medical College and Hospital of Philadelphia. From then to the turn of the century, the school and faculty held their own among medical colleges in Philadelphia, responding to the changing educational landscape by recognizing the need for well-trained professionals. No doubt competition with the city's rival institutions lay behind many of the changes. Among the six homeopathic schools established before the Civil War and the dozens that opened, merged, reorganized, or closed before the end of the century, the Hahnemann Medical College and Hospital of Philadelphia was America's premier homeopathic institution.[40] Between 1887 and 1905 six buildings were constructed, including a medical college, a dispensary and general hospital, a women's hospital, and a residence for student nurses.[41]

NEW YORK AND NEW ENGLAND COLLEGIALITY

New York's entry into the ranks of homeopathic education arrived several decades after Pennsylvania due to its tradition of greater diversity and accommodation between homeopaths and regulars. Nevertheless, as hostilities grew, owing in part to the popularity of homeopathy among New York's urban elite, the pressure for separate schools increased. At a meeting of the Homeopathic Medical Society of the State of New York in Albany in February 1853, Dr. H. D. Paine offered a resolution authorizing the president and secretary of the society to establish a homeopathic medical college in New York City. The resolution approved, the president appointed a committee to nominate a board of trustees, procure a charter, and raise the needed funds.[42] In its deliberations, the committee considered that most homeopathic physicians were converts from Old School medicine and that European homeopaths had not, so far, founded their own medical colleges. They also discussed the potential impact of a new homeopathic college on existing schools and whether enough students were enrolled. With the encouragement of nearly 400 practitioners across the state, the committee announced that the opening of a new school represented an "honorable exertion and wholesome competition" to existing medical colleges. The committee concluded they had the patronage, the funds, and the moral influence to support 100 students at a college.[43]

The migration of disgruntled faculty from the Homeopathic Medical College of Philadelphia contributed to the establishment of the New York college, but the college's staunchest supporter was poet and journalist William Cullen Bryant. A man of letters, not medicine, he worked tirelessly on behalf of homeopathy to which he converted in the late 1830s. In 1841, Bryant was elected president of the New York Homeopathic Medical Society, a clear sign of the role that lay homeopaths played in the early years. Moreover, he used the pages of his *Evening Post* to expand on homeopathic doctrines. In 1846, Bryant publicly advocated a charter for a homeopathic college in New York, believing that Allentown Academy and the subsequent Philadelphia college were insufficient to meet the country's needs.[44]

In the meantime, by an act of the legislature on April 13, 1857, New York acknowledged the existence of homeopathy in law, endowing it with the same privileges as regular medicine. Homeopaths interpreted the law as entitling them to half the wards in the state's public hospitals, including Bellevue Hospital.[45] In response, the hospital's board of governors appointed a three-member committee to consider setting aside half of the institution for the practice of homeopathy. Among the supporters of the idea were editors Horace Greeley of the *New York Tribune* and Charles Dana of the *New York Sun*. The committee's majority report, prepared by Washington Smith and P. G. Moloney, recommended against the change, citing failed experiments in Europe over the previous twenty years and, by inference, connecting homeopathy with Perkins' Tractoration and similar quackish movements. A minority report written by Benjamin F. Pinckney explained that homeopathy was no longer an experiment since its adherents were found in every part of the world.[46] Pinckney noted that homeopathic doctors numbered in the thousands (including nearly 150 in New York City and its suburbs) and were protected by legislation in most states. More recently, homeopaths had been placed in charge of numerous private charities in New York, including the Protestant Half-Orphan Asylum. Following a review of both reports, and under intense pressure from regulars, the hospital's board of governors voted to deny homeopaths access to the wards.[47]

On April 12, 1860, the legislature incorporated the Homeopathic Medical College of the State of New York under the supervision of the State Board of Regents.[48] The college, located at 116 East 20th Street near Gramercy Park in the center of the business district, opened on October 15, 1860, with an address by its president, former New York City mayor Daniel F. Tieman—a clear and unmistakable sign of homeopathy's power and connections.[49] Initially, the school had the right to award only the doctor of homeopathic medicine degree, but its charter was later revised to include the doctor of medicine.[50]

In 1869, the trustees amended the charter to rename the school the New York Homeopathic Medical College. The trustees also directed that the faculty consist of at least six professors, and that a board of censors of not less than three (none of whom could be a professor in the college) would examine each candidate for the degree of medicine. A year later, the trustees enlarged the faculty and appointed Carroll Dunham (1828-1877) as dean. They also authorized the school to require applicants to pass an admission examination that embraced a "thorough English education, chemistry, botany, and the rudiments of Latin." Only graduates of academies or liberal arts colleges were excused from the exam. In addition, the trustees authorized the faculty to adopt a three-year graduated course of study: the first year comprised the basic sciences; the second and third years included the more advanced and practical side of the medical sciences. Finally, they directed the faculty to introduce microscopes into the laboratory experience and to examine students on subjects taught during the first and second terms. The examination for the degree of doctor of medicine was to be conducted in public and in the presence of a board of censors, each of whom held membership in the American Institute of Homeopathy. These were higher standards than those maintained by the majority of medical schools—regular or sectarian—and represented a distinctive pattern of pedagogical reform evident among the stronger homeopathic colleges in the United States.[51] The three-year curriculum proved so satisfactory to faculty and students that it became obligatory in 1878, well ahead of most other medical schools.[52]

From 1867 through 1872, the college was housed at 151 East 20th Street; it then relocated to Third Avenue and 23rd Street, sharing space with the New York Ophthalmic Hospital. There it raised admission criteria once again, added to the curriculum, lengthened the term of study to six months, and organized an alumni association.[53] Applicants for admission were now required to present a diploma from a college or high school, or a first-grade teachers' certificate. If they had no diploma, they were required to pass an entrance examination in English composition, elementary physics, geography, and mathematics.[54]

In 1872, the college obtained teaching privileges at both the New York Ophthalmic Hospital and Ward's Island Inebriate Hospital. Three years later, the hospital was renamed Ward's Island Homeopathic Hospital and became the college's primary clinical site. This was a singular accomplishment for the faculty and trustees, and it gave clinical instruction a more central focus in the college's curriculum. In 1894, the hospital was shifted to Blackwell's Island and renamed Metropolitan Hospital.[55]

The location of Metropolitan Hospital, however, posed a continuing problem for the faculty and students, and by 1886 the trustees were once again looking for a new site, supported in their endeavor by John D. Rockefeller and David Dows, each of whom contributed

$25,000. With a site identified at 64th Street and what is now York Avenue and with a generous donation from Congressman (later Governor) Roswell P. Flower, construction began in 1888. Once again the name changed, this time to the New York Homeopathic Medical College and Hospital. In 1894, the college lengthened its course of study to four years of seven months each, and in 1908, it became the New York Homeopathic Medical College and Flower Hospital.[56]

The college and hospital prospered until 1935 when the American Medical Association's Council on Medical Education resolved that, after July 1, 1938, it would no longer approve sectarian schools. In response, the school dropped *homeopathic* from its title to become the New York Medical College, Flower and Fifth Avenue Hospitals.[57]

One of the lingering frustrations among the faculty, students, and alumni was the failure of the school to receive support through the private philanthropy of John D. Rockefeller (1839-1937) and his son, John Jr. (1874-1960). The two Rockefellers, along with Andrew Carnegie (1835-1918), left an imprint on medical education in both North America and in Europe that no amount of public funding before or since has quite equaled. Rockefeller Sr. had made his fortune in oil and, guided in his giving by Frederick T. Gates (1853-1929), a former Baptist minister, directed the philanthropic investments of the Rockefeller Foundation and the General Education Board to build and sustain the most promising medical schools, most of which had been identified by Abraham Flexner. As Kenneth Ludmerer recounted in *Learning to Heal: The Development of American Medical Education,* while Rockefeller Sr.'s personal choice of medicine was homeopathy and he urged its support, John Jr. and Gates derided New School medicine and directed that the millions of dollars in medical philanthropy go to support scientific medicine, not fading systems.[58]

Even though the Massachusetts legislature granted a charter in 1869 authorizing a homeopathic medical school, not until 1873 did the trustees of Boston University, an institution supported by the generous contributions of Isaac Rich, express interest in establishing such a college. At the time, the Boston Female Medical College, founded in 1848 through the guiding efforts of Dr. Samuel Gregory, was attempting to solve its financial difficulties by seeking a homeopathic hospital and wealthy patrons to assume responsibility for its debts. Boston University expressed interest in the college's proposal and was able to handle the financial arrangements, including its debts. In March 1873, a group of the city's leading homeopathic physicians established the Boston University Medical College, and along with it, the Homeopathic Association of Boston University.[59] In the fall of 1873, Boston University Medical College opened its doors to both men and women, with an eight-month, three-year graded course of study, and with students required to pass an examination in each year's study before moving to the next level. By 1876, the college had 172 matriculants and was graduating an average of 30 students annually. In 1900, the school moved to a four-year graded course of study.[60] In 1918, the college announced that its curriculum had been made as broad and as inclusive as was consistent with medical science by establishing a chair of Old School materia medica and therapeutics. The change was significant since it meant that the college was no longer required to register as sectarian.[61]

Women's Medical Education

When Elizabeth Blackwell (1821-1910) sought admission to a half dozen established medical colleges in the mid-1840s, she faced formidable obstacles, including the belief that medical education went counter to woman's intellectual capacity as well as would affect her femininity and morality. At best, woman's role was limited to nursing and midwifery. Undeterred by rejections, Blackwell applied to a number of smaller schools. Both the Eclectic Medical Institute of Cincinnati and the Central Medical College in New York offered her the opportunity to study. Instead, she chose Geneva Medical College in rural western New York. Founded in 1835, the college had a student body of 150 and two four-month courses of lectures. Blackwell enrolled in November 1847 and, between sessions, spent her time at Blockley Almshouse in Philadelphia where she observed treatment of the city's sick and insane. Upon awarding her degree in 1849, the school followed the lead of the more established regular colleges by closing its doors to any additional women applicants. By contrast, the eclectic colleges in Worcester, Syracuse, Rochester, and Cincinnati kept their doors open to women applicants. The same applied to Boston Female Medical College, formed in 1848 by Samuel and George Gregory, and renamed New England Female Medical College in 1850; the Female Medical College of Pennsylvania, founded in 1850; and the Women's Medical College of the New York Infirmary for Women and Children, founded in 1863.

Orthodoxy's opposition to women physicians carried with it several unintended consequences. Most important, women were forced by orthodoxy's prejudices to seek sectarian schools whereupon regulars criticized not only their choice of school but also the character of the schools that accepted them. Ultimately, sectarian colleges found it easier to gain legitimacy (or at least tolerance) by following the lead taken by regular colleges in choosing to exclude women from their ranks. In this manner, women's medical education unwittingly became a handicap to the efforts undertaken by sectarian schools to win public approval. Thus, by the time of the Civil War, many of the very schools that had opened their doors to women now closed them. Although not opposing the medical education of women, the consensus among regulars and sectarians was that women should attend medical schools established exclusively for their benefit. This conservative mentality continued until 1872 when New York Homeopathic, followed by Boston University Homeopathic College, Cleveland Homeopathic Hospital College, St. Louis Homeopathic, Detroit Homeopathic, and the Hahnemann Medical College in Chicago, opened their doors to women. Although the American Institute of Homeopathy opened its membership to women in 1870, not until six years later did the American Medical Association take a similar step.

In April 1863, in response to petitions from suffragette Elizabeth Cady Stanton (1815-1902), Dr. Clemence Sophia Lozier (1813-1888), and others, the New York legislature endorsed the establishment of the New York Medical College for Women (regular), one of two colleges in the English-speaking world where women could receive a medical education among their own sex. Lozier, dean of the college, opened the first course of lectures for seven students at 724 Broadway, New York City. The leaders of the college included Mrs. Maria C. Ewen, first president of its board of trustees; Elizabeth Cady Stanton, secretary and lay homeopath; and board members Carroll Dunham, Timothy F. Allen, William Guernsey, Edmund Carleton, Henry Ward Beecher, Julia Ward Howe, and Clara Barton.[62]

At the college's first graduation ceremony in 1864, Beecher, Stanton, and Lucretia Mott delivered speeches. That same year, the legislature amended its charter to include a hospital and, in 1866, the school became the New York Medical College and Hospital for Women. Although the school was not *officially* homeopathic in philosophy, several of its professors were graduates of the New York Homeopathic Medical College. These included Timothy F. Allen, Carroll Dunham, H. M. Dearborn, William T. Helmuth, E. Carleton, and Rosalie Stolz. A subtle but visible division soon occurred within the faculty and led to the eventual departure of regulars and the creation of a separate Women's College of Physicians and Surgeons (regular) with Lozier as its head. However, Lozier found that her loyalties were to her former college, which was now openly homeopathic; on returning, she became professor of diseases of women and children, and later president, and dean for twenty-five years.[63]

In 1868, the New York Medical College and Hospital for Women moved to new quarters at the corner of Second Avenue and 12th Street. Here the Lozier Memorial Training School for Nurses organized. With forty-five students graduating during the first six years of the school's existence, the trustees decided in 1874 to purchase property for further expansion of the institution. The effort proved premature and financial difficulties forced the college to sell the property and relocate temporarily to Lexington Avenue. In 1880, the college moved to Clarendon Hall on 13th Street and then, in 1881, leased new space on West 54th Street, between Broadway and 7th Avenue, where it remained for the next twenty years. With the death of Clemence Lozier in 1888, Phoebe J. B. Waite, an 1871 graduate of the college and chair of obstetrics, became dean of the college. Waite served as dean from 1888 to 1896, followed by Jennie de la Montagnie Lozier (1896-1898), M. Belle Brown (1898-1905), Helen C. Palmer, Emily C. Charles, and Cornelia Chase Brant.[64]

In 1893, the New York Medical College and Hospital for Women adopted a four-year graded course of study, and in 1895 became part of the University of the State of New York. In 1897, the college moved to 101st Street, west of Central Park, where, following a successful fund-raising drive, a new college and hospital was built. In 1918, the college merged with the New York Homeopathic Medical College and Flower Hospital, later called the New York Medical College, thus creating a fully coeducational school.[65]

On the surface, homeopathic medical schools appeared to welcome the change since homeopathic identity was linked to the women's rights movement and women's medical education. Besides, nineteenth-century women felt a special affinity for homeopathy. Part of this was because Hahnemann placed greater emphasis on symptomatology rather than physical examination. Although never raised to the level of public ideology, the symbolic implications of this were discernable in homeopathy's physician-patient relationship which recognized woman's more delicate temperament and spirituality, her interests in diet and hygiene, and her preference for milder medicines. With parents, especially mothers, preferring milder therapies for their children, and with the popularity of homeopathy among middle- and upper-class families, women were quick to convert from regular medicine.

In 1880, nine of the eleven homeopathic colleges admitted women. However, one of those nine was Pulte, where coeducation had become such a divisive issue that it nearly destroyed the school. In 1878, the feud spilled into the public arena with the press reporting it as the "Homeopathic War." Before the dust settled, there were resignations from the faculty and trustees, personal vendettas among faculty members, and legal suits charging libel and slander. The issue paralleled a national debate on the same subject, prompted by the publication of Harvard medical professor Edward H. Clarke's *Sex in Education; Or a Fair Chance for Girls* (1873) which suggested physiological and psychological reasons why coeducation was detrimental to woman's mental and physical well-being. The faculty and trustees were divided on the issue, and despite Pulte's own support for coeducation the doors remained shut to women matriculants. With the trustees unable to resolve the issue, the faculty finally broke the impasse by establishing a separate track for women students in anatomy, obstetrics, gynecology, and clinics. By 1883-1884, however, women accounted for 31 percent of the students in homeopathic colleges and 19 percent of the graduates.[66] By the turn of the century, women constituted 17 percent of homeopathic physicians as compared with only 6 percent of regular physicians.[67]

Hybrid Schools

On the fringes of homeopathic medical education in the East were two schools that taught the principles of Hahnemann as part of an effort to assemble all medical philosophies without prejudice, and give students the opportunity to investigate and to choose those elements that would make the practice of medicine more successful. Both fit within the eclectic tradition of medical education by accepting the universality of medical science, leaving no theory or technique untested. The first was Albany Medical College in New York, founded in 1838; the other was Penn Medical University in Philadelphia, chartered by the Pennsylvania legislature on February 2, 1853.

Unlike the New York Medical College and Hospital for Women which, over time, came under the influence of a predominantly homeopathic faculty, Albany Medical College became the first allopathic medical school in the country to openly fill some of its chairs with teachers of homeopathic theory and practice. Support for this decision came from several trustees known to be homeopaths, and from the Honorable Ira Harris (1802-1875), a state legislator (1845-1846), justice of the New York Supreme Court (1847-1859), and U.S. senator (1861-1867). A firm believer in homeopathy, he became a professor at Albany Law School and filled the chair of medical jurisprudence at the medical college.[68]

The other school to offer homeopathy as a part of its curriculum was Penn Medical University, the creation of Dr. Joseph S. Longshore. With the help of Lucretia Mott, Horace Mann, James Flowers, and others, Longshore hoped to remedy the deficiencies in the art of medicine by building a more rational therapeutics around the periodicity and changes of body temperature (Chrono-Thermal system) discovered by Samuel Dickson (1802-1869) of London.[69] Penn announced that it adhered to no single system of medicine but would dedicate itself to all truths, wherever they may derive. The school, led by Dean Abraham Livezey, opened its doors to what was termed "co-coordinate" medical education, i.e., women students were accepted in the fall term and men in the spring. Both had access to the same subject matter and the same teachers, except in practical anatomy where women were given their own demonstrator. Interestingly, Penn became the first American medical college to offer a graded course of instruction. The curriculum, which extended through four progressive courses of four months, was divided into lectures designated as *philosophical, physiological, pathological,* and *practical.* Rather than have students attend two courses of lectures in order to qualify for the degree, the second simply a repetition of the first, Penn required a sequential program of study that brought students together in the mornings for four hours of daily lectures, and in the afternoons for practical matters such as dissecting, botanical excursions, laboratory or clinic work, and hospital experience. In 1858, the American Medical Association, whose Committee on Education had pushed for curricular reform, gave its approval of the school's changes and recommended other schools adopt them.[70]

Unlike the curriculum for which Penn could rightfully be proud, the school's facilities were less than adequate. The first session was given in Franklin Hall on Sixth Street, below Arch. In 1854, the college moved to Thirteenth and Arch Streets, and a year later, to 419 Market Street. In 1857, the college moved once again, this time to Twelfth and Chestnut Streets, and the following year to 910 Arch Street. The Civil War sapped the school of its vitality and it closed following the 1863-1864 winter course of lectures. Over the ten years of its existence, eighty men and forty-five women received degrees.[71]

In 1873, after a suspension of nearly a decade, Longshore brought together a new faculty at 1131 Brown Street. Although continuing the principles of earlier years, the school suffered from the decline in the influence of eclectic philosophy and the effects of Longshore's debilitating illness. By 1881, the school was extinct, but not before establishing its reputation for a progressive, graded curriculum.[72]

MIDWESTERN PRIDE

Midwestern homeopaths did not stand idly by as schools organized in the East. First in Ohio, then in Illinois, Kentucky, Missouri, Michigan, Iowa, and Minnesota, New School reformers proudly organized colleges that rivaled the denominational character of their Eastern cousins. With confidence in their beliefs, they became a formidable force in the states and territories, seeking charters and demanding equal protection before the courts and inclusion of their faculty and students in publicly funded hospitals. In some states, they even convinced legislatures to establish homeopathic departments in state-supported universities. Undaunted by the obstacles before them, they expressed an optimism and authentic freshness that won them friends and followers.

In June 1849, homeopathic physicians from northern Ohio met in Cleveland to hear Professor Benjamin L. Hill (1813-1871) of the Eclectic Medical Institute (EMI) in Cincinnati speak about medical reform.[73] Hill reported that his faculty, in keeping with their commitment as eclectics to teach the best from all schools of medical thought, desired to "enlarge the circle of instruction in medical science" by including in their curriculum the principles and practice of New School reform. Homeopathy, they concluded, represented an important source of ideas and practices that should be added to the armamentarium of the medical art. Hill then offered a "full, free, and equal" professorship in homeopathy at EMI.[74]

Ohio homeopaths accepted the offer and selected Dr. Storm Rosa (1791-1864) as chair of principles and practice at the school. Rosa had studied medicine with several allopathic physicians and graduated with a doctor of medicine degree in 1816 before moving to Madison, Ohio, then to Painesville, where he opened a practice. He was persuaded to study homeopathy by Joseph H. Pulte of Cincinnati and Samuel B. Barlow of New York in 1841, and adopted the system three years later.[75]

Because as yet no homeopathic colleges were found west of Pennsylvania, supporters of EMI's offer agreed to encourage interested students to attend the school's lectures. A circular described the school's decision to include "whatever great truth might be found lying in their pathway, up the hill of science," and that homeopathy was considered one of those "great truths." It also praised the school's dean, Joseph Rodes Buchanan, for correctly representing the views of homeopathy to his classes and for urging students to investigate the system, and reminded readers that Buchanan had addressed the Ohio legislature on medical reform and the right of both eclectic and homeopathic physicians to practice at the Commercial Hospital in Cincinnati.[76]

The authors of the circular (B. W. Richmond, John Wheeler, David Shepard, C. D. Williams, and A. Plympton) intended it to pacify Eastern homeopaths who felt that accepting a professorship in an eclectic school was a rejection of the new Homeopathic Medical College of Pennsylvania. "We feel a deep interest in the welfare of that school," the authors wrote, "and know that the friends at the east have the men, the money, and the students to sustain it." They hoped that Eastern homeopaths would not interpret their action as an indication of sectional strife or as an effort to distance themselves. Instead, it was important to recognize that most students in the West were practical people who had neither the time nor the money to attend schools far away. Besides, the West was itself "an Empire" and should not depend on the East to provide medical instruction. Self-reliance was a notable characteristic of Westerners, and the time would soon come when the only things they needed from the East were "fashions and oysters." In fact, efforts were already under way to establish a medical college in Cleveland. With this in mind, "shall we halt and shrink back at the thought of a single professorship in our wide spread Republic? We trust not."[77]

Dean Buchanan was obviously pleased with the inclusion of homeopathy in EMI's curriculum and in its journal. For one thing, it quelled pressure for a separate homeopathic college in Ohio. Articles on homeopathy in the *Eclectic Medical Journal* recognized the extraordinary effects of remedies prepared in high triturations. For eclectics, the study of homeopathic books and the trial use of homeopathic remedies was deemed timely and useful. "Much of our current Eclectic practice is Homeopathic . . . although the doses are not of the attenuated character of those commonly used by the followers of Hahnemann," wrote Buchanan in 1849. The experiences of homeopathic physicians had taught him the importance of reducing doses where the remedy had a proper specific relation to the disease.[78]

As a member of the school's faculty, Storm Rosa took every opportunity to pronounce homeopathy above all other methods of cure and the "only true philosophical method." He thanked his colleagues for their generosity and promised to be open-minded to all systems, including eclecticism, provided they were "willing to compare notes and facts, and abide the result." Unwittingly, the eclectics had given him a forum from which he proclaimed to the world the superior doctrines of Hahnemann. This braggadocio was a backhanded slap to his eclectic patrons, and it did not go unnoticed or unpunished.[79]

Rosa's 1850 lectures at the college were popular and well attended, but instead of being considered additions to the canon of eclectic thinking, they resulted in a half dozen students graduating with degrees in both homeopathy and eclectic medicine.[80] The faculty soon realized they had placed themselves in the awkward position of advocating eclecticism as the best of all systems, while awarding a special role to homeopathy. Homeopathy's unique relationship soon became a burden and an embarrassment, with both homeopaths and eclectics demanding a clarification of the school's intentions. Subscribers to the *Eclectic Medical Journal* were not opposed to a homeopathic professor at the school, or even a homeopathic section in the pages of the journal, but they pointedly remarked that such liberality was "not intended to make Homeopathics out of Eclectic physicians."[81]

At the close of the 1849-1850 session, the faculty voted to abolish the school's special relationship. In justifying their change of heart to the trustees, Dean Buchanan explained that the homeopathic system contained "practical errors, delusions and false philosophy," hindered the progress of medical science, and, finally, was just a "more subtle modern form of medical hunkerism."[82] Resigning in disgust, Rosa accepted the chair of obstetrics and diseases of women in 1851-1852 at the newly organized Western College of Homeopathic Medicine in Cleveland. When the St. Louis Homeopathic College organized, he was offered the chair of theory and practice but preferred to retire instead. Rosa's influence on EMI had been far-reaching; into the late 1850s and 1860s, the Cincinnati eclectics saw a continued migration of their graduates to the homeopathic camp.[83]

In March 1850, spurned by EMI's decision to end its relationship with Rosa, homeopathic physicians in northern Ohio seized the opportunity to obtain a charter for the Western College of Homeopathic Medicine.[84] The college began auspiciously with a larger than predicted class. Fifteen candidates received their degrees following the first session in 1850-1851. Women were welcomed, and the first woman to receive the MD degree graduated at the end of the second session. During that same course of lectures, the college faced a severe test of faith when rumors spread that the faculty and students had "resurrected" the daughter of a local citizen for dissection. Enraged by the accusation, townspeople marched on the college with axes in hand. Initially held in check by the faculty and students, the rioters soon forced their way into the building. Finding the remains of several corpses and concluding that one of them was the missing daughter, they set fire to the building, destroying the library and much of the faculty's private collections. The mob then descended on the home of one of the professors but was turned away by an armed force of soldiers who threatened to shoot the rioters.[85] Neither the mayor and his police force nor the governor and two militia companies were able to protect the school's property, and despite the vigorous denials by the faculty of having dissected the body of the young woman, the school was never reimbursed for the mob's destructive acts.[86]

In February 1852, the faculty solicited support to equip a new college building. On May 1, 1852, the college was incorporated as the Western College of Homeopathic Medicine, and by August of that year, property on Ohio Street was deeded to the trustees and preparations were undertaken for the new session.[87] In 1857, the college changed its name to the Western Homeopathic College, and then to the Cleveland Homeopathic Medical College. In 1859, the faculty secured use of the county hospital, giving students the advantage of a large surgical and medical hospital experience.[88] By 1861, 257 students had graduated, including 12 women.[89]

In 1864, the session included twenty-one students from Ohio, five from Michigan, four from New York, three from Pennsylvania, two from Illinois, several from other states, and nine from Canada. Among the twenty-two who graduated, three were women, the last to receive a diploma from the college.[90] Although not opposed in principle to the medical education of women, the faculty, with the strong encouragement of Seth R. Beckwith, chair of surgical and pathological anatomy, were "convinced by observation and experience that the association of both sexes in the same medical school [was] detrimental to both."[91] As a result, a compromise was struck that admitted women to the lectures but prohibited them from graduating with a degree.[92]

In 1867-1868, the faculty once again debated the role of women in the college but, failing consensus, agreed to support the chartering of a separate Homeopathic College for Women. Soon after the school opened its doors, the faculty of the two schools merged and, in 1870, the combined board changed the name to Homeopathic Hospital College.[93] The method of instruction at the college differed from others in that student proficiency was tested daily on prepared forms. At the twenty-first commencement exercises, among the thirty-two graduates were four women.[94]

During the 1879-1880 session, a local "resurrectionist" arranged to supply bodies for the medical college. The contract specified that all dissecting material would come from outside the state. Unfortunately, the dealer found it easier to obtain his material locally by robbing graves in the East Cleveland Cemetery, the contents of which he transported to nearby colleges. The school took possession of one such corpse, along with a certified statement that it had come from New York. The next day, the dean and the professor of anatomy were arrested for possession of the body of "one of our best citizens and a patient and friend of the Dean." As friends and family would admit no apologies, the matter ended in the courts and the incident became a costly lesson.[95]

While Cleveland rightfully claimed the first homeopathic college in the West, Cincinnati was not far behind. In 1872, Pulte Medical College opened, named after Joseph H. Pulte (1811-1884) of Germany who immigrated in 1834, worked with Hering at the Allentown Academy, and moved to Cincinnati in 1840 where he built his reputation during the cholera epidemic of 1849. He was author of *Organon der Weltgeschichte* (1846); followed by *Homeopathic Domestic Practice* (1850) which, by 1900, had gone through seven editions, was reprinted in England, and had been translated into Spanish. He also authored *Women's Medical Guide* (1853); *Household Homeopathist; or, Mother's Guide to Practice* (1859); *Letters on Diphtheria* (1860); and *Asiatic Cholera* (1866).[96] From the time the college opened its doors, the faculty used a graded system; those students who completed three years of study and passed an examination received a special degree of Fellow Pulte College (FPC). Ten men graduated at the first session of 1872-1873, and by 1876 an average of twenty-seven students were graduating annually.[97] Through its free dispensary, the college focused much of its attention on clinical teaching, which took up nineteen of the thirty-nine weekly lectures. A dedicated board of trustees served the college, and its influence was so great that the college seldom lacked for resources.[98]

In 1910 Pulte merged with the Cleveland Homeopathic Medical College, forming the Cleveland-Pulte Medical College. Classes graduated each year until 1914 when the school and its property were transferred to Ohio State University in Columbus and became the Ohio State University College of Homeopathic Medicine.[99]

Efforts to establish a homeopathic college in Kentucky began in 1892 with the support of an active state association and thirty practicing homeopaths in Louisville. A charter, modeled after the New York and Philadelphia colleges, was drafted and incorporated as the Southwestern Homeopathic College and Hospital of Louisville. Supporters purchased $20,000 in capital stock and bought a residence on Sixth Street for the college's home. The first course of lectures was given in 1893-1894 and efforts were immediately begun to obtain clinical access to the 500-bed Louisville City Hospital. This was accomplished in April 1895 through the efforts of Mayor Henry Tyler and several other city officials who supported homeopathy. With their encouragement, the college received equal access to the City Hospital where every fifth patient was designated for homeopathic treatment. Permission was also granted for placement of an intern in the hospital and access to weekly clinics in the hospital's amphitheater. By 1895, City Hospital supported five allopathic colleges, a Negro medical college, and a homeopathic college.[100]

In 1903, the college moved to new quarters at the corner of Floyd and Walnut Streets, one block from City Hospital. There, students had access to daily clinics at their own college hospital, a weekly clinic at City Hospital, and clinics at nearby allopathic colleges as well. Medical licensing was controlled by a state board of medical examiners that contained three allopathic, one eclectic, one homeopathic, and one osteopathic physician. In 1910, the college merged with Hahnemann of Chicago, with several of the Louisville faculty joining the staff.[101]

Further west, the Chicago Board of Health assigned a portion of the new City Hospital to homeopathy in 1857, appointing a homeopathic board of physicians and surgeons in equal numbers to a similar allopathic board. The board of health based its decision on the endorsement of homeopathy from many of the city's most prominent citizens; the numbers of patients seeking admission to hospitals who preferred homeopathic treatment; and the fact that the Chicago Homeopathic Hospital, under the superintendence of Dr. George E. Shipman since 1854, had willingly treated many of the city's charity patients. Those supporting the decision also believed the division of labor between regulars and homeopaths would provide a statistically accurate foundation on which to measure the comparative value of the two systems and would also allow "simple justice" for those desiring the benefit of the system employed within their own families.[102] Opposition, however, from regular physicians in the city and from the American Medical Association, whose national offices were located in Chicago, forced the board to rescind its action and deny homeopaths access to the city's wards. One unanticipated consequence was that the city lost control of its hospital, which was then leased to regular doctors to operate.[103]

The hostility of the American Medical Association toward homeopathy did not extend to the city's more affluent citizens. Through the efforts of the Honorable J. Y. Scammon, a wealthy and public-spirited philanthropist who had been the first layperson known to have received homeopathic treatment in the city, Illinois incorporated the Hahnemann Medical College of Chicago in 1855. Scammon's doctor was David S. Smith (1816-1891), the first practicing homeo-path in Illinois.[104] The college opened with nine junior and eleven se-nior students in October 1860 in rented rooms above the homeopathic pharmacy of Halsey and King on South Clark Street. The course of study involved five daily lectures, including one daily clinical lecture, over a period of eighteen weeks.[105]

In 1868, the college moved to South State Street between 12th and 13th Streets where it occupied the upper floors of a vinegar factory. By 1870, the college had its own building at the corner of 28th Street and Cottage Grove where fifty-one students, including eight women, enrolled in lectures. At its tenth commencement in February 1870, there were seventy-nine students in the entering class, and nineteen graduates, including one woman, Clara Youmans.[106]

In 1873, the college changed its name to the Hahnemann Medical College and Hospital of Chicago and the faculty adopted a graded curriculum after the manner of Harvard and several other schools. The graded course extended through three sessions, two of which were obligatory. This meant students could enter their senior course

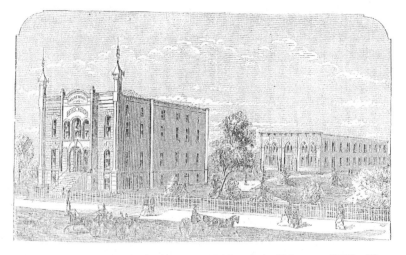

The Hahnemann Medical College and Hospital, Chicago, 1874. (*Source:* Courtesy of the Lloyd Library and Museum, Cincinnati.)

only after they passed examinations in the other two courses. The curricular change had an unfortunate effect on enrollments, and for two years the dean levied assessments on the faculty to cover the revenue shortfall.[107]

In 1881, the Cook County commissioners designated one-fourth of the beds at Cook County Hospital for homeopathic use. This represented a reversal in the hospital's policy of 1857. By 1882, Hahnemann Medical College and Hospital boasted a class of 263 students from 22 states. Of that number, thirty-seven had come from other colleges to complete their education and forty-one had come from the East, a particularly comforting statistic given regional prejudices.[108] In 1920, the medical department of Valparaiso University in northwest Indiana became affiliated with the college. A year later, Hahnemann Medical College and Hospital was reorganized, with the college separating from the hospital. In that same year, the AMA classified the college as "B," the only school so classified in Illinois except for a poorly equipped night college.[109]

During this time, the college came under increased criticism from conservatives. Noting that several of the faculty were no longer homeopaths, the editor of the *Journal of the American Institute of Homeopathy* questioned whether the college should be identified as homeopathic. "Lukewarm and antagonistic professors have no proper place on the faculty of any denominational college," the editor wrote. Unless the college had the "right tempered faculty," it was useless for it to continue.[110] The college closed in 1924, by which time it was known as the General Medical College. It had graduated nearly 5,000 medical doctors.[111]

Chicago was also home to the Chicago Homeopathic Medical College, a result of a feud between the liberal and conservative elements within the Hahnemann Medical College of Chicago. The break occurred when the majority of faculty seceded and went to the west side to establish Chicago Homeopathic. Incorporated in 1876, the college opened the same year, graduating its first class of eleven in 1877. With the faculty as the sole stockholders, the school was not subject to control by a board of trustees as were most other schools. The college was located on the second floor of a building at 200 Michigan Avenue. In 1881, it moved to Wood and York Streets across from Cook County Charity Hospital where it remained until 1905.[112]

Much to the dismay of state's homeopaths, a war ensued between the city's two colleges. "Not that the vast North-West is not extensive enough to support two homeopathic colleges in her central city," wrote one critic, "but this is not the best time for such an enterprise." Another college was appropriate only when two could flourish in an environment of "noble emulation" rather than "bickering contention." Hahnemann Medical College already had fifteen chairs, all of whom were well-respected teachers and practitioners.[113] The institution finally merged with Hahnemann Medical College in 1904. Under the merger, A. C. Cowperthwaite, dean of the Chicago Homeopathic Medical College, was added to the board of trustees. By the time of the merger, the college had graduated nearly 1,200 students.[114]

During the 1876 Centennial Exposition in Philadelphia, at a joint session of the American Institute of Homeopathy and the International Homeopathic Congress, conservative members lamented the failure of homeopaths to grasp fully the significance of Hahnemann's principles and expressed the hope that a college might be established to sustain those principles in their purest form. One result of that discussion was the creation in 1880 of the International Hahnemannian Association to protect the interests of conservatives among New School reformers. Two other outcomes were the establishment in 1890 of the Post-Graduate School of Homeopathics in Philadelphia under the tutelage of James Tyler Kent (1849-1916), and the opening of Hering Medical College and Hospital in Chicago in 1891 by Henry C. Allen (1830-1909), one of the founding members of the International Hahnemannian Association and editor of *Medical Advance,* devoted to the preservation of strict homeopathic practice along the lines expounded in Hahnemann's *Organon* (1833 edition) and *Chronic Diseases.*[115]

The Post-Graduate School of Homeopathics had the strong financial backing of John Pitcairn, a prominent businessman and devout Swedenborgian. The object of the school was to teach pure homeopathy as the universal application in disease, using the 1833 edition of the *Organon.* This included instruction in the single remedy in the single dose in the minimum quantity; a combination of didactic and clinical teaching; and a thorough grounding in the homeopathic philosophy. Instruction focused on seven distinct departments: materia medica and philosophy of homeopathy, clinical medicine, diseases of women, diseases of children, obstetrics, diseases of the eye and ear, and surgery.[116] The school was intended as a fifth year of instruction to what, by 1900, had become a four-year curriculum in most medical colleges. Kent's lectures included a strong dose of New Church metaphysics, leading graduate A. S. Ironside to call it a "Swedenborgian School." This charge was vigorously denied by the school's trustees who demanded that Ironside return his diploma. Over the course of its brief history, the school awarded thirty students the master of homeopathics.[117]

Hering Medical College and Hospital's first announcement, issued in 1892, stated that the college intended to teach and demonstrate the principles of *pure* homeopathy. Although the school promised to teach all the disciplines, the faculty would be homeopaths first and specialists second. An important feature of the college was its connection with neighboring hospitals including the Chicago Baptist Hospital, the National Temperance Hospital, the Women's Christian Temperance Union Hospital, and Cook County Hospital. The college also had access to the botany, zoology, anatomy, and physiology laboratories at the University of Chicago, which extended privileges to Hering College students.[118]

From the beginning, the school was open to men and women on equal terms, including the filling of faculty positions. With the first lectures in October 1892, sixty-nine students matriculated. The first class graduated in 1893, including two women. By the third year, ninety-seven were in attendance, including students from eighteen other states, plus Bohemia, Canada, Denmark, England, and India.[119] According to historian Anne Kirschmann, with the exception of Hahnemann Medical College of Chicago, Hering graduated the largest number of women of any homeopathic college in the West.[120]

In 1895, heated differences within the faculty at Hering Medical College caused a schism and the subsequent chartering of Dunham Medical College of Chicago, which was dedicated as well to the original principles of homeopathy. Named after the much-revered American homeopathic physician Carroll Dunham (1828-1877), former dean of faculty at the New York Homeopathic Medical College and president of the American Institute of Homeopathy, the college promised to adhere to the purity of Hahnemann's healing art and not to lower standards by adopting new fads, medicines, or surgeries.[121] All too often, doctors were graduating with skills in microscopy, bacteriology, serum therapy, chemistry, and electrotherapeutics, but were

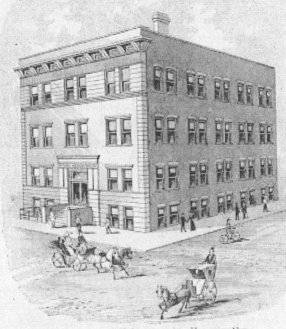

Hering Medical College.
3832 and 3834 Rhodes Ave., Chicago, Ill.

The True Representative of Hahnemannian Homeopathy.

BETTER CLINICS, NEW BUILDING, NEW LOCATION, INCREASED FACILITIES, LARGER FACULTY.

H. C. ALLEN, M. D.,   W. W. STAFFORD, M. D.,
            DEAN.   REGISTRAR, 100 State St.

United Faculty, Superior Clinical Instruction, especially in Homeopathic Therapeutics. Thorough Training of Students in Correct Homeopathic Prescribing.

Send For Catalogue.

"If our School ever gives up the strict inductive method of Hahnemann we are lost, and deserve only to be mentioned as a caricature in the history of medicine."—CONSTANTINE HERING.

Advertisement for Hering Medical College, Chicago, 1898. (*Source:* Courtesy of the Lloyd Library and Museum, Cincinnati.)

weak in the principles of homeopathic healing. Although these fields were important, they could not replace symptomatology and proper treatment of disease.[122]

In 1900, James Tyler Kent moved his Post-Graduate School of Homeopathics to Chicago where it affiliated with the Dunham Medical College. At the same time, a portion of the faculty and student body of the National Medical College of Chicago joined with the Dunham college. These two acquisitions strengthened both student enrollment, which reached approximately 100, and the quality of the faculty. Notwithstanding these mergers, Chicago could not sustain two homeopathic colleges dedicated to the same mission, and in the summer of 1902 Dunham and Hering merged, making it the most orthodox school in the teaching of pure homeopathy. With this merger, Kent's Post-Graduate School of Homeopathics closed its doors and Kent became dean of the newly organized Department of Materia Medica.[123] Meager in equipment and supporting a small dispensary, the merged school struggled unsuccessfully to maintain its existence and closed in 1913.[124]

Missouri Schisms

Farther west, the Missouri legislature incorporated the Homeopathic Medical College of Missouri in St. Louis in November 1857. Two years later, prominent homeopaths in the Western states and territories were invited by the trustees to organize the college. Five former Cleveland faculty members joined in the endeavor.[125] The school's most prominent faculty member was William Tod Helmuth (1833-1902), who moved to St. Louis from Philadelphia in 1858. A graduate of the Homeopathic Medical College of Pennsylvania, he was for two years professor of anatomy at his alma mater where he published *Surgery, and Its Adaptation to Homeopathic Practice* (1855) before joining the Missouri college as chair of anatomy, registrar, and in 1865 as chair of theory and practice. In 1864, he started the *Western Homeopathic Observer,* a monthly journal that he edited until 1870. Believing that much of the country had been "over-run by quacks and eclectics," Helmuth promised that St. Louis would become the center for homeopathy in the West.[126]

The Civil War caused a severe drop in the college's enrollment, forcing the trustees to close the doors from 1861 through 1863. The

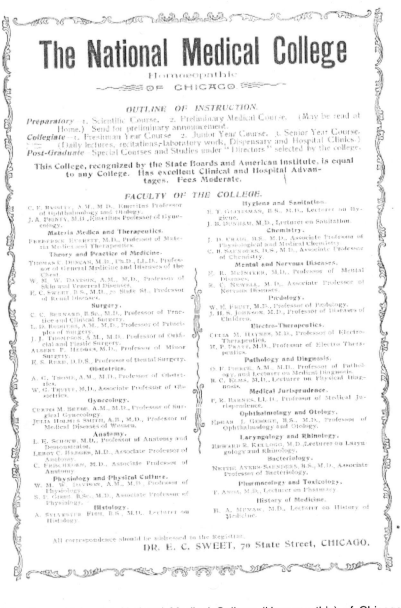

Advertisement for the National Medical College (Homeopathic) of Chicago, 1897. (*Source:* Courtesy of the Lloyd Library and Museum, Cincinnati.)

school opened again in 1864 with G. S. Walker in obstetrics and diseases of women; E. C. Franklin in civil and military surgery; T. J. Vastine in clinical medicine; John Hartman in physiology; and G. B. L. Clay in theory and practice. Franklin, grandnephew of Benjamin Franklin and former student of Valentine Mott, MD, of New York, served as a surgeon in the U.S. Army and in 1864 was appointed chair of surgery in the Medical College of Missouri. He authored *The Science and Art of Surgery* (1867) and later became surgeon of the Good Samaritan Hospital, president of the Western Academy of Homeopathy, and vice president of the American Institute of Homeopathy.[127]

In addition to a strong curriculum, students had access to the Good Samaritan Hospital, which operated on homeopathic principles.[128] They also had the opportunity to witness surgical operations and clinical treatment under the supervision of their own professors at the Colored Orphan's Home and at the Post Hospital at Benton Barracks.[129]

In 1871, eleven graduates, including one woman, graduated from the Homeopathic College of Missouri. Mrs. M. E. Munsey, of Virden, Illinois, was reputedly the first female graduate west of the Mississippi to receive the MD degree.[130]

St. Louis was home to several other homeopathic institutions, most of which were short-lived. In the fall of 1869, as a result of internal bickering between the conservative and liberal factions of the faculty, Helmuth left and organized the St. Louis College of Homeopathic Physicians and Surgeons that lasted for two sessions before closing its doors in 1870. In 1872, another college, the Homeopathic College of Medicine and Surgery, promised to be free from all "eclecticism," even though one of its professors, Dr. Benjamin L. Hill, was once a faculty member at the Eclectic Medical Institute in Cincinnati.[131] The college closed before offering its first course of lectures. The Homeopathic Medical College of St. Louis organized in 1873 but suspended operations two years later. Others included Hering Medical College, organized in 1880; the St. Louis College of Homeopathic Physicians and Surgeons (revived by a portion of the Homeopathic Medical College of Missouri faculty), which opened in 1880 and held only two sessions; and the Women's Medical College, which opened in 1883 and closed a year later.

These stillborn efforts reflected the internal dissension within homeopathy during the 1870s and the escalating tensions between lib-

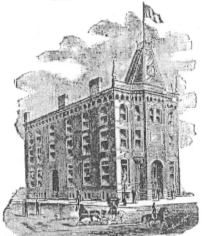
Advertisement for the Homeopathic Medical College of Missouri, St. Louis, 1897. (*Source:* Courtesy of the Lloyd Library and Museum, Cincinnati.)

eral and conservative trustees and faculty. Teaching posts changed almost yearly at the colleges until 1882 when the St. Louis College of Homeopathic Physicians and Surgeons and the Hering Medical College merged with the Homeopathic Medical College of Missouri. By 1906, the consolidated college offered a four-year graded curriculum and had a student population of forty-five and a faculty of twenty. Under mounting pressure for curricular reform and facing severe financial challenges, the college closed its doors in 1909 following a visit by the American Institute of Homeopathy's own Council on Medical Education which inspected eighteen homeopathic, eclectic, and osteopathic schools using a rating system adopted in 1907.[132]

In western Missouri, the Kansas City Homeopathic Medical College was chartered on May 19, 1888. With ill-defined admission requirements, "lax methods of teaching," and only two years required for the diploma, the school provided a marginal educational program at best. In 1892, the state board of health required all medical colleges to provide laboratory facilities to supplement didactic teaching. To meet these new standards, the faculty and trustees of the Kansas City Homeopathic Medical College managed to purchase new and larger facilities. The building, which opened September 1892, contained an amphitheater capable of seating 100 students; recitation rooms; chemical, histological and bacteriological laboratories; dissecting rooms; and administrative and faculty offices. At the same time, the college, in deference to the new requirements of the American Institute of Homeopathy, expanded to a four-year curriculum. By 1898, however, differences among the faculty over the policies and direction of the college resulted in a decline in students and dissolution of the charter following the 1901-1902 session. It then merged with the College of Homeopathic Medicine and Surgery of Kansas City University, an institution incorporated in 1896 and operated by the Methodist Church. With consolidation, the combined institution became known as the Kansas City Hahnemann Medical College.[133]

State Schools

In 1837, the year Michigan became a state, the legislature chartered a state university at Ann Arbor, to include a literary college and schools of medicine and law. Although the university opened in 1841, not until 1850 did the medical department offer its first course of lec-

tures.[134] In 1855, in response to petitions from the state's homeopathic population, the legislature directed the university's governing
board to establish, teach, and maintain the specific philosophies of
regular and homeopathic medicine. The law read as follows:

> The Regents shall have power to enact ordinances, by-laws, and
> regulations for the government of the University; to elect a Pres-
> ident; to fix, increase and reduce the regular number of profes-
> sors and tutors; and to appoint the same, and to determine the
> amount of their salaries; *provided that there shall always be at
> least one professor of homeopathy in the Department of Medi-
> cine.*[135]

The action of the legislature to include homeopathic teaching
sounded an "alarm" bell through the ranks of regulars who began efforts almost immediately to reverse the decision, claiming that it violated the independence of the regents. The leaders of the American
Medical Association pledged to fight the action as well.[136] Accordingly, the regents saw no reason to comply with the amended revenue
act but did accept the legislature's suggestion to examine ways to
connect homeopathy to the existing school of medicine. Not surprisingly, the regents found no precedent in other states and concluded
that the legislature had no power to force the university to make such
an arrangement. The legislature had only advisory power because the
state constitution vested control of the university in a board of regents
elected by popular vote for six-year terms.

Michigan homeopaths took issue with the decision, arguing that
the control of the university by the regents was limited since their tenure of office, mode of appointment, right of appeal, and budget lay
within the power of the legislature. Should the regents decline to provide the inhabitants of the state with the means of acquiring knowledge of the arts and sciences, or should they "limit the advantages of
the institution to our colored population alone," the legislature could
compel the university to act differently. It was therefore contrary to
the spirit of the constitution and the purposes of the state to exclude
instruction of any of the recognized branches of science.[137]

Ten years passed without action by the regents. Year after year, and
at numerous sessions of the legislature, the matter continued to be
discussed and debated, and motions were made to enforce the
amended act. Even when A. I. Sawyer, MD, president of the State

Homeopathic Society, offered to soften homeopathy's position lest the university suffer at the hands of the legislature, the regents remained firm and unmoved. For their part, Michigan homeopaths viewed the board's intransigence as an "unnecessary and willful delay"—a conscious and purposeful evasion of the law. With homeopathy recognized as a legitimate branch of medical science by many European governments, and with homeopaths holding professorships in schools in Scotland, Austria, and Prussia, it was wrong, they argued, to deny the same to the university. They estimated that of the 800 physicians in Michigan, between 250 and 300 were homeopathic, serving a clientele of 200,000 to 300,000 citizens.[138]

In 1867, the legislature sought to resolve the impasse by providing additional revenue to the university through a one-twentieth mill levy on each dollar of taxable property, provided the regents appoint at least one professor of homeopathy to the Department of Medicine. Until this was done, the state treasurer was directed to pay the university none of the revenue acquired by the tax.

At a meeting in April 1867, the regents discussed the appropriation, and the medical faculty attacked it as a barbarous interference in the internal governance of the university.[139] Regent Edward C. Walker offered a resolution explaining the university's opposition to the conditions attached to the tax, pointing out that placing a homeopath in the department would destroy what had been "built up at so much expense and with so much labor, and with such distinguished success." Because of the problems created by the proviso, Walker urged his colleagues to explain their reasons to the public and to the legislature for not appointing a homeopathic professor and the "absolute necessity" for the university to receive its share of state dollars. Following Walker's advice, the board appealed to the legislature to modify the conditions of the act by establishing a homeopathic school separate and distinct from the medical department, at a location other than Ann Arbor.[140]

Some of Michigan's homeopaths sought a compromise in the form of a separate school in Detroit. The regents came to view this as a potential solution to their dilemma, but there was no consensus among the state's homeopaths. Those who had fought for the original law regarded the separate school option as nothing less than capitulation. As a result, homeopaths within and without the state embarked on a "conversation" regarding the virtues of a separate medical school.[141]

At the August 1871 university board of regents meeting, homeo-pathic physicians E. R. Ellis and Lancelot Younghusband presented a plan proposing Detroit for the university's branch medical depart-ment in homeopathy. They explained that Detroit, which had one-eighth of the state's population, had superior hospital advantages but no state educational institution. While they asked the board to estab-lish a medical department, they requested no money, explaining that the state's homeopaths would provide the necessary funds. A month later, the regents acted on the recommendation, adopting a resolution offered by Walker to establish a homeopathic medical school at De-troit, "to be eventually connected with the University."[142] Following approval of Walker's resolution, circulars announcing the establish-ment of a homeopathic college in Detroit were distributed to the state's 300 practicing homeopaths. The Homeopathic Medical Col-lege of Detroit held its first session March through July 1872.[143]

Not to be outmaneuvered, a competing group of homeopaths an-nounced the opening of the Michigan Homeopathic Medical College in Lansing, a rival school whose organizers hoped it would become the homeopathic branch of the university's medical department.[144] The college graduated sixteen students in its first session of 1871-1872.[145]

The state's homeopaths were now divided into three camps: those supporting the college at Lansing, those supporting the college in De-troit, and those who still argued for a medical department at Ann Ar-bor.[146] All three groups sought eventual recognition by the university as well as legislative support. Two state homeopathic medical societ-ies eventually formed out of the rivalry, each championing homeopa-thy under the supervision of the state university, but differing on location.

Not surprisingly, many of the state's homeopaths were troubled by the competing school initiatives, believing this represented a division within their ranks that would bring defeat and ridicule. Elijah H. Drake (1821-1874), editor of the *American Homeopathic Observer,* resolved to oppose the Detroit Homeopathic Medical College, noting that the school's faculty were "vendors and prescribers of quack med-icines" who followed "disreputable practices." Announcing that the college had no authority to confer degrees or grant diplomas, Drake repudiated the college and denied that the school's faculty were "qualified or authorized to represent the sentiments or wishes of the homeopathic profession."[147]

Drake's criticisms were not without merit. Two of the school's supposed advocates, doctors George H. Palmer and O. P. Baer, claimed that their names had been willfully misrepresented as supporting the school when, in fact, they were not connected with it in any manner. Andrew B. Spinney, MD, listed as chair of anatomy and physiology, was not a physician at all but a spiritualist who sold "Spinney's Homeopathic Specific—Ague Pills."[148] Another member of the faculty, a Reuben H. Chase, had come to the city as an insurance agent before beginning to practice medicine.[149] Chase had sold insurance in Bangor, Maine, before moving to Kansas where he read medicine and practiced for eleven months. He then moved to the Detroit Homeopathic College where he attended lectures and joined the faculty upon graduation.[150]

Drake's harshest criticisms were directed at Dr. Lancelot Younghusband, president and dean of the college who claimed to hold an AM, MD, and LLD, and advertised himself in the newspapers as "one of the foremost physicians in the West."[151] Although there was no evidence of an AM degree, he had been a teacher of Latin and Greek in a private high school in the village of St. Thomas in Upper Canada (now Ontario). From there, he attended the New York Hydropathic and Hygienic Institute on Laight Street near St. John's Park. Founded by Russell Thatcher Trall (1812-1877), editor of the popular *Water Cure Journal,* the institute taught the principles of hygienic medicine and treated patients by these measures alone.[152] Until 1857, the institute was unchartered and lacked any legal basis for granting degrees. Younghusband also possessed a special degree (without attendance) from the Homeopathic Medical College of Pennsylvania in 1866, signed by Lippe, Hering, and Raue. Special degrees were typically conferred on those who were already graduates of a medical college. But Younghusband had no earned medical degree at the time he received his special degree.[153] H. N. Guernsey, dean of the college, admitted that Younghusband had been granted a diploma "on account of a recommendation that he was a regular A.M., MD, and a gentleman of good standing in the profession. He DID NOT ATTEND at our school, nor was he examined by us." All he had at the time was a certificate from the Laight Street New York Water Cure.[154] Younghusband also listed himself among the graduates of the Philadelphia University of

Medicine and Surgery in 1868 and 1869. The charter for this institution, a notorious diploma mill, was later annulled by the Pennsylvania Legislature for disreputable and criminal practices.[155]

In May 1875, the regents met at Ann Arbor to consider a resolution calling for a separate two-person homeopathic college to be established in Ann Arbor, with appointments in materia medica and theory and practice of medicine. The resolution further stated that the students would pay the same fees and be subject to the same regulations as other students at the university; that the students entering the Homeopathic Medical College should receive instruction in the existing medical department in all branches except in the two established chairs; and that all persons graduating from the homeopathic college would be furnished with a diploma from the university. After much discussion, the resolution was unanimously approved, and Dr. Samuel A. Jones of Englewood, New Jersey (materia medica), and Dr. John C. Morgan of Philadelphia (homeopathic theory and practice) were appointed to fill the chairs. University president James B. Angell then appointed Jones to be dean of the new college. Along with this decision came an announcement that the Detroit Homeopathic Medical College would close on May 6, 1875, so that its students, along with those at the Lansing school, might enroll at Ann Arbor. By this time, the Detroit school had graduated eighty-two physicians.[156]

The Ann Arbor medical faculty accepted the action of the legislature and the decision of the regents. They understood that the homeopathic college would be entirely separate from their own, and that they would not be required to sign homeopathic diplomas, nor in any way be forced to recognize the new department.[157] However, the decision angered the Michigan State Medical Society, which adopted a resolution in June 1875 announcing a state of crisis between itself and the university. Cooler heads prevailed, and the resolution was laid aside for another requesting the regents to make a full three-year graded course of study and lectures obligatory upon all students.[158] Dean Abram Sager of the medical faculty took more direct action by resigning his position. Viewing the act of the regents as a "disaster" and a "disgrace," Sager considered it his duty "to withdraw from any alliance or affiliation tending to defame, demoralize, and finally, to crush out a hitherto loved and cherished institution."[159]

Professor Samuel Gross, a prominent anatomist and president of the American Medical Association, tersely commented on the actions of the Michigan legislature and the university's board of regents. "The American Medical Association, and all our colleges," he stated, "would unquestionably place the Medical Department of your University under the ban, and cease to recognize your pupils."[160]

In spite of these threats and dire predictions, many of the early fears about the relationship between the two departments proved false. The homeopathic professors were not members of the existing department of medicine; nor were the allopathic professors members of the faculty of the homeopathic college. The schools had separate statutory authority and were distinct and separate departments.[161] Students in the homeopathic college took their examinations on materia medica and practice from homeopathic professors, and from the regular faculty in the other branches. To their credit, the allopathic faculty chose not to allow partisanship to raise its head in the sciences.[162]

In the fall semester, twenty-four students, including several women, were admitted into the new school and a course of lectures began according to the plan agreed to by the regents and the Michigan Board of Education. Homeopathic students attended all classes with regular students with the exception of materia medica and theory and practice. For those lectures, they crossed the campus to the homeopathic college. Women's classes in both schools occurred at the same time, an hour after the lectures to male students. As a further sign of their separateness, the University Hospital at Ann Arbor contained two twenty-five-bed clinics, one on each side of the campus, for allopaths and homeopaths.[163]

The matter was eventually debated at the AMA convention in Atlanta in 1879 and resumed in Richmond in 1881 where delegates argued and postured. After all was said and done, however, the Ann Arbor regular faculty was spared the embarrassment of censure. Although they continued to instruct homeopathic students, they were uninvolved in either their admission or the awarding of their diplomas and certificates of proficiency. With this as the outcome, the AMA seemed satisfied. However, instead of celebrating their victory, the state's homeopaths began to worry. Had they compromised their principles? Were there other options to consider? Watching events unfold in Iowa and Illinois, some wondered whether they had settled for too little.[164]

The answers to these questions were provided in 1921 when the regents voted to merge the two departments, reasoning that the cost of educating forty-seven homeopathic students represented an unnecessary duplication of resources. In place of the former department, the regents approved the summer offering of two postgraduate courses—a didactic course in the principles of homeopathy and a laboratory course in drug action.[165]

Similar to the efforts at the University of Michigan in Ann Arbor, the Hahnemann Medical Association in Iowa sought in 1873 to include the teaching of homeopathy in the state university at Iowa City. Dr. E. A. Guilbert of the state homeopathic society asked the board of regents to establish a homeopathic department in the university and appoint two professorships to support instruction. Arguing the lack of funds, the board did not act on the recommendation but promised to ask the legislature to increase the university's appropriation to permit the granting of the petition.[166]

In 1874, and again in 1876, bills to accommodate the change were drafted for the Iowa general assembly only to be defeated on floor votes. Finally, after much lobbying and a petition that bore approximately 10,000 signatures, the state's homeopaths secured a rider to the university's appropriation bill in 1877, directing the board to establish a department of homeopathy with equipment and two chairs (materia medica and theory and practice) at $950 per year. The official name was the Homeopathic Medical Department of the State University of Iowa. In response, the regular medical faculty threatened mass resignation unless the regents established a completely separate homeopathic program. The regents, however, preferred a mixed program where homeopathic students received training from the regular medical faculty in all of the noncontroversial disciplines. Except for materia medica and theory and practice, students in the department were instructed together with students in the regular medical department.[167]

With the enabling legislation now completed, the Hahnemann Medical Association of Iowa then lobbied for space. In October 1877, the first class of eight students met in rented rooms over a store in the city. A year later the regents authorized construction of a two-story brick building on university property. However, because of space limitations, the department had no available operating room, nor opportunity for obstetrics, and patients in the department's small clinic had to be seen outdoors. The regents did permit Dr. A. E. Rockey to serve as surgeon gratis but, due to lack of space, supplies, and patients, the position was soon abolished. With the department existing on a shoestring budget and a less than optimal learning environment, it was not surprising that, as late as 1888, graduates of the homeopathic department were denied licenses in Illinois, Minnesota, and California.[168]

When the department was first established, there were no entrance requirements except "good moral character." Everything else was vouched for by the student's preceptor. Not until 1884-1885 were any requirements listed in the department's annual announcements.[169] Recognizing deficiencies in the program and knowing the importance of preparing the next generation of the state's homeopathic doctors, the Hahnemann Medical Association of Iowa created a committee to monitor the needs of the department and provide assistance. The committee met with the regents and asked for two additional professorships in surgery (1885) and obstetrics and diseases of women (1888). The regents approved the positions but failed to support them with sufficient clinical space. Undaunted, the committee and the association solicited donations and rented space for a ten-bed "dwelling-house" hospital. With the operating room on the ground floor and beds on the second floor, patients were carried up the stairs on the students' shoulders after surgery. The hospital continued until 1890 when the association voted to build an addition to the department's building and turn it over to the university to manage.[170]

In 1896, the homeopathic department moved into new quarters at the northwest corner of the public square in Iowa City. The building had room for fifty-four beds, an amphitheater, kitchen, offices for five faculty and their assistants, a lecture room, and student rooms. The facility was the result of a now-strong relationship among the regents, the legislature, and the Hahnemann Medical Association of Iowa. During the years of the department's existence, Governor James Grimes and two of the four university presidents (Christian Slagle and Josiah Pickard) were patrons of homeopathy.[171]

Advances in bacteriology seriously challenged homeopathic principles and the faculty found themselves defending their vitalistic principles against the laboratory experiments of germ theorists.

Moreover, the program faculty continued to emphasize drug provings even though there was little scientific rigor in their activity. Laboratory research on the chemical and physiological action of drugs was painfully deficient.[172]

Concerned with the quality of the program, George E. MacLean, the newly appointed president of the university, began a process of consolidation in 1900 by forming colleges from departments and delegating to a university examiner the authority to decide the qualifications of applicants. At the same time, the university's admission standards changed, requiring students not only to have a high school diploma but to have fulfilled all the requirements for entrance into the university's College of Liberal Arts.[173] Unfortunately, because of waived admission requirements in the areas of chemistry, physics, and biology, students in the homeopathic program were ill prepared for the rigor demanded of them and quickly reverted to second-class citizens within the university community. As part of his reforms, MacLean required Dean Allen C. Cowperthwaite and his faculty to explain in their catalog the precise relationship their program enjoyed with the regular medical program and their clear dependence on it for the education of homeopathic students in the basic disciplines. This forced Cowperthwaite to acknowledge the advances in medical science and concede the need to narrow the universality and applicability of Hahnemann's laws.[174] In 1912, the university trustees consolidated several chairs on grounds of redundancy. Enrollments continued to drop and the homeopathic department eventually closed in 1919. In that year, the General Assembly passed House Bill 454 replacing the College of Homeopathic Medicine with a Department of Homeopathic Materia Medica and Therapeutics.[175]

In neighboring Minnesota, the number of homeopaths grew from 1 physician in 1852 to 130 by 1886. A group of the state's homeopaths in January 1886 voted to start a college. The majority favored a college in Minneapolis in a department of the state university. A committee of five was then appointed to take the steps necessary for incorporation, organization, and implementation. The committee secured a building within three blocks of the Minneapolis Homeopathic Hospital, and in October 1886, the Homeopathic Medical College opened with twenty matriculants and a six-month course of study.[176]

In the meantime, the University of Minnesota College of Medicine and Surgery (regular) organized in 1883 and began a slow but steady effort to absorb all medical schools in the state. In April 1888, homeopaths appealed to the regents of the University of Minnesota, promising to waive their school's charter and cease teaching provided that homeopathy be represented in the medical department of the state university. The regents agreed and appointed a committee to nominate faculty for the department. By summer, the faculty were selected and the catalog of the university announced a new department of medicine consisting of fourteen faculty. The students of the Minnesota Homeopathic Medical College were admitted to the medical department without entrance examinations and were given advanced standing. The curriculum covered three years, with each year comprising a six-month course of lectures. Homeopathic students attended lectures with other university students in anatomy, physiology, chemistry, pathology, histology, hygiene, and medical jurisprudence.[177] Within two years, the homeopathic college was strongly tied to the university and its rules. In the basic sciences, students in the allopathic and homeopathic departments received instruction from the same professors. The faculty even shared rooms in three buildings known as Medical Hall, Laboratory of Medical Sciences, and Laboratory of Chemistry.[178]

Beginning with the 1895-1896 course of lectures, the college added an additional year to the program, with classes commencing in October and lasting until the end of May. When the homeopathic faculty presented a plan to the regents for their own separate building, the regents refused the request because of the relatively small size of the program. The number of graduates was never large: two in 1887; four in 1888; four in 1889; two in 1890; four in 1891; four in 1892; eight in 1893; three in 1894; five in 1895; eight in 1896; eleven in 1897; none in 1898; four in 1899; and seven in 1900.[179]

In 1903, at a meeting of the Minnesota State Homeopathic Institute, the issue of low enrollment led to a general discussion of the department's weakened condition. The regents proposed to abolish the college and in its place establish two homeopathic professorships in materia medica and therapeutics within the general college of medicine, a move that would give students the opportunity to choose between the two schools of medicine. The state's homeopaths opposed the change, and there matters stood until 1909, when the university's College of Medicine and Surgery absorbed all other medical schools in the state, including the homeopathic department of the university.[180]

THE SOUTH

Homeopathy's inroads into the South came later than other regions of the country due primarily to the lack of population centers and the more conservative nature of the people. In Maryland, the Reverend Jacob Geiger, a German pastor with eight separate congregations in Carroll County, took an interest in the system following the death of his wife. Eventually nine of his descendants graduated from homeopathic colleges and practiced in the South. Other Maryland pioneers included Dr. Felix R. McManus who opened a practice in 1837; Dr. Adolph F. Haynel, a pupil of Hahnemann, who located in Baltimore in 1839; and Dr. Amelia A. Hastings, who established the first homeopathic pharmacy in the state in 1862. In 1874, the Homeopathic Society of Baltimore City formed, followed by the establishment of a free dispensary. A year later, the Maryland Homeopathic State Society formed, and in 1881 the members of the Medical Investigation Club took up the study of the materia medica. From this group also came suggestions for a college and hospital.[181]

Discussions began as early as 1884 to establish a college, but not until 1890 did these become serious. By that time there were sixty practitioners in Baltimore. In 1891, the state authorized articles of incorporation for the Southern Homeopathic Medical College and Hospital of Baltimore City (also known as Atlantic Medical College). The provisions of the articles were written broadly to encompass a medical, dental, pharmaceutical, and veterinary school. The hospital opened in October 1890 at 323 North Paca Street. By December, a constitution and bylaws were adopted. Shares of capital stock in the college, each worth $25, were divided almost equally among faculty and laypeople. A search for suitable facilities resulted in the purchase of Old Calvert Hall, a three-story Roman Catholic school on Saratoga Street.[182]

With a staff of fourteen chosen by the trustees, and a curriculum requiring three years of six-month terms, the first session opened in October 1891 with nineteen students: six third-year students; one second-year student; and twelve first-year students. Following the 1894-1895 session, the faculty adopted a four-year course of study.[183] By 1909, when Abraham Flexner visited the school as part of his review of medical education in the United States and Canada, it had "passed through many vicissitudes" and had become nonsectarian.[184]

THE FAR WEST

With nearly 200 practicing homeopaths practicing in California, and with the state's Medical Practice Act of 1878 permitting homeopaths their own board of examiners, a group of homeopaths met in January 1881 at the San Francisco office of Dr. J. A. Albertson to establish their own college. Nine trustees were subsequently elected for the Hahnemann Medical College of San Francisco. Capital stock was fixed at $5,000 and shares at $25 each. Although the organizers hoped to begin the first course of lectures in 1882, financial problems prevented this. In 1883, the trustees increased the capital stock to $25,000 in shares of $100 each. This produced the needed resources and the trustees purchased a former Baptist church at Stockton and Geary Streets to become the college's new home. The first set of lectures began June 3, 1884, with a class of sixteen students. The college later moved to Haight Street in a building formerly owned by the medical department of the University of the Pacific, which had changed from hydropathy to allopathy. Marginal at best, the college was ill adapted for medical education and was most remembered as "cold, cheerless, dark and unsanitary." Its library began with a nucleus of twenty volumes and eventually grew to several thousand. Clinical opportunities were provided by the Pacific Homeopathic Dispensary that affiliated with the college. However, efforts to obtain clinical access to the city and county hospital failed due to opposition from regular medicine.[185]

In 1894, as the college was struggling to define itself and its curriculum, the American Institute of Homeopathy recommended a four-year course of study for all homeopathic schools. The trustees opposed the change, believing the cost would be detrimental to small colleges, but they were forced to comply. Lacking its own hospital, and without privileges in the city and county hospitals, the college struggled on. During this time, the management of the college even considered repudiating homeopathy and affiliating with a regular college. In 1896, there were open discussions about whether to close the college. Not only did class size remain small (the largest graduating class being nineteen in 1897), the school's financial condition was abysmal and debts were met only by assessing the stockholders. Requests to affiliate with the University of California were defeated following aggressive opposition from regulars in the state.[186]

Rather than being discouraged, homeopaths began construction of a new college building in 1899. After an initial flurry of support, only $7,500 in pledges was realized, far short of what was needed. Had it not been for the contractor who was an ardent homeopath and his willingness to work without remuneration, the facility might not have been built. The building stood at the corner of Maple and Sacramento Streets and had sufficient land for a hospital. With completion came gifts that helped to stock the library, maintain the school's laboratories, and support curricular changes demanded for accreditation by the Illinois and Michigan state boards of health that were spearheading national medical reform. However, changes in curriculum as well as extension of sessions imposed heavy costs on the college. In 1902, the Hahnemann Hospital College gave up its charter to become a nonstock corporation called the Hahnemann Medical College of the Pacific.[187]

On July 1, 1918, the Hahnemann Medical College was united with the University of California Medical School. The assets of the college were accepted by the University of California and teaching was now carried out in a Department of Homeopathic Instruction. A year later, Hahnemann Hospital also passed into the hands of the university. The school appointed William Boericke as its first homeopathic lecturer. Instruction in homeopathy continued until 1939 when the school dropped it from the curriculum.[188]

SUMMARY

On balance, the profiles of homeopathic colleges in the Eastern and Western states show several interesting patterns and characteristics. As noted earlier, homeopathic education had its beginnings in Pennsylvania and New York where each state's homeopaths chose somewhat different instructional paths. Pennsylvania homeopaths favored a more exclusive arrangement that, on occasion, invited discord and even schism, while New York homeopaths seemed more intuitively inclined to collegial cooperation. With few exceptions, the plan of instruction in these schools paralleled the better regular medical colleges. And, like regulars, homeopaths invariably chose the proprietary school model that not only suited the impatience of American society for meeting the demand for more doctors, but fit society's taste with respect to standards, licensing, and a market-driven educational system. Overall, homeopathic colleges in the Eastern states had a farsighted sense of mission and carried a perception of rightness that, with few lapses, seldom became self-righteous. Although jealous of regular medicine's trappings, they maintained a dignified aloofness that became a mark of both their maturity and civility. Backed by many of society's most educated, genteel, and affluent citizens, they successfully competed with regular colleges for the public's trust, and in their politics possessed a shrewdness and practicality that won them many distinctions.

In both Eastern and Western schools, eclectics and homeopaths maintained a close but acrimonious relationship, joining forces when it was politically expedient to do so, and equally dismissive of the other when the opportunity presented itself. In both sections of the country, the specter of collaboration with medical eclecticism was always an explosive issue, a no-man's-land between purists seeking to retain Hahnemann's principles in their entirety and liberals urging a more open-ended approach to homeopathic theory and practice. Both regions were also conscious of their competition, a factor that weighed heavily on the breadth and depth of the curriculum and the length of term. On the other hand, Western schools were usually more cost conscious, fearful of the impact of higher standards and longer terms on student supply and demand. And although both sections of the country showed great pride in their respective alma maters, Westerners were more regionally conscious and, at times, even jingoistic, prone to celebrate the numbers of Eastern students who traveled west for their education.

From another perspective, Western homeopaths seemed more willing to incorporate coeducation and competing "isms" without great contentiousness. When problems did arise, their individual and corporate differences were often solved by schism rather than by consensus building. Like the frontier which served to accommodate society's more dissident individualists, Western schools were able to absorb the tumultuous energies of homeopathy's more vigorous libertarians as well as Hahnemann's extreme metaphysicians. As a result, many more colleges organized, merged, and closed in the Western states than in the East.

Finally, Western homeopathy garnered more positive sentiment from the general public, a factor that helped in efforts to gain entry into four state universities and access to public tax dollars. In the East, by contrast, New School reformers were beholden to wealthy patrons who, in the absence of state tax dollars, came to the support of home-opathy's private schools through gifts and endowment. Compared to homeopathic schools in the Midwest that proudly claimed a spirit of freedom and independence, including the endorsement of hydro-pathic and other nonhomeopathic remedies in the treatment of dis-ease, Eastern schools were more reticent in showing their diversity of practice. Some Eastern schools even tried to refuse diplomas from Western schools as "not being good homeopathic documents." The attempts failed, but not before leaving a chilling effect on East-West relations. "We should not think it strange if Philadelphia became the general headquarters of foggyism in medicine, and Ohio the center of liberalism," wrote one Western critic. The further eastward, he ex-plained, "the deeper is the darkness of bigotry." Was New Jersey not the "darkest spot" because it was the last state to repeal its medical laws? And beyond New Jersey, there was London, Rome, St. Peters-burg, Constantinople, Asia Minor, Persia, China, and Japan.[189]

Chapter 6

Incivilities

1838, New York physician James McNaughton, a regular and president of the Medical Society of the State of New York, addressed his society by placing Samuel Hahnemann within the mainstream of medical thinking, suggesting that the profession should more closely examine the system which had already spread from Germany to nearly every part of Europe and America. He acknowledged that Hahnemann made no claim of originating the principle of similars; in fact, he had identified numerous predecessors who had investigated the effects of medicines upon themselves and others. However, he added, no one could deny Hahnemann's perseverance in his investigations, the diligence of his followers, their reasoned arguments for smaller doses, or the avoidance of mixtures and combinations.[1] McNaughton felt that the good sense and propriety of Hahnemann's injunctions, including the assertion that his New School remedies did no harm, could not be denied, although physicians might disagree with his having transformed the principle of similars into a "grand axiom." The influence of friction in imparting energy to medicines certainly seemed improbable to McNaughton; on the other hand, "it may nevertheless be true." Given the known effects of electricity, galvanism, and electromagnetism, he urged the medical profession to ascertain the veracity of Hahnemann's claim, and determine as well the efficacy of belladonna to prevent scarlet fever; dorsera as a specific in whooping cough; the odor of gold to cure melancholy; and aconite to treat inflammatory fevers.[2]

McNaughton admitted to prescribing homeopathic medicines in "less urgent complaints" when his patients requested them. However, the results were not such as "to give me any great respect for the system, or any desire to abandon the old practice, without some further proof of the superior efficacy of the new," he admitted. Nevertheless, he was struck by the rapid recovery of many of his patients. It was time, therefore, to assess the comparative merits of the two schools in an American hospital environment and under the auspices of an impartial set of judges. Although he had no hesitation in condemning the charlatanism practiced in the name of homeopathy, and criticizing clergy who were unabashedly zealous in its support, he concluded that the time was ripe to make an honest examination of New School claims.[3]

Nine months later, homeopath William Channing, MD (1800-1855), a convert from regular medicine who represented the earliest strict or purist view of homeopathy in the United States, delivered an address before the New York Physicians' Society that challenged those like McNaughton who were seeking common ground between the two schools. A native of Massachusetts, Channing graduated from Rutgers College and served as a censor for the Medical Society of the County of New York where he first met Hans Burch Gram and Abraham D. Wilson, took part in their discussions on reform practice, and joined with them to advocate the public examination of all candidates for the license to practice medicine. With the outbreak of the 1832 cholera epidemic, Channing tested Hahnemann's choice of camphor, veratrum, and cuprum, and was so pleased with the results that he published his findings in the *New York Commercial Advertiser*.[4] Because of family connections (he was cousin to Unitarian William Ellery Channing of Boston) as well as his appeal to the benevolence and progressive tendencies in the laws of nature, his break from regular practice had a decided effect on colleagues and the prospects for homeopathy in America. Unlike most of his contemporaries who struggled to find a middle ground between Old and New School practices, Channing became a thorough Hahnemannian, as did other like-minded converts in the 1840s and 1850s. When Hahnemann adopted the potentizing theory, Channing immediately followed suit and became one of its strongest advocates.[5]

Channing urged promoting the medical sciences, elevating medical ethics, and cultivating a spirit of friendship among all members of the profession. He explained that from the time of Hippocrates to the days of Benjamin Rush, system builders had put forth one theory after another on the causation of fever. Despite pretenses, none of these efforts proved to be more than "vain-glorious distinctions of scholastic hypotheses." It was time, therefore, for the profession to awaken to the truths of inductive philosophy, the only true basis for genuine medical education. Without it, the medical license was "little better than a legal license to destroy."[6] In support of his argument, he fondly referred to Samuel Jackson at the University of Pennsylvania whose "Lecture on Medical Education Introductory to the Course of the Institutes of Medicine" in 1833 had urged reform of the profession since Jackson saw little difference between regular practice and empiricism.[7] Noting that true reformations seldom originated within institutions rife with error and abuse, Channing explained that, with the rise of homeopathy, medicine had finally become a science based on an uncomplicated general law. Thus fortified, New School reform had carried the medical arts into an era of scientific precision in less than fifty years. Admittedly, homeopathy could not yet boast a "full and perfect development," so Channing encouraged medical institutions in the United States to adopt the principle of free and open competition.[8]

However sympathetic the remarks of McNaughton, few regulars were willing to vouch for Channing's scientific claims. Hahnemann emphasized that his New School principles should sit on bedrock, removed from Old School pretensions, and few American medical societies were willing to countenance such arrogance. With lines drawn, neither side accepted the claims of the other. One became a caricature of "old physic," and the other a combination of German mysticism and protestant perfectionism.

AMERICAN INSTITUTE OF HOMEOPATHY

The American Institute of Homeopathy (AIH) originated at a July 1843 meeting of the New York Homeopathic Physicians' Society which invited all homeopaths to meet in New York City to form a national society. The convention, held at the Lyceum of Natural History in April 1844, established the institute and elected Constantine Hering of Philadelphia as president; Josiah F. Flagg of Boston and William Channing of New York as vice presidents; Henry G. Dunnell, secretary; J. F. Gray, general secretary; and S. R. Kirby, treasurer. The AIH became the second oldest national medical association in the United States (after the Friendly Thomsonian Botanic Society that formed in 1832), and drew its charter members from Illinois, Indiana, Kentucky, Massachusetts, Michigan, New York, Ohio, Pennsylvania, and Rhode Island.[9] The largest number came from Ohio (especially the cities of Cleveland and Cincinnati), followed by Pennsylvania, New York, and New Jersey.[10] Criteria for membership required applicants to have pursued a course of medical studies (either regular or homeopathic) and to have obtained a certificate signed by three members of the association affirming good moral character, and qualification in the theory and practice of homeopathy.[11]

As explained by Martin Kaufman in *Homeopathy in America: The Rise and Fall of a Medical Heresy,* the purpose behind the organization was not to launch an assault on orthodoxy but, instead, to ensure competency in the principles and practices of homeopathy through legitimate reform, investigating drug action, and discrediting pretenders.[12] Accordingly, the association's earliest activities included a monthly journal, a volume on drug provings, a publication on topographical anatomy, and an annual meeting of members.

William A. Gardiner of the *North American Homeopathic Journal* urged all homeopaths to become active patrons of the institute. "Let selfishness, indifference, and indolence . . . be abolished, or, rather, let them be banished; and let no duty be left undone," he urged readers.[13] In keeping with this advice, the AIH recommended the formation of state and county societies; provided advice on their formation; and supervised their provings of medicines.[14] These local societies consisted of both academically trained physicians and laypersons, the latter of whom served principally in small towns and rural districts. Here again, the structure resembled the Thomsonian Friendly Botanic Societies of the 1830s and 1840s, which lobbied for equality before the law along with helping communities cope with cholera, yellow fever, and other epidemic diseases.

In 1853, the AIH strengthened its criteria for membership by requiring all applicants to provide the name of the medical college from which they had graduated. This had the effect of distinguishing the academic homeopath from the lay advocate. That same year at their meeting in Cleveland, AIH delegates appointed a committee to ascertain the names and residences of all homeopathic physicians in the United States and to make the report public at the next annual meeting. The delegates also established a Central Homeopathic Pharmacy under the control of the association.[15] When the AIH met a year later at Albany, New York, the delegates reaffirmed the homeopathic law of similars as "co-extensive with disease."[16] The association also re-affirmed a higher standard of education for homeopathic physicians and a determination to test and identify all potentially beneficial medicines.

In 1855, the society turned its attention to charges of irregularities in the practice of one of its members, Dr. Frederick Humphreys (1816-1900), an 1850 graduate of the Homeopathic Medical College of Pennsylvania and author of *Manual of Specific Homeopathy* (1855). The committee investigating the charges recommended that the society refuse to countenance the sale of Humphreys's book and urge the author to resign or face expulsion. In his defense, Humphreys argued that the AIH lacked the authority to expel any of its members. Moreover, he claimed not to have departed from the objectives of the association (i.e., "the improvement of the science of medicine") but rather to have discovered a newer method for preparing and dispensing remedies. In the committee's defense, Dr. Samuel Gregg of Boston explained that every society had the right to expel members found acting detrimental to its interests. Furthermore, no medical society would ever permit a member in good standing to engage in the manufacture and sale of nostrums or patent medicines.[17] Doctor Jabez P. Dake, president of the AIH in 1857 and later coauthor of *Cyclopedia of Drug Pathogenesy* (1886), went further, claiming that Humphreys had not only violated the trust of the association but had broken homeopathic law by combining several medicines in one pill (the compound action of which was unknown), and providing only the name instead of the symptoms of a diseased condition.[18]

The AIH was usually guarded in its public references to regular medicine, lest it be categorized with other sectarian groups. Most of the members had been educated in regular schools and therefore considered themselves equal in education to their allopathic peers. Besides, because many viewed homeopathy as a specialty within medicine, requiring additional training in materia medica and therapeutics, they considered education in regular medical schools preferable to their own colleges. Accordingly, the AIH passed frequent resolutions urging dignity in speeches and writing, refusing to resort to "black-guardism" and other actions unbecoming members of a scientific profession.[19] For example, in June 1858, in an address before the assembled delegates meeting in Brooklyn, Dake extended an olive branch to regular and eclectic medicine, noting that "the selfish and

bitter manner" in which the different schools carried on their communication was "disgraceful to men, gentlemen, and Christians." Although he could not control how the dominant school treated homeopaths, especially those opposed to high dilutions, he did feel that
homeopaths had much to learn from the works of Carl Rokitansky,
Robert James Graves, William Stokes, Sir James Mackenzie, Sir
James Young Simson, and other noted regulars. "We can never expect
charitable and kindly treatment from others unless we exhibit it ourselves," Dake observed.[20]

These conciliatory gestures reflected, in part, a growing rift within
homeopathy between the high and low dilutionists and an effort by
the latter to build closer ties with those outside their ranks. In 1859,
the AIH met at Mercantile Hall in Boston where Dr. J. A. Ward of
New York, representing the high dilutionists, a Hahnemannian fac-
tion within the organization, presented a communication signed by
thirty-four members expressing alarm at these efforts. This petition
condemned those who used the pages of the *North American Homeopathic Journal* to openly dissent from the strict theory and practice of
homeopathy; those who urged the adoption of certain allopathic and
antipathic measures; and those who encouraged merger with the
eclectic school of medicine. All such tendencies, explained Ward,
were anathema to true homeopathy and should be ended. Referring to
the *North American Homeopathic Journal,* Ward called it a "stray
plank" in the false employ of homeopathy. Although the journal
claimed to be trustworthy and reliable, he accused it of carrying on
"insidious opposition" to the cause of New School reform.[21] Despite
Ward's remarks, the Hahnemannians failed to win control of the convention or curb the efforts of its more liberal members.[22]

In June 1860, however, during the last meeting of the AIH before
the outbreak of the Civil War, a core of forty Hahnemannian delegates presented a much-disputed Declaration of Principles:[23]

> *Resolved,* That this Institute do now adopt, and order to be
> printed annually in the journal of its proceedings, the following
> brief declaration of principles.

> *Resolved,* That the law of cure discovered by Hahnemann, and
> set forth in the terms 'Similia Similibus Curantur,' is universal in
> its control of medicinal dynamical forces.

Resolved, That the law requires a materia medica furnished by the strict proving of such forces upon persons in health.

Resolved, That the nature of the means indicated, and the relationship to the diseases for which they are prescribed, require the least doses that experience proves to be efficiently curative.

Resolved, That all medicines should be administered singly.

Resolved, That all other principles or practical rules concerned in the use of such medicinal forces must be subservient to those already stated.

Resolved, That homeopathy not only allows, but calls for the cultivation of all those branches of science which can be tributary to the art of healing.[24]

John Fitzgibbon Geary resented the fact that the delegates who prepared the declaration presumed to speak for the entire membership of the organization. Worse still, they had "thrown together such a confused system of metaphysics, having neither order, clearness, nor connection in its component parts." He insisted that Hahnemann did not *discover* the law of similars as stated in the second resolution, nor did he ever claim its discovery. Geary likewise objected to the terms *spiritual essence, vital power,* and *dynamic forces* in Hahnemann's *Organon,* believing that references to the soul, the mind, or the spirit were inappropriate. If the soul was part of the Divine essence, it was pure, ethereal, and immortal, and not subject to disease or death. Even if Hahnemann had referenced these terms simply to designate the life force that pervaded nature, Geary thought them ill-used. "We cannot see the 'spiritual essence,' nor yet the 'vital power,'" he wrote, therefore "we have no means of learning how the material human body is influenced by them." Incensed by the arrogance of the resolution, he urged that whenever the association intended to bring forward any new law, regulation, rule, or doctrine, by which all would be bound, every member should have the opportunity to exercise his vote.[25]

Actually, much of the hostility among members of the AIH was simply a reflection of the internecine feuds taking place between liberals and conservatives in the state and local societies. Exemplary was the fifth annual session of the Illinois State Homeopathic Medical Association held in November 1859 when an amendment to its constitution was to open the doors of the society to allopathic physicians who were either favorably disposed to homeopathy or partial converts. Those who supported the amendment felt that it was time for the followers of homeopathy to drop the title *homeopath* from their lexicon in a display of liberality. Reaction to the amendment was strong and forceful, with opponents arguing that the change would "fatally injure" the homeopathic cause, lower standards, and inaugurate a reign of "mongrelism" and "eclecticism" within their ranks. Ultimately, the members rejected the amendment, stating that the society did not wish to accept members who would be "sometimes on one side of the field and sometimes on the other."[26]

AMERICAN MEDICAL ASSOCIATION

It was not the repeal of licensure laws in the states or even the threat of homeopathy that led to a meeting of concerned physicians in the spring of 1846 in New York. Rather, it was, as Martin Kaufman explained in his *Homeopathy in America: The Rise and Fall of a Medical Heresy,* the *condition* of medicine which had caused it to lose both its prestige and its following.[27] This in turn led to a call for a broader assemblage of physicians the following year to look into such matters as standards of medical knowledge, the elevation of the science, and professional qualifications—concerns that were strikingly similar to the reasoning behind the founding of the AIH. Behind these issues were other heartfelt concerns: more practitioners than necessary for the population; the lack of fair remuneration; medical education failed to meet the needs of a liberal profession; and fears that quacks and empirics had captured the public's eye and pocketbook.[28] With twenty-nine regular medical schools issuing diplomas in 1846, with legislatures having decided to make no distinction between regular and irregular schools in licensing, and with Thomsonians (1832) and homeopaths (1844) already having formed national organizations, critics such as Samuel Jackson of the University of Pennsylvania correctly recognized there was no common standard for the conferring of the doctor of medicine, much less fixed standards for admission to practice. So serious was the deterioration in the title of "doctor" in the public's eye that it ceased to be a title of distinction. Recognizing that the federal government lacked the power to interfere and that the states and territories could not provide uniform legislation, Jackson urged the medical community to undertake self-regulation. To achieve this, the medical community had to reform its ranks, formulate a code of ethics, institute positive regulations, elevate the moral and scientific tone of the profession, and return the title of the doctor of medicine to its original high worth.[29]

Moderates in the homeopathic and regular camps voiced hopes for some type of recognition or accommodation in the newly formed organization, but the American Medical Association would have none of it. Instead, it chose to draw strict boundaries —both legal and ethical—between orthodoxy and so-called sectarianism. Professional identity, weak as it was, would initially rest on such tentative matters as society membership and consultation. While it would be wrong to assert that the American Medical Association was founded principally to fight homeopathy, it was nonetheless structured in such a way as to more effectively counteract homeopathy's growing influence. The AMA's Code of Ethics, adopted in May 1847, included language that effectively excluded consultation between sectarians and orthodox practitioners. The consultation clause quickly became the dividing line between homeopaths and regulars, aggravated by rhetoric that tended to exaggerate their respective differences. Symptomatic of this, at the 1855 meeting of the AMA in Philadelphia, the delegates approved a resolution offered by J. L. Atlee that formalized orthodox sentiment:

> *Resolved,* That any such unnatural union as the mingling of an exclusive system, such as Homeopathy with Scientific Medicine, in a School, setting aside all questions of its untruthfulness, cannot fail, by the destruction of union and confidence, and the production of confusion and disorder, unsettling and distracting the minds of the learners, to so far impair the usefulness of teaching as to render any School adopting such a policy unworthy the support of the profession.[30]

Homeopaths condemned the resolution as "vile," "inaccurate," and so "ill-arranged" as to be "devoid of the signs even of a decent elementary education in a common school." John F. Geary considered it the product of "the boot-boy of some hotel." He viewed the resolution as gratuitous since no homeopath had even sought such a union. Besides, since legislatures in the South and West had recognized the success of homeopathic practice by appointing homeopathic physicians to administer their public hospitals, this was evidence enough of New School strength.[31] But the resolution was neither forgotten nor forgiven by homeopaths as they bristled at the assumptions of its drafters. Noting that educated scholars, philosophers, and politicians from the capitals of Europe had placed themselves under the standard of New School reform, they preferred to let the facts speak for themselves in contrast to regular medicine's arrogance and conceit.[32]

Not all orthodox physicians agreed with the position being formulated by the American Medical Association. Perhaps the most significant communication on this matter came from the pen of Dr. James Jackson, professor of theory and practice at Harvard. Criticized by several of his professional colleagues for having consulted with a homeopathic member of the Massachusetts Medical Society, he responded that his conduct had been in accordance with the laws of the society. Although not a proponent of homeopathy, he drew a line when it came to persecuting persons holding opinions different from his own. He considered it as improper to refuse consultations with fellows of his own society who adopted homeopathic principles as it was to refuse to consult with an advocate of the Brunonian system. "To that system [Brunonian] I was as much opposed as I am to homeopathy . . . for it did much positive harm to the sick, while homeopathy only fails to do them good," Jackson observed. His rule was to meet with any fellow of the Massachusetts Medical Society "unless there is something objectionable in his character." More to the point, he considered many orthodox doctors more dangerous to their patients than homeopaths. "I cannot believe that the black sheep are found in one flock only," he concluded.[33]

UNCIVIL ACTS

The earliest hostilities between regulars and homeopaths in the United States began behind the closed doors of county and state medical societies and escalated from there into the courts. In 1843, in one of the earliest civil trials at Fort Plain, New York, the Montgomery County Medical Society accused one of its members, Elias P. Phelps, MD, of practicing homeopathy, publishing articles derogatory to regular practice, and acting in "gross professional ignorance and misconduct." The judges in the trial found no evidence substantiating the society's allegations and ordered it to restore Phelps' rights and privileges as a practicing physician and surgeon.[34] That same year, homeopaths Amos G. Hull (1810-1859) and Phineus P. Wells (1808-1891) applied for membership in the Kings County Medical Society of New York and were turned down. Hull, a well-educated physician, challenged his rejection in the courts, claiming that he had met all of the requisite formalities for acceptance into the society. Before the court could act on the suit, the New York legislature passed a law in 1844 disbarring all sectarians, declaring any practitioner who was not a member of a county medical society or who had not received a diploma from an incorporated medical college to be unlicensed and therefore liable to prosecution. Hull's lawsuit bounced in and out of the legal system for sixteen years before the court finally ruled in his favor. After the society grudgingly paid the costs of the lengthy court actions and reluctantly invited Hull to join, he declined the honor. His decision was based on an April 13, 1857, act passed by the New York legislature legalizing homeopathy by allowing the incorporation of homeopathic county medical societies. Hull died two years later.[35]

In Massachusetts, trouble between the two schools of thought began in May 1850 when homeopath Isaac Colby announced his resignation from the Massachusetts Medical Society because it had deliberately withheld from him all professional courtesies attached to membership in the society. After Colby left, the society ruled that a homeopathic diploma would no longer be accepted as evidence of a medical education, nor would the society's censors regard attendance at homeopathic lectures as entitling candidates to an examination for a license to practice. Clearly, the die had been cast in fostering a concept of orthodox professional identity among those who adhered to the AMA's Code of Ethics and viewing homeopathy as an exclusive system unworthy of the honors and privileges of recognition. However sincere in their motives, homeopaths were viewed as adhering to a dogma that rendered them outside the privileges of membership.[36]

That same year, following deliberations on how best to rid the association of errant members, the Massachusetts Medical Society took formal steps to arraign Dr. Ira Barrows on grounds of professional dishonesty, in other words, practicing homeopathy. Found guilty and expelled from the society, Barrows brought suit. Despite a multitude of political and legal maneuverings, much of which turned the public against the society, the court refused to reinstate Barrows's membership. Nevertheless, over the next twenty years, homeopathy grew in the state, and rather than challenge applicants suspected of practicing New School medicine, the society chose to quietly bury the issue. In an attempt to minimize the public relations damage it had received, the society embarked on a unwritten policy: "Don't ask. Don't tell." This lasted until 1870 when the American Medical Association refused to receive the society's delegates until it purged itself of all homeopathic members.[37]

Besides these early examples of discrimination within medical societies, homeopaths were disappointed with the exaggerated credence extended to allopathic testimony in cases of civil and criminal law. Given the multiplicity of opinions that defined the art and science of medicine in midcentury, regulars assumed powers and prerogatives they had little claim to and where none was deserved. In some instances, they managed to elevate themselves to the role of an umpire "from whose imperial decisions there is no appeal." This was a bitter pill for such men as William Gardiner, MD, who accused allopathy of intolerance and ill-gotten pride. "Homeopathy has been knocking at the door for the last fifty years, asking only for an honest, impartial hearing," he complained bitterly in 1852, "but, as yet, without a single exception, admittance, even on trial of its merits, has been denied."[38]

Exemplary of regular medicine's prejudice and presumption of wrongdoing by homeopaths was the case in 1854 of Agnes Lottimer, aged twelve, whose untimely death was diagnosed by homeopathic physicians Phineus P. Wells and Carroll Dunham as intermittent fever complicated by mumps. Troubled by the diagnosis, the parents allowed their daughter's body to be examined by Dr. James R. Wood, a regular surgeon, assisted by colleagues Willard Parker and C. R. Gilman. After analyzing the contents of the girl's stomach for traces of poison (none was found), they lobbied for a coroner's jury to determine whether the girl died of malpractice. Wells, the attending physician, and a graduate of New Hampshire Medical College in 1833, had practiced for seven years as a regular before turning to homeopathy. During the inquest, he was queried for six and a half hours on topics mainly irrelevant to the case. In its verdict, the jury reported that the girl had died from a hemorrhage of the lungs; that her treatment had been homeopathic; and that the remedies used to treat her were high dilutions. Whether the remedies were useful or not, the jury refused to speculate. In general, juries were more tolerant of homeopaths and less inclined to accept the accusations made against them by regular doctors and their societies.[39]

In June 1855, Silas S. Brooks resigned from the Philadelphia County Medical Society, an association of regular physicians and surgeons, on grounds that his homeopathic practice conflicted with the constitution and bylaws of the society. Following his letter of resignation, Brooks published the results of his investigation into homeopathy and his reasons for converting to New School reform. In response, the society's board of censors summoned Brooks to appear on the charge of violating the American Medical Association's Code of Ethics. Viewing the summons as unauthorized, he refused to obey, stating that the society had no authority to question his actions since he was no longer a member. The censors ignored his letter of resignation and, instead, expelled him for adhering to an "exclusive dogma as the basis of his practice."[40]

Also typical of the regular profession's behavior was the expulsion of J. S. Curtis, MD, of Hartford, Connecticut, for having consulted with two physicians who, although they had obtained their medical education and degrees from regular schools, practiced according to the principles of Hahnemann. Upon learning of the incident, the state medical society sought Curtis's promise not to consult with the two individuals again. When he refused, both the city and county medical societies expelled him in absentia. He attended a meeting of the state medical society to defend his position, but the society refused him permission to speak.[41]

By the 1860s, the proponents of homeopathy had become publicly incensed by the continuing saga of discrimination. Most knew that the influence upon orthodoxy of New School reforms had been profound and permanent. In the past thirty years, medicine had changed and homeopathy could claim a share of the new ideas and practices. These included the disuse of bleeding, cups, setons, and issues; smaller doses of medicines in general practice; a more relaxed physician-patient relationship; greater emphasis on diet and the body's vital powers; and reducing the practice of mixing medicines. While advocates of high potencies continued to stake their claims and spoil the public's image of New School reform, the majority of American homeopaths adopted the lower dilutions, taking pains to distinguish Hahnemann's law of cure from his more metaphysical pronouncements.[42]

American Civil War

At the outbreak of the Civil War, regular physicians and surgeons held all 115 positions in the U.S. Army's Medical Department. Under no circumstance did the Army Medical Board knowingly permit homeopaths or other sectarians to take any of these positions. Arrogating to itself full authority over all medical and sanitary departments, the Medical Department enforced a uniform system of medicine despite the fact that Union soldiers were not, in their public and private beliefs, all patrons of allopathic medicine. Many, in fact, preferred homeopathic, eclectic, or botanic medicine, and when they could get it they paid for it themselves.[43] It was not at all uncommon for soldiers on both sides to carry domestic books and kits containing their favorite medicines. The homeopathic kits included arnica for soreness following hard marches and contusions; rhus to counter the effects of wet weather; and calendula to treat lacerated wounds. These remedies were distinctly different from regular practice and seldom prescribed except by homeopathic physicians.[44]

Homeopaths such as T. P. Wilson, professor of anatomy and physiology at the Cleveland Homeopathic College, rejected the notion that the U.S. government should recognize only one medical system any more than it should recognize one religious sect exclusively, or patronize one political party. The hospitals of the Army and Navy ought to be open to all properly qualified medical doctors without regard to their particular medical philosophy.[45] Surely there were no specific guarantees or licenses given to regular medical schools under the U.S. Constitution or the laws of the states. It stood to reason, therefore, that legally chartered medical colleges should be allowed to send their graduates anywhere they could benefit the Army. "Thousands in the hospitals have suffered," complained Wilson, "not because the men were not to be found who were willing and able to meet this want, but because a medical dog-in-the-manger policy ruled the day."[46] And so he reasoned: "If it be true that this war is of, and by, and for the people, no class of persons can . . . be excluded from bringing their sacrifice to the common altar of the country." Soldiers should have equal access to their homeopathic, eclectic, and allopathic physicians, whose colleges were chartered under the laws of the states. Despite this reasoning, the Medical Department would not budge.[47] "No matter how well qualified a candidate might be," complained Wilson, every homeopath was "set aside" without benefit of judge or jury. "Just why one school of medicine should assume to monopolize this department," he opined, "none but the partisans of that school can see."[48] He urged an end to this "shameless" monopoly, for surely the government could not refuse its citizens the benefit of "true medical reform."[49] Wilson noted that in every war, ten soldiers fell by the effects of disease for every one slain on the battlefield. The time had come for the Union to provide its patriotic soldiers with the best weapons, along with the most appropriate sanitary regulations and medical treatment available. The instruments of medicine should be equal to the instruments of war.[50]

Consistent with this reasoning, Senator James Wilson Grimes (1816-1872) of Iowa introduced Senate Bill 188 in 1862, placing some military hospitals in the nation's capital under homeopathic administration. It also gave the president authority to make appointments from among the volunteer surgeons to expand the Medical Department. Regulars reacted harshly to the proposal, arguing that sick and wounded soldiers should not be made the basis of experiments to test the worthiness of medical sectarians. If such was the intent, then why not test the theories of the botanics, hydropaths, eclectics, mesmerists, spiritualists, rappers, and others as well? Surely, explained the editors of the *American Medical Times,* the welfare of the soldiers stood above any legislative desire to test the "false pretensions" of these crass pretenders.[51]

Lincoln signed the bill into law, but it did not result in an influx of homeopaths into the military. As a consequence, pressure continued, and in the spring of 1862 the Massachusetts Homeopathic Medical Society petitioned Congress for the immediate inclusion of homeopathy in every military hospital, believing that this would afford the Army a practical alternative by giving sick and wounded soldiers an option in treatment. The society based its appeal on information gathered during the cholera epidemic in 1831-1832; hospital statistics for 1847-1849; yellow fever statistics in the United States for 1853; and numerous statistical comparisons carried out in Eastern and Western Europe.[52] The petition, signed by more than 30,000 voters, included individuals of wealth and position. Noting that homeopathy was an accepted system in Europe and practiced by more than 3,500 physicians in the United States, with five chartered medical colleges and numerous hospitals and dispensaries, the society appealed to the Army Medical Board to respect the wants and needs of its loyal citizens. The petition included the following propositions:

> Whenever any considerable portion of the officers and soldiers of any brigade desire to have a homeopathic surgeon attached to the brigade, such additional surgeon shall be appointed.

> Whenever a majority of any regiment desire a homeopathic surgeon and assistant surgeon, such appointments shall be made.

> Whenever army hospitals are established, a fair proportion of them shall be devoted to homeopathic treatment.

> As allopathic surgeons are by their education and position necessarily disqualified for intelligently examining candidates in homeopathic medicine, an additional Examining Board shall be appointed for this purpose, composed of surgeons skilled in homeopathic medicine.[53]

The U.S. government received similar resolutions from the Miami Homeopathic Medical Association and the Western Institute of Homeopathy asking it to recognize homeopathic physicians and to grant them a proportion of the medical and surgical cases in the Army and Navy during the course of the war and into the future.[54] Nevertheless, the Army Medical Board held firm, prohibiting homeopaths from taking an examination for the office of surgeon or assistant surgeon in the Army or Navy.[55]

But rules were not always followed and reality was not always what it seemed. Beneath the ranks of surgeons and assistant surgeons of the U.S. Army were layers of other doctors whose credentials were not closely checked. These included the brigade surgeons and assistant surgeons of the volunteers; regimental surgeons and staff surgeons commissioned by the state governors; acting assistant surgeons in the U.S. Army, many of whom were "contract" surgeons; medical officers of the veterans corps; acting staff surgeons; and surgeons and assistant surgeons of the African-American troops. In all, more than 12,000 physicians were retained in service to the Union troops.[56]

In May 1862, the Ohio Senate passed a bill removing all restrictions to the appointment of sectarian doctors to medical positions in the state militia. Although the state medical society questioned the qualifications of doctors whose credentials were suspect, many irregular and sectarian physicians found their way into volunteer regiments.[57] In 1862, John King, editor of the *Eclectic Medical Journal*, the official organ of the Eclectic Medical Institute in Cincinnati and of eclectic medical philosophy, announced that twenty-two graduates of the school had garnered commissions in the Union Army. A year later, the number increased to fifty, including two who were professors at the institute.[58]

The Mound City General Hospital, near Cairo, Illinois, was administered by volunteer physician and homeopath E. C. Franklin of St. Louis, who reported a mortality rate of 7.9 percent among 8,078 patients. Although the treatment of patients was not entirely homeopathic, the hospital reported a mortality rate that was significantly lower than City General Hospital (14.5 percent), Good Samaritan Hospital (12.4 percent), Jefferson Barracks Hospital (11.5 percent), Lawson Hospital (25.9 percent), and the Military Prison Hospital (14.7 percent), all of which were under regular medical supervision. Franklin, assisted by two homeopathic contract physicians (Drs. Pratt and Wales), treated patients at the hospital, including some whom were considered beyond hope of recovery. After Horace R. Wirtz, medical director of the Army of the Tennessee, learned that contract homeopaths were managing the hospital, he relieved Franklin of his duties and ordered the resignations of the assisting contract physicians.[59]

When Franklin later took charge of the General Hospital in Springfield, Missouri, Medical Director G. G. J. DeCamp of the Department of the West informed him that the Army would not interfere with his providing homeopathic care to the men. However, the director made it clear that should Franklin appear on the *Register* as an Army surgeon, his appointment would be rejected unless he renounced homeopathy in a formal letter to the board of examiners. Franklin took issue with the director, pointing out that "as you have not superintended the regimental hospital under my charge, nor investigated the results of my practice, it is manifest you cannot be a proper judge of my professional attainments."[60] Furthermore, having been accused of not possessing the proper qualifications for treating the sick, Franklin reminded DeCamp that he was a graduate of the University of New York and had been a private pupil of Valentine Mott and thus *did* possess proper qualifications for treating the sick. He challenged the director to investigate his practice, including the time he had been in charge of the Mound City Hospital. The results of such an investigation, he predicted, would show that he had saved soldiers' lives by lowering the pernicious doses of calomel and quinine.[61]

Circular Order No. 6

On May 4, 1863, William A. Hammond, the reform-minded surgeon general appointed by Secretary of War Edwin M. Stanton, signed Circular Order No. 6 calling for the prompt end by military surgeons to the indiscriminate use of calomel. To achieve this, he directed that calomel (mercurous chloride) be struck from the supply table and that medical directors make no further requisitions. Hammond's decision was based on pathological reports that "proved the impropriety of the use of Mercury in very many of those diseases in which it was formerly unfailingly administered."[62] Hammond arrived at a similar conclusion with tartar emetic (tartrate of antimony and potassa) which he also ordered struck from the supply table.

The reaction to Hammond's decision was immediate and vocal, escalating to a clarion call among regulars for a recession of the order. Believing that the decision represented an attack on the foundations of orthodox medicine, regular physicians campaigned against the surgeon general by seeking his removal from office. A meeting of regulars at the Medical College of Ohio on May 27 resulted in the following resolution:

> *Resolved,* That the removal of W. A. HAMMOND from his position as Surgeon-General, would meet the approbation of the profession, be of advantage to our soldiers, and credible to the government.[63]

A more diplomatic but no less draconian resolution passed the Ohio State Medical Association:

Resolved, That Dr. W. A. Hammond be requested to revoke circular No. 6, and place Calomel and Tartar Emetic again on the supply table.

Resolved, That this Society will not be satisfied with anything less than a revocation of the order.

Resolved, That in the event of the refusal of the Surgeon-General to comply with this request, *he is hereby requested to resign.*[64]

When the American Medical Association convened its fourteenth annual meeting in Chicago in 1863, the principal piece of business was the surgeon general's order and its presumed insult to professional judgment. The association appointed a committee to respond to Hammond's Circular No. 6. The majority report, written by Dr. L. M. Lawson of Cincinnati, urged the continued use of calomel and tartar emetic in the army, while a strong minority report, written by Dr. J. M. Woodworth of Indiana, endorsed the surgeon general's decision. Upon receiving the majority report, the president of the American Medical Association submitted a set of resolutions to the delegates aimed at attacking the infamous Order No. 6 and its originator.[65]

In their public rhetoric, regulars accused Hammond of having conspired with the Thomsonians, eclectics, homeopaths, and other "Anti-Mineral knaves and fools." By contrast, reform-minded regulars and almost all sectarians were elated with the decision. In the August 1863 issue of the *North American Journal of Homeopathy,* the editors reported examples of mouth gangrene resulting from the effect of mercurial salivation in young children between their first and second dentitions.[66] Other longtime critics of calomel and tartar emetic, including many regulars, supported Hammond's decision. The real reason behind Circular Order No. 6, they argued, was the humiliating realization that Army physicians had fallen into the habit of administering these medicines for nearly every ailment.[67] Nevertheless, Hammond's decision left a bitter taste among Old School doctors and confirmed their belief that he was in league with the enemies of regular medicine. During the postwar years, homeopathy would bear the brunt of this hostility—one that would serve to intensify the ill will between regulars and homeopaths.

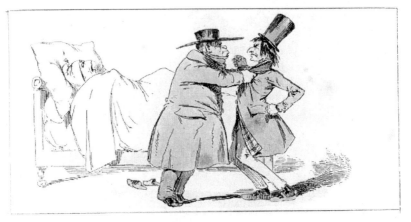

Lithograph depiction of homeopath and allopath arguing the virtues of their medical systems over the bed of the patient (183?). By Henri Monnier (1805-1877). (*Source:* Courtesy of the National Library of Medicine.)

Feelings continued to fester and, during the annual meeting of the American Medical Association in 1865, speakers threw heated insults at homeopathy and harshly criticized the consultation by Surgeon General Joseph K. Barnes (Hammond's replacement) with Secretary of State William Seward's homeopathic family physician, Dr. Tullio S. Verdi, following the knife attack on the secretary the night of Lincoln's assassination. Allowing Verdi to prescribe for Seward had given unwarranted recognition to the sect and reputedly had caused "a demoralizing effect" on the profession. William H. Mussey, vice president of the American Medical Association, insisted that Barnes be censured for associating with the "quack" Verdi. Wisely, the association's delegates chose not to follow Mussey's advice. Instead, they left the matter alone, fearing that by criticizing Barnes for his judgment they would be condemned in the public arena.[68]

In 1865, Dr. N. F. Cooke, professor of theory and practice at Hahnemann Medical College, accused Old School physicians of suffering from the disease *veriphobia,* or fear of truth. Using their combined strength, regulars had brought pressure on medical colleges to "loathe and detest" the very name of homeopathy. Deciding it was important to shun homeopaths as pariahs of the profession, they urged medical schools to require their graduates to pledge not to consult with homeopaths. Expulsion from their offices and medical societies and even forfeiture of their medical degrees were penalties they would face. The same "veriphobia" had affected congresspersons and military officers who excluded homeopaths from public hospitals and the Army; it had also caused Hammond's dismissal by Secretary of War Stanton in November 1863 and his discharge from the service a year later. "Who believes that justice would have been so swift and sure" upon the surgeon general, queried Cooke, "but for his famous anti-mercury and tartar emetic order? Here, veriphobia shivered to its very roots!"[69]

MORE UNCIVIL ACTS

In the postwar years, homeopaths became more resolute in demanding equal treatment from the state and federal governments. With their sizeable numbers of physicians, hospitals, dispensaries, and periodicals, homeopaths thought it absurd for examining boards to act in defiance of the laws by refusing licensure to comparably educated physicians and surgeons. "Was a clergyman, otherwise qualified, ever refused a position as chaplain of a regiment during the late war because he was an Episcopalian, a Presbyterian, a Unitarian, or a Catholic?" asked Dr. William H. Watson, president of the New York State Homeopathic Medical Society in 1869. Americans should not be enslaved by a state system of religion or one of medicine. He reminded delegates in his annual address:

> The Homeopathic branch of the medical profession raises no arrogant or puerile claim of exclusive legitimacy. It seeks not to monopolize all the charitable institutions of this country, as the Allopathic school has done, and still seeks to do. We ask nothing but simple justice. We wish only as many appointments as we are justly titled to by our numbers and intelligence.[70]

He urged his colleagues to be catholic in their thinking and in their practice. He hoped, too, that regular doctors would relent from rules that forbade consultations with homeopaths.[71]

When, in 1870, newly elected president Ulysses S. Grant appointed Dr. Henry Van Aernam, a regular, as U.S. Commissioner of Pensions in New York, replacing Christopher C. Cox, relations between the two schools of medical thought once again turned sour. At

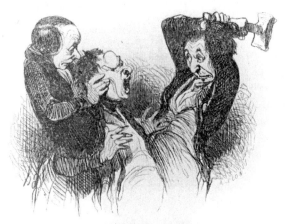

Similia similibus, or like cures like, as depicted by Daumier from his illustrations for Fabre, 1841. (*Source:* Courtesy of the National Library of Medicine.)

the suggestion of the surgeon general, Van Aernam "discovered" several homeopaths among his pension surgeons and challenged their education and practice. Fearing that continued employment of the surgeons in the bureau would give unintended recognition to New School principles and beliefs, he announced that "all Examining Surgeons should belong to one school and adopt one theory of medicine."[72]

Following this edict, the medical society for the District of Columbia appointed a committee consisting of doctors Thomas Antisell, Thomas Miller, Louis Mack, and Joseph M. Toner to consider "the claims of homeopaths and other irregular practitioners for professional recognition in the medical service of the United States Government." In its report, the committee claimed that the qualifications for surgeons in the Pension Bureau had been lax, to the point that all kinds of irregulars were on its rolls—from eclectics and Thomsonians, to Indian doctors, herbalists, hydropaths, homeopaths, and abortionists. Because the American Medical Association was the only legitimate medical governing body in the country, this organization should define the qualifications for a physician. The report concluded that regular medicine alone should serve the government, and that homeopathy and other irregular theories of medicine, "no matter how numerous or influential, politically or otherwise, they may be, should not be represented in such situations."[73]

Angered by these conclusions, the Homeopathic State Medical Society of New York appointed a political action committee to take the issue directly to President Grant. The state's eclectic medical society appointed a deputation of Alexander Wilder, M. M. Fenner, and J. Edwin Danelson to do the same. Wilder, an eclectic and historian of American sectarian medicine, bristled at the audacity of the report and the authority it relegated to the American Medical Association. The "genius of Protestantism," he pointed out, was its refusal to countenance the arbitrary or pontifical authority to prescribe a ritual, creed, or formula. Americans "will tolerate no such endeavor to dominate the conscience of men." No code or statute had conferred on the American Medical Association the exclusive right to govern the body of medicine.[74]

Of the 1,350 pension surgeons holding government appointments, 38 were subject to the audit, 19 of whom were homeopaths. In June 1870, Van Aernam dismissed pension surgeon Dr. Stilman Spooner of Oneida on grounds that he practiced homeopathy. Similar actions were carried out against doctors S. C. Card, Courtland Hoppin, A. T. Bull, and several other sectarians. Spooner challenged the decision, claiming that he had practiced allopathy for twenty years before turning to homeopathy, and that he carried all the credentials of a practicing physician. State and county homeopathic societies, along with the press, joined in the fight and demanded the dismissal of Van Aernam and the reinstatement of Spooner and the other victimized doctors.[75] Pressure mounted and, as a result of the acrimonious political fallout, including a bill introduced by Representative James Garfield that would have prohibited the dismissal of homeopaths from the Pension Bureau, Van Aernam resigned and the Senate replaced him with General James H. Baker. With Baker's appointment, the affected homeopaths were reinstated and the threats subsided. Baker even appointed several new homeopaths to posts in the Pension Bureau.[76]

In 1871, the Maine legislature introduced a bill regulating the qualifications of all practitioners and requiring each physician to register and be examined by a board consisting of seven members, two of whom were selected by the trustees of the Maine Medical School (regular), two by the Maine Medical Association (regular), two by the governor, and the seventh (who would also serve as president of the board) by the other six appointees. Realizing that no homeopath could be registered under this bill, the state's homeopaths went before the Judiciary Committee to protest the bill and seek amendments to it. Undeterred by their arguments, the committee reported the bill out, but it subsequently died because of protests from across the state. As testament to homeopathy's power and public recognition, the Maine legislature then granted a charter for a state homeopathic hospital at Portland. In addition, various municipal authorities within the state appointed homeopaths as city physicians, and placed the Soldiers and Sailors' Orphan Asylum under homeopathic care.[77]

The assault on sectarian medicine did not end with Van Aernam's replacement or with the Maine legislature's failed effort at regulation. In November 1871, after a nearly twenty-year policy of "Don't ask. Don't tell," Samuel A. Fisk, president of the Massachusetts Medical Society, sent letters to eight members who were also leading homeopathic physicians in the state (Drs. William Bushnell, Milton Fuller, William Gregg, H. F. H. Hoffendahl, George Russell, Israel T. Talbot, David Thayer, and Benjamin West), directing them to appear before a board to answer the charge of "practicing or professing to practice according to an exclusive theory or dogma, and by belonging to a Society whose purpose is at variance with the principles of and tends to disorganize the Massachusetts Medical Society."[78] Homeopathy was not mentioned in the notice, but the intent was clear to all, including the local newspapers, which took exception to the action.

The catalysts for Fisk's action were the objections raised by Boston gynecologists John L. Sullivan and Horatio R. Storer to the seating of the Massachusetts Medical Society delegates at the 1870 convention of the American Medical Association. Having tolerated homeopaths within its ranks for several decades, the society, it seemed to Sullivan and Storer, had flaunted the code of medical ethics. The convention delegates approved a subsequent committee report recommending that the Massachusetts Medical Society purge itself of its irregular members, and the onus fell on the society to respond.[79]

In response to the AMA committee report, the society established a council of five to preside over the trial. The eight accused members objected to the proceedings, but the board refused their appeal, stating that its only function was to determine whether they had practiced homeopathy and were members of a homeopathic society. Protesting the right of the society to act in such a high-handed manner, the accused members obtained an injunction forbidding their expulsion. Of the eight, several were graduates of Harvard and all were members in good standing with the society. Immediately following the injunction, the press, which had felt ill treated by the society's refusal to allow their presence at the trial, depicted the proceedings as a shabby inquisition. At the same time, homeopaths around the state took advantage of the delay to raise $80,000 to establish the Massachusetts Homeopathic Hospital. Most significant of all, the trustees of Boston University in February 1873 decided to organize a homeopathic medical department and dispensary.[80] As for the Massachusetts Medical Society, it used the injunction and the postponement of the trial as an opportunity to withdraw "before a gun was fired." Homeopaths claimed victory.[81]

The court eventually agreed to hear arguments on the injunction, but it did so without ruling on the powers of the society under its charter. Dr. Oliver Wendell Holmes advised against the trial on grounds that it would only make martyrs of the accused. The leadership of the society, however, disregarded his advice, and the in-house trial proceeded in April 1873. The defendants requested that the trial be held in public; the press be allowed to attend; they be permitted legal counsel; a stenographic reporter be appointed by mutual consent; and they be given the right to challenge members of the board. The board denied all of the requests.[82] In his arguments against the doctors, George C. Shattock, president of the Massachusetts Medical Society, charged them with attempting to "disorganize and destroy" the society by having joined the Massachusetts Homeopathic Medical Society; practicing medicine "according to a certain exclusive theory or dogma known as homeopathy"; and "conduct unbecoming and unworthy an honorable physician."[83]

SUMMARY

Clearly, both camps had embarked on campaigns of demonization, crusades that seemed to echo the times. Occasionally, as in the case of the Pensions Bureau, homeopaths were able to win back their positions. Nevertheless, in the confrontations, particularly when they involved the federal government or the AMA, homeopaths faced repeated defeats. By contrast, in local matters where homeopaths could rely on personal relationships and the power and prestige of supportive patrons, their successes were more evident.

Although members of the two schools found frequent opportunities to consult with each other, particularly specialists practicing in urban areas, the public stereotype not only polarized the two schools but forced each to defend its respective therapies, no matter how inaccurate, dated, or limited they had become. Regulars seemed to go out of their way in their public statements to portray homeopaths as doctrinaire in their allegiance to Hahnemann's most spiritualistic speculations. Similarly, New School reformers deliberately chose to emphasize bloodletting and other depletive measures as the only true symbols of orthodox practice. Exemplary was the following poem published in the *North American Journal of Homeopathy.*

> Ah! What a dreaded warrior was he
> Who came with lancet sharp hung at his side
> And from his breast-plate glittering you could see
> The cupping instrument full often tried.
> Then, too, behold, the blisters at his back
> And from his shoulders all his plasters hung
> The seton needle there and, yes, alack!
> The skeins of silk all round in order strung.
> The issue peas form bracelets for his arms,
> A bag of mustard on his body see,
> Tartar emetic ointment with its charms
> Hang down in tubules from his awful knee.
> A match box, cotton and a lamp to burn
> (And make the moxa on the simple fool),
> Peep from beneath his armor in their turn
> Fit emblems for an antiquated school.
> Thus then in truth ye used to march along,
> Admiring crowds in wonder stood aside—
> But now they change the tenor of their song
> And look on all as humbug, and deride.[84]

The often arresting images used to describe homeopaths and regulars did little to explain the broader lens of contemporary medical practice and culture. As explained by historian John Harley Warner, "the threat sectarianism posed to regular physicians is best understood against the backdrop of the social and economic realities of medical practice."[85] The various and intimate contexts in which the two opposing schools practiced seems overlooked in the range of rich but superficial material that both groups sported in their public representations of each other. Thus, although there was no end of rhetorical diatribes, caricatures, and literary and artistic satires, few do justice to the complexity of the physician-patient relationship or the range of physician-physician contacts that belied their more publicized encounters. Homeopaths attended some of the most prominent members of American society, including oil magnate John D. Rockefeller, Indiana politician and Vice President Schulyer Colfax, psychologist William James, poet Henry Wadsworth Longfellow, Secretary of State William Seward, journalist Horace Greeley, abolitionist William Lloyd Garrison, author Louisa May Alcott, and President James Garfield. Imbedded in their patronage of homeopathy was a tangled set of relationships that, despite allopathy's periodic pogroms and contentious legal cases, succeeded in providing lucrative and successful practices for well-connected doctors.

As the next chapter will show, the most controversial relations between homeopaths and allopaths were not to be found in their day-to-day dealings but those which played out most overtly in print. This is where homeopathy became subject to public criticism and ridicule, and where the campaign against its beliefs was realized in its most powerful and pervasive form.

Chapter 7

The Four Horsemen

Through most of the nineteenth century, regular medicine publicly manifested disdain, skepticism, and outright arrogance toward the principles and practices of homeopathy. Enterprising critics deridingly calculated infinitesimal potencies and attributed patients' deaths to homicide. With article titles such as "Homeopathic Wrath," "The Homeopathic Tribe," "Quackery Rampant," "Frauds of Homeopathy," "Craven Knaves," and "Medical Renegades Who Prostitute the Title of MD," allopathic journals contributed to the rhetorical feeding frenzy against medical sectarianism. This hardened position did not coalesce immediately, but gradually, as homeopaths found strong advocates and healthy remuneration among society's more elite families. The realization that homeopathy had become a successful rival was a hard blow to regulars, who saw their pocketbooks and their influence wane in the presence of what they considered little more than metaphysical healing combined with expectant medicine. Stung by homeopathy's success, regulars proceeded to challenge New School reformers in their county and state medical societies; in the granting of military commissions; in the passage of tougher licensing laws; and in public support of homeopathic hospitals and dispensaries. Along with these efforts came the publication of four books intended for both the public and the profession. These works, written over a period of eleven years, differed from earlier texts in that they more directly attacked homeopathy's credibility, revealing an arsenal of vivid images of homeopathy's more controversial principles and predicting its eventual demise.

OLIVER WENDELL HOLMES

The opening salvo came in 1842 when Oliver Wendell Holmes (1809-1894), professor of anatomy at Harvard Medical School, delivered two lectures before the Boston Society for the Diffusion of Useful Knowledge on the subject of "Homeopathy and Its Kindred Delusions." The lectures, quickly published, came as a thunderclap to proponents of New School reform and to those from both schools who had worked out amicable relationships with each other. Known for his wit and his command of the King's English, Holmes presented a devastating portrayal of Samuel Hahnemann's "delusions." He explained that homeopathy had originated during a period of "eclecticism" when many honest minds were turning to new theories and practices, hoping to find something of value. But Holmes felt the results of this reform thinking had not been worth the effort; in fact, most only encouraged "ignorance, error, or deception in a profession that deals with the life and health of our fellow creatures."[1]

Recounting earlier histories of the royal cure for the King's Evil (scrofula), Weapon Ointment (unguentum armarium), the virtues of Bishop Berkeley's tar-water treatment, and Dr. Elisha Perkins's patented Metallic Tractors, Holmes laid the groundwork for a public examination into the doctrines of Hahnemann and his disciples. Although he promised to treat the topic with "good temper" and "peaceable language," like many contemporary physicians he took exception to Hahnemann's unilateral decision to apply the term *allopathy* to all of orthodox medicine since Hippocrates and designating all regular physicians as allopathists in heart and deed. Holmes felt homeopaths had deliberately chosen to draw a line between themselves and the rest of the profession by creating this unwelcomed designation. Further, having also announced several universal doctrines in medical science based on the slimmest evidence, and having erroneously claimed a significant difference in mortality between patients attended by regular doctors and those treated homeopathically, New School reformers now, according to Holmes, must face a "sober examination" of their principles and claims.[2]

Holmes explained without comment or exaggeration his interpretation of the three cardinal doctrines of Hahnemann's *Organon* and treatise on *The Chronic Diseases*. These were the law of similars, the importance of infinitesimal doses, and the origin of most chronic diseases in psora. He also recounted Hahnemann's lesser principles: giving little power to the curative efforts of nature; administering medicinal substances in a state of purity and uncombined with any other; admitting the medicinal powers of substances thought to be inert; recognizing diseases by their collection of symptoms; and describing symptoms of any complaint with exactness.[3]

Holmes addressed the first of Hahnemann's doctrines, agreeing that under certain circumstances diseases yielded to remedies capable of producing like symptoms, a factor recognized since the days of Hippocrates. However, resemblances between the effects of a remedy and the symptoms of disease occurred in only a small number of cases. "Nor has it ever been considered as an established truth," he reminded his audience, "that the efficacy of even those few remedies was in any definite ratio to their power of producing symptoms more or less like those they cured." To transform what applied to only a few remedies into an irrefutable and universal law applicable to all medicines was a "pregnant novelty" and the equivalent of basing a religion on the rumor of one miracle.[4]

Holmes asked his listeners to consider the power of one drop of tincture of chamomile given in the quantity ordered by Jahr's *Manual*. The imagined powers of infinitesimal doses, he noted, were guaranteed to tax the very foundations of credulity.

> For the first dilution it would take 100 drops of alcohol. For the second dilution it would take 10,000 drops, or about a pint. For the third dilution it would take 100 pints. For the fourth dilution it would take 10,000 pints, or more than 1,000 gallons, and so on to the ninth dilution, which would take ten billion gallons, which {Dr. Panvini} computed would fill the basin of Lake Agnano, a body of water two miles in circumference. The twelfth dilution would of course fill a million such lakes. By the time the seventeenth degree of dilution should be reached, the alcohol required would equal in quantity the waters of ten thousand Adriatic seas. Trifling errors must be expected, but they are as likely to be on one side as the other, and any little matter like Lake Superior or the Caspian would be but a drop in the bucket.[5]

When discussing symptoms, Holmes borrowed liberally from Hahnemann and G. H. G. Jahr, who recounted the sensations that occurred in the minutes, hours, days, and weeks following a single dose of medicine. He thought it strange, if not ridiculous, that every sensation of mind and body (e.g., sighing, pimples, wakefulness, dreams, tickling) was annotated and ascribed to the medicine.[6]

Holmes then turned to the tests carried out on healthy subjects, noting results that were very different from those claimed by Hahnemann and his disciples. Gabriel Andral, professor of medicine in the School of Paris, who once was touted by homeopaths as an "eminent and very enlightened allopathist," had carried out hospital experiments testing the effects of aconite, arnica, cinchona, sulphur, and other favorite homeopathic remedies on healthy persons. He concluded in his report to the Academy of Medicine that, after years of tests, none of the medicines produced anything similar to the symptoms attributed by homeopathy. Holmes also referred to Paris medical writer F. J. Double who had reached similar conclusions with extensive tests on cinchona in 1801, long before he had even heard of homeopathy. Similarly, Bonnet, President of the Royal Society of Medicine of Bordeaux, had prescribed cinchona for various medical conditions during the Peninsular War (1808-1814) but "never found it to produce the pretended paroxysms" claimed by Hahnemann. Louis Fleury made similar tests and, although taking additional precautions as to diet and regimen, discovered no evidence to confirm a universal law of similars. From these examples, Holmes concluded that the catalogs of symptoms developed by Hahnemann and Jahr to explain the influence of drugs upon healthy persons were "not titled to any confidence."[7]

Because Hahnemann had relied on numerous ancient authors to confirm points in his doctrines, Holmes next sought to verify the referenced passages and found several to be misquoted or grossly misrepresentative of the original author's intent. He concluded from this that the doctrine of similars was based on a "pretended science" that was nothing more than "a mingled mass of perverse ingenuity, of tensile erudition, of imbecile credulity, and of artful misrepresentation."[8]

Holmes reported that Hahnemann's so-called doctrine of psora, or the itch, tested the faith of the founder's most ardent disciples. Refusing to waste time with "this excrescence," he judged it wholly without merit—both within and outside homeopathy—and observed that the theory's lack of influence in mainstream homeopathy explained why there had been no schism when Hahnemann first announced it.[9]

Holmes predicted that after the novelty of homeopathy wore off, most of its high dilution practitioners would "gradually withdraw from the rotten half" of New School reform and return to the more "visible doses" of the low dilutionists. He was less optimistic concerning the ultrahomeopathists who clung faithfully to Hahnemann's every word. These believers would either have to recant before rejoining their colleagues or move further afield to embrace other "equally extravagant doctrines."[10]

Homeopaths quickly responded to Holmes's attack. Charles Neidhard of Philadelphia prepared the initial rebuttal, followed by Robert Wesselhoeft of Cambridge, Massachusetts, and Abraham H. Okie of Providence, Rhode Island. Otis Clapp, who sold an assortment of homeopathic books, medicine chests, and single remedies in Boston, published all three rejoinders.[11]

In *An Answer to the Homeopathic Delusions, of Dr. Oliver Wendell Holmes* (1842), Charles Neidhard proclaimed that homeopathy had won the respect of numerous physicians of the Old School. Had Holmes studied the homeopathic method in greater detail and tested its principles, Neidhard felt his lectures would have taken a different turn. Had Holmes given a "logical and faithful history" of homeopathic doctrines, separating the main doctrines from Hahnemann's lesser theories, and properly accounting for the "changes and reformations" in homeopathic thought, he would have come to different conclusions. Denying himself that opportunity, Holmes was forced to rely on the trials, proofs, and assertions of others.[12]

Neidhard's refutation represented one of homeopathy's earliest revisionist dialogues with allopathy. Instead of referring to Hahnemann for clarification of legitimate practice, Neidhard allied himself with a newer generation of more liberal practitioners who attempted to steer a less combative and less pretentious course. For these reformers, the differences between allopathic and homeopathic medicine were matters of degree, not kind. Neidhard made no attempt to replace the old doctrines of medicine, merely claiming the discovery of a new law that provided a "surer foundation to the materia medica and the practice of medicine." Moreover, he admitted that the law of similars was "by no means perfectly understood." Enlightened homeopaths were continually "enlarging the boundaries of medicine," and while the two schools were traveling in different directions, they would eventually arrive at common ground.[13]

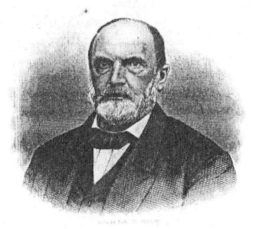

Charles Neidhard (1809-1895), founder of the American Institute of Homeopathy. (*Source:* Courtesy of the Lloyd Library and Museum, Cincinnati.)

Neidhard admitted that the principle of infinitesimal dosages had been a "great stumbling block" for regular physicians, a situation made even more confusing by Hahemann's peculiar explanations. However, physicist and mathematician Christian Johann Doppler (1803-1853) of Prague had provided a more plausible rationale. His work suggested that the active strength of a medicine should not be judged by its gross weight but by the size of the surface area which increased with each trituration. Furthermore, the electricity that was manifested as a result of a medicine's attenuation increased the drug's power in a ratio equal to the increase in surface.[14]

In defending the drug trials carried out by Hahnemann and his disciples on healthy persons, Neidhard admitted to the "folly" of recording symptoms that had sprung from causes other than the remedy. He further admitted that homeopaths were well aware of the "imperfect state" of their trials. These problems aside, the fact remained that provings on healthy persons raised the materia medica from its once "shadowy" existence. As for Gabriel Andral, Victor Baillie, F. J. Double, Louis Fleury, and Léon Simon, who declared the drug effects on healthy patients worthless, Neidhard reminded readers that none of these men knew anything of the system they had endeavored to refute. Hahnemann never claimed that bark would produce an intermittent fever in *any* person, "only that the symptoms collected from a number of persons, would correspond to a particular kind of intermittent fever." This applied to other drugs as well. And, argued Neidhard, "the remedy and the disease must only be alike in certain characteristic symptoms, whilst in others, they may be unlike, and yet a cure be effected."[15] Clearly, Neidhard spoke a language differing in substance and degree from fellow homeopaths, particularly those who had taken Hahnemann literally in his desire to be medicine's revolutionary and not simply its reformer. Rather than relying on Hahnemann's theory of infinitesimal doses, or regarding psora as the cause of chronic diseases, Neidhard urged critics to take a closer look at the homeopathic law of similars and the maxim of giving one medicine at a time. These, he asserted, were the "main principles" of homeopathy and upon which "the whole science depends."[16]

Robert Wesselhoeft, a recent immigrant from Germany, added to homeopathy's response in a series of letters published under the title *Some Remarks on Dr. O. W. Holmes's Lectures on Homeopathy and Its Kindred Delusions; Communicated to a Friend* (1842). After giving deference to Holmes and his skillful use of the English language, he likened him to the new set of writers called "young Europe" or "young France" who, with their witticisms and sophistry, made sport of their fellow man. Wesselhoeft found nothing significant in Holmes's arguments and analogies. His ridicule, like that from these writers, represented little more than Old School medicine's continued scorn for reform.[17]

Wesselhoeft stood by Hahnemann's law of similars but admitted that many homeopaths had rejected the theory of psora as not legitimately homeopathic doctrine. He also tried to deflect Holmes's criticism of minute dosages by stressing the "medical virtue" in every drug and emphasizing the right of each practitioner to determine the proper level of dosage.[18] Yet when he attempted to explain what he called the *dynamic virtue* in homeopathic medicines, his German and English seemed to collide, and incoherency resulted.

> When, by a proper process, the quantitative element of gravity, called the parenchyma of a drug, is removed, in order to gain its true quality, we effect a free development of the dynamic virtue. Annihilating the molecules, and their power to make the solid substances coherent, in the peculiar manner discovered by

Hahnemann, by the extension of the superficies we increase the development of the dynamic quality. For this means the enfranchisement of the bound qualities is thus favored, that they are enabled to surpass the limits of their own substratum.[19]

A proponent of Hahnemann's earliest thinking, Wesselhoeft explained that homeopathy cared nothing for pathology. It sought the cause of disease in neither the nerves, blood, lymphatic system, irritation, nor stheny. He likewise disapproved of "shameless bodily examinations" that had been the cause of "much alarm and anxiety" among female patients. Surely, doctors could now substitute remedies that produced in a healthy person symptoms similar to those found in a sick patient. In other words, symptomatology rather than pathology was all that mattered in New School medicine.[20]

Finally, Abraham Howard Okie responded to Holmes's critique in a pamphlet titled *Homeopathy with Particular Reference to a Lecture by O. W. Holmes, MD* (1842). In it, he made a detailed response to the arguments and observations recounted by Holmes. Instead of testing the system himself, Okie said, Holmes had focused his attention on Hahnemann's theory of infinitesimals. But Okie defended infinitesimals and based his support on the known effects of magnetism, electricity, and galvanism; the infectious but imperceptible environment surrounding persons sick with smallpox; and Rush's claim that certain odors could produce insanity. He likewise countered Holmes's criticism of the psoric doctrine with references to Xavier Bichat, Benjamin Rush, and other revered Old School physicians who had written about attacks of "the itch" and its suppressed or latent relationship with diseases designated as chronic.[21]

Ironically, the slow pace of medical reform continued to trouble Holmes. In 1857, responding to the attraction of homeopathic medicines for treating babies and young children, Holmes remarked that, unlike regular medicine, homeopathy "does not offend the palate, and so spares the nursery those scenes of single combat in which infants were wont to yield at length to the pressure of the spoon and the imminence of asphyxia."[22] By the 1870s, he had made several additional admissions of regular medicine's failures, not the least of which concerned the materia medica: "I firmly believe that if the materia medica, as now used, could be sunk to the bottom of the sea, it would be better for mankind, and all the worse for the fishes." Although his criticism came late, the frustration evident in Holmes's comments were greeted favorably by New School advocates who, while refusing to forgive him for his earlier comments on homeopathy, seemed more tolerant of his later admissions.[23]

JOHN FORBES

In 1846, four years after Holmes's lectures, John Forbes (1787-1861), editor of the *British and Foreign Medical Review,* published *Homeopathy, Allopathy, and "Young Physic."* Now that homeopathy was "openly advocated" by professor William Henderson of Edinburgh, he said, the time had come for a full examination of it as a system of medical doctrine and practice. Forbes recognized Hahnemann as a "very extraordinary man" by any definition, and one whose name would remain permanently in the history of medicine. In fact, Forbes was willing to admit that homeopathy had caused "more important fundamental changes in the practice of the healing art, than have resulted from any promulgated since the days of Galen himself." Nevertheless, the ideas propounded by Hahnemann had raised concerns among members of the medical profession, all the more so by the "seemingly monstrous extravagance" of the principle of infinitesimal doses, which he found to be "abhorrent" to common sense. Believing that Hahnemann and his followers were "sincere, honest, and learned men," he urged the profession to undertake an investigation of the evidence and to judge it fairly.[24]

Forbes recounted the story of Hahnemann's discovery of the principle of similars and the rationale for the cures he effected, noting that the doctrine of infinitesimal doses had never been part of his original system. He went on to explain that the medical profession regarded Hahnemann's principle of infinitesimal doses as "incomprehensible posology," treating it as a marvelous fiction which they garnished with playful exaggeration. Thus when Hahnemann explained that a sextillionth of a grain of carbonate of ammonia could act beneficially on the body for up to thirty-six days when prepared by specific frictions and shakings, even the fair-minded found it difficult not to be judgmental.[25]

Forbes identified a series of claims that homeopathy had made over the years which he felt to be undocumented:

1. Hahnemann's preferred medicines were incapable of exciting artificial diseases or the symptoms of diseases in the healthy body, beginning with the very medicine that gave rise to his doctrine, namely cincona.
2. The majority of symptoms recorded in homeopathic trials bore no relation to or consequence from the medicines taken by healthy persons. To be valid, the so-called consequences had to be different from a parallel group of healthy persons who recorded all of their sensations after taking no medicine. The 1,090 symptoms recorded as the effects of calcarea (oyster shells), the 590 symptoms produced by plumbago, and the 1,242 symptoms produced by the sepia (cuttlefish) suffice to demonstrate "the absurdity of the conclusions drawn."
3. In those instances when a medicine produced specific effects on a healthy body, there was no evidence that the effects bore any resemblance to a natural malady or its symptoms.
4. While it was true that a new artificial action could destroy an existing morbid condition, this was "as good and rational a theory as most of our orthodox medical theories."
5. To admit the special potency of infinitesimal amounts of homeopathic medicines shaken in a vial or rubbed in a mortar defied all reason.[26]

These objections were enough, argued Forbes, to prove the "unsoundness" of Hahnemann's theory and make it useless "to waste more time in the discussion of its merits." No theoretical doctrine, however appealing, could have credence if it were little more than "poetical speculation."[27] Forbes conceded that allopathy had limited powers for curing disease in that nature or *vis medicatrix naturae* had reduced the art of medicine to only a few diseases. At best, the physician could remove obstacles and prepare the body for nature's remedial powers. Similarly, the perceived "triumphs" of homeopathy were really attributable to the power of nature. Here, he felt, was the nexus for a true "reformation" in medical thinking. Society was just beginning to recognize and appreciate the power of nature in freeing the body from disease. When the power to fight nature conflicted with belief in the healing power of nature, homeopathy gratified the feelings of those who wanted changes in practice but were unwilling to concede the power of nature. Nevertheless, *vis medicatrix naturae* was sufficient to explain the past and present triumphs of homeopathy.[28]

Having proposed that the reputed successes of homeopathy arose not from its therapeutics and materia medica but through the inherent powers of nature, Forbes had to admit that homeopathy did expose the sorry history of heroic medicine. While homeopathy's successes came from acts of omission (e.g., providing little or no medicine), allopathy's reputation had been based on acts of commission (i.e., employing intrusive medicines). Not by intention, homeopathy relied on the powers of nature to relieve and remove disease. Forbes concluded from this that allopathic physicians often hindered, rather than assisted, nature's curative abilities. He suggested that in many diseased conditions, patients would be better off "if all remedies, at least all active remedies, especially drugs, were abandoned." While accepting this restriction, he nonetheless felt that allopathy had more to contribute than homeopathy since it "is, or may be made, in its exercise, consonant with the principles of science, and is capable of indefinite improvement."[29]

Clearly, the history of therapeutics suggested that regular medicine's use of bloodletting, along with its drugs of choice, principally calomel and antimony, had been singularly disappointing and even injurious. From Louis's *Recherches sur les Effets de la Saignée* (1835), practitioners learned that none of these remedies had served their intended purpose. Although believing that medicine was neither a science nor an art, Forbes insisted that it was a noble and glorious calling, "even in its present most imperfect state." Great progress had occurred in physiology, pathology, and diagnosis, and many improvements had been made in the general mode of treating patients. Doctors were now less guided by theory and tradition and less insistent on meddling. In addition, doctors had profited from "humbler notions" and "milder practices" in the treatment of disease, having learned more of the morbid processes within the body. Doctors had thus grown "more trustful" of nature and a "little less trustful" of medical intervention. Believing therapeutics to be in its "merest infancy," Forbes urged colleagues to recognize that there was as yet no certainty in medicine.[30]

According to Forbes, the medical profession had much to learn from homeopathy, including the need for thorough reform in practical therapeutics. This meant a greater knowledge of the natural history of diseases; better understanding of medicines as therapeutic agents; establishing which diseases benefited from medical treatment and which did not; an appreciation of the difference between *post hoc* and *propter hoc;* and the adoption of the numerical method in recording medical information. Forbes urged doctors to give nature "the best chance of doing the work herself" and to abandon polypharmacy for a more simple and more intelligent system of medicine. In achieving these objectives, he suggested they give greater attention to hygiene; choose an "expectant" rather than a "heroic" system of treatment; oppose powerful medication unless definite evidence supported its beneficial effect; oppose large doses of medicines; and encourage the greater use of placebos "for the satisfaction of the patient's mind." Above all, he urged simplicity in medical prescriptions and cautioned physicians to avoid the habit of "prescribing certain determinate remedies . . . merely because the prescriber has been taught to do so, and on no better grounds than conventional wisdom." Doctors, he felt, should give greater value to diet, temperature, clothing, air purity, mental and bodily exercise, baths, and occupation than ever before. This would produce a more comprehensive system of nosology in chronic diseases and teach medical students to be more knowledgeable about the elements of medical science and more skeptical of past medical beliefs and practices. Finally, Forbes encouraged physicians to build a stronger patient-doctor relationship, reconcile patients to simpler and milder forms of treatment, avoid the practice of preparing and selling medicines, and improve the overall education of the medical practitioner.[31]

William Henderson, professor of medicine and general pathology at the University of Edinburgh, responded to Forbes in the *British Journal of Homeopathy* in 1846; his response was published by William Radde as *An Inquiry into the Homeopathic Practice of Medicine* that same year. Noting that Forbes was the first opponent who had treated homeopathy "with the courtesy of a gentleman," Henderson thanked him for his review but indicated that there was still much to correct in his account. Forbes's depiction of homeopathy had all the appearance of fairness, but his misuse of statistical information and his insistence on dismissing homeopathic practice as simply the result of nature's inherent power over the body represented a failure of nerve.[32] Henderson admitted that Hahnemann had erred "on the safe side" by recording "trivial occurrences" among the symptoms identified after taking medicines. Nevertheless, he and his followers had tested the truths of their medicinal substances, while allopaths simply based their practices on tradition, and this was reason enough to acknowledge the significance of homeopathic remedies.[33]

Henderson accused Forbes of reading only Hahnemann's works and to be unacquainted with the beliefs and practices of later homeopaths. In fact, Forbes never seemed to have considered that the practice of homeopathy could differ from its originator over a period of twenty or thirty years. This was as unfair as believing Laennec the sole authority on auscultation. Henderson explained that many of the customs and doctrines of Hahnemann had been abandoned. These included his psoric theory of chronic diseases; his dynamization hypothesis in which medicines increased in their potential through triturations and shakings; the use of higher attenuations in acute diseases; and his belief in long intervals between doses. As early as 1824, Gottlieb M. W. L. Rau had dissented from the Hahnemannian dogma of higher attenuations, preferring lower ones, especially the original or mother tinctures administered at short intervals. Rau also discarded the psoric theory and the theory of dynamization. Instead, he stressed the significance of *similia similibus* as the only homeopathic principle, as well as the practical importance of pathology and careful diagnosis. Anatomy and physiology were now necessary to the pathologist and to homeopathic practice, as were botany and chemistry. Indeed, modern homeopathy gladly took advantage of the most recent allopathic discoveries. Since both homeopathy and allopathy now had the same respect for pathology, physiology, botany, and the other medical sciences, their only differences were in therapeutics. And this, Henderson explained, stemmed in large measure from allopathy's reverence for the past, which left it with a trail of senseless empiricisms. Homeopathy, on the other hand, was barely fifty years old and adhered to a more regulated method of empiricism. As Forbes had already admitted, the testimony of the previous 2,000 years of medicine amounted to very little given the clinical research of Louis and others. Therefore physicians reasonably could give greater credence to the more recent discoveries in the medical sciences.[34]

WORTHINGTON HOOKER

In 1851, the Rhode Island Medical Society awarded Worthington Hooker, MD (1806-1867), the Fisk Prize for his dissertation titled *Homeopathy: So Called, Its History and Refutation.* In a subsequent edition titled *Homeopathy: An Examination of Its Doctrines and Evidences,* Hooker made little effort to conceal his antagonism toward New School reform. His characterizations of Hahnemann included sobriquets such as "medical fanatic," "wild dreamer in science," "absurd theorizer," "scientific fool," "flimsy reasoner," "prone to delusion," "quack," "mongrel," and "radical." To Hahnemann's followers, Hooker applied similar descriptions: "quack imposter," "ignoramus," "dreamers," "scientific fools," "loose analyzers," "cheats," "uneducated," and "irresponsible." Hooker broke new ground in presenting regular medicine's position toward homeopathy. Unlike Holmes and Forbes, he took a strident and far more venomous approach that underscored regular medicine's rising animosity.[35]

Hooker introduced homeopathy to his readers as "a wordy and fine spun theory, built upon the loosest analogies" and accompanied "with all forms of delusion and quackery." He intended for his investigation of the system to expose readers to its delusions, identify its errors, and refute its claims of evidence. He promised not to make homeopathy responsible for everything that had been claimed by its many advocates; rather, he chose to rely only on the works of prominent homeopaths who had contributed significantly to its canon. Notwithstanding this caveat, he admitted having difficulty in understanding why so many intelligent and influential members of the nonmedical community favored a system he believed was so "absurd."[36]

Despite the circumstantial manner in which Hahnemann introduced the idea of infinitesimal doses, Hooker explained that disciples quickly transformed the concept into Hahnemann's most singular achievement. However, the arithmetic calculations went beyond anything intelligible or comprehensible, leaving rational persons "in a chaos of undefined entities, or nonentities, we know not which." He went on, "We fancy that we grasp the reality, and then it instantly vanishes as a phantom, even beyond the sphere of imagination itself."[37] Hooker reported that the homeopath's doses jumped from the millions and billions to even trillions of an attenuated grain—doses so minute and mysterious as to defy explanation. This "adventurous" mathematics was too much for Hooker, who reprinted in his book a popular caricature that had appeared in a contemporary newspaper. The poem represented a prescription for a homeopathic rum cordial.

> Take a little rum,
> The less you take the better;
> Pour it in the lakes
> Of Wener and of Wetter.
> Dip a spoonful out,
> Mind you don't get groggy,
> Pour it in the lake
> Winnipissiogee.
> Stir the mixture well,
> Lest it prove inferior,
> Then put half a drop
> Into Lake Superior.
> Every other day
> Take a drop in water,
> You'll be better soon,
> Or at least you ought to.[38]

As if dynamized medicines were not difficult enough to conceptualize, Hooker pointed out that even the smell of certain medicines was deemed detrimental to overly sensitive persons. He reported on a homeopath whose wife forced him to live in the basement for several days because the smell of camphor on his injured limb interfered with the recovery of his children who were sick in another part of the house. Proudly explaining that regular medicine consisted mainly of "*material-headed* reasoners," Hooker announced that the profession dismissed the etherialized, spiritualized, and dynamized medicines of homeopathy as utter nonsense.[39]

Hooker focused considerable attention on Hahnemann's doctrine of similars, arguing that if it was the *sole* law of cure as homeopaths contended, then they must prove beyond question that cures were never effected by any other cause. He also explained that if camphor could cure cholera, the same dose given to a healthy person should produce the symptoms of cholera. But this was not the case. He also criticized Hahnemann for his poor opinion of the curative powers of nature even though it was the real reason behind his success.[40] In all,

Hooker concluded that if Hahnemann's "great central doctrine" was true, it applied to only a "very small range of phenomena" and "the treatment of disease based upon this mode of observation must therefore be utterly absurd."[41]

Hooker identified four lessons learned from the errors in homeopathy. First, he listed the problems plaguing physicians and scientists who preferred "flights of theory" to the tough regimen of observation and induction. He accused Hahnemann of being so far under the dominion of the "theorizing spirit" that in his delusions he lost sight of truth.[42] Having noted that Hahnemann encouraged both mesmerism and clairvoyance, Hooker was convinced that he would have accepted the grossest claims, including the spiritual world of "rappings" had he been aware of them.[43] Admittedly, the same evidence that rejected homeopathic theory would also reject a large number of theories and practices of regular medicine. In truth, too much had been taken upon trust and the "gross errors" of homeopathy would serve "to direct the attention of medical men to their own lesser errors, and to the cautions that are requisite in estimating the effects of remedies." Medicine had nothing to fear from "pushing the rules of evidence to their strictest application." However, for homeopathy, it had become both an example and a warning.[44]

The second lesson learned from homeopathy was the importance of nature in the effort to remove disease. Like John Forbes before him, Hooker believed that the cures claimed by homeopathy had actually been effected by nature. This lesson had already been learned from study of the expectant mode of treatment, long popular in France and Germany. It was also obvious in the treatment of smallpox where the profession had moved away from "indiscriminate heroic medication." Hooker credited homeopathy with indirectly influencing this change in medical thinking.[45]

The third lesson Hooker noted was that regulars were still careless about the effects of their medicines and in their readiness to try any new remedy before it was fully tested. Certainly homeopaths had actively pointed this out. However, the errors of allopathic medicine did not make homeopathy valid. Finally, Hooker hoped that the history of homeopathy and other past delusions would serve as a lesson for medicine and guard it against "yielding a ready credence to those of the present day." All too often, however, medicine failed to learn this lesson, which is why the "absurd delusion" of homeopathy was so much in vogue.[46] Homeopathy, Hooker felt, attacked both the science and the profession of medicine. Although lofty in its claims, its true aim was to destroy the profession and "to substitute in its place a mere sect, bound together by an ephemeral folly, and founded by one who began his career as an open and unblushing quack."[47]

The *Philadelphia Journal of Homeopathy* rebuked Hooker for his "stale wit, sophistry, false statements, and ignorance."[48] Another rebuke came from Erastus E. Marcy (1822-1901), editor of the *North American Homeopathic Journal* for fifteen years, who published a 143-page response titled *Homeopathy and Allopathy: Reply* (1852). Marcy accused Hooker of presenting a "tissue of misrepresentations . . . and artifices" intended "to mislead the ignorant and unthinking" from homeopathy's real doctrines. Not one to mince words, he called Hooker a "pettifogging perverter of facts" and a "panderer to the hate, malice, and medical demagogueism of the more contemptible of his school." Endeavoring to injure the reputation of Hahnemann, Hooker had become little more than a "Tom Thumb challenging Lord Bacon."[49]

What particularly infuriated Marcy was Hooker's effort to discredit homeopathy through witty characterizations of the system's higher attenuations while failing to account for nature's own attenuated and imponderable substances such as miasmata, the contagious particles of smallpox, scarlet fever, measles, and typhus, as well as the invisible energy units in magnetism, electricity, light, and caloric. Since Hooker had concluded that Hahnemann's attenuations were absurd, Marcy wondered if the Connecticut seer was willing to apply the same judgment to these other imponderables. Sufficient evidence existed from observation that substances of infinitesimal size, either in nature or produced in the laboratory, could still be of considerable consequence. Notwithstanding this fact, Marcy emphasized that Hahnemann considered the question of infinitesimal doses wholly distinct from his principle of similars, alluding to the subject only in his *Organon*, in notes apart from the text.[50]

Marcy laid out ten "incontrovertible" precepts of homeopathy and urged Old School doctors to examine them carefully:

1. The conservative forces of the organism are always brought to bear against all deleterious influences acting upon the tissues. If the disturbing cause be slight, nature alone suffices to bring about a cura-

tive reaction; but when the morbific impression is so intense as to re-
sist the restorative efforts of nature, the homeopath deems it necessary to call in the aid of medicines.

2. In his remedial measures the homeopath recognizes but one law
of cure, viz., *similia similibus curantur.*

3. The only real cures ever made by drugs are accomplished in accordance with the homeopathic law, whether made by physicians of
the old or the new school—by crude drugs or by dilutions.

4. No two diseases, whether morbific or medicinal, can affect the
same structure at the same time.

5. The vital force reacts with much less power against impressions
made by morbific agents than against those caused by specific medicinal influences. Disorders . . . caused by the former, tend to run on to
the disorganization of the affected parts, while those produced by the
latter, speedily result in spontaneous recoveries.

6. Homeopathic medicines expend their entire forces upon those
parts alone which are actually diseased; and it is for this reason that
very minute doses are adequate to produce those impressions which
result in spontaneous curative reactions.

7. A medicinal action, sufficient to cure disease, may be produced
either by the tincture or by a dilution of the appropriate remedy—our
only object being to substitute a healthy drug action in the place of a
morbid one. Experience, however, has amply demonstrated, that in a
majority of instances diluted drugs act more mildly, more speedily
and more safely in provoking curative reactions, than crude medicines, the first impressions of which are more active than is absolutely necessary for curing, although not usually so active as to give
rise to serious results.

8. Drugs never lose their identity, individuality, or specific modes
of action, whatever may be the form they are made to assume. . . . It is
for this reason that homeopathists, from the time of Hahnemann to
the present day, have employed, in their provings of drugs, every variety of form and dose, and numerous experimenters of different ages,
sexes, temperaments, countries, and occupations, in order that the
most complete pathogeneses might be obtained.

9. The susceptibilities of the tissues of the organism to medicinal
impressions, are proportionate to the amount of inflammation, irritation, or nervous erethism present in each case; and as no two maladies
or groups of symptoms ever correspond precisely in all respects, it

follows that a great variety of strengths may be employed with advantage in our remedial applications.

10. In regard to doses, the homeopath has but one object in view, viz., the selection of that strength or attenuation which will most safely, mildly and speedily cure the disease. As this is purely a matter of experience and of facts, and not at all connected with the homeopathic theory of cure, its entire reasonableness must commend itself to the judgments of candid men.[51]

Marcy was both a homeopath and a gifted musician and used his skills in both to win friends and cultivate a large practice. He published much during his professional career, but his reply to Hooker was perhaps his most significant work. When homeopaths were criticized for not having sought to integrate their principles with regular medicine, Marcy explained that it was for the same reason Christians never amalgamated with Muhammadanism: they refused to mix truth with error.[52] While Hooker sneered at the administration of medicines to the healthy, Marcy was quick to explain the importance of such tests and their recognition by Robley Dunglison (1798-1869) of Jefferson Medical College, as well as by Jonathan Pereira (1804-1853). Similarly, when Hooker accused homeopaths of neglecting the study of anatomy, physiology, and pathology, Marcy offered to wager $1,000 that four or more of the city's youngest homeopaths could outmatch any four regulars chosen by Hooker, with the results of their knowledge of medicine judged by three impartial scholars. "We do not believe that a single homeopathic physician can be found . . . who does not esteem a knowledge of Anatomy, Physiology, and Pathology, not merely important, but absolutely essential to a proper appreciation and practice of his profession," countered Marcy. Once an enemy of clinical pathology, homeopathy had learned much from the findings of the Paris clinics.[53]

JAMES Y. SIMPSON

When James Y. Simpson (1811-1870) of the University of Edinburgh took on the role of homeopathy's executioner, proponents of New School reform regarded him as a "fool of a doctor," thinking himself capable of destroying their faith with a single publication.[54] When the dust cleared, however, Simpson's *Homeopathy: Its Tenets and Tendencies, Theoretical, Theological, and Therapeutical* (1853) had dealt a near-lethal blow. A professor of midwifery at the university and physician accoucheur (obstetrician) to the Queen of Scotland, Simpson posed questions and criticisms that resounded across Europe and America, forcing a rethinking of many homeopathic tenets.

Simpson was no novice in medicine. President of the Medico-Chirurgical Society, former president of the Royal College of Physicians, former president of the Royal Medical Society, and member of the Imperial Academy of Medicine of France, as well as societies in Berlin, Copenhagen, Ghent, and Stockholm, he stood first among peers in both reputation and experience.[55] Thus, when he reported that the Royal College of Physicians and the Royal College of Surgeons of Edinburgh, along with the Faculty of Physicians and Surgeons of Glasgow, the Medical Society of London, the Provincial Medical Association of England, and numerous other medical societies, had passed resolutions prohibiting their members from meeting professionally with homeopaths, his notice had a significant impact in medical circles. Although not intended to interfere with the right of British subjects to patronize homeopathic physicians, the resolutions represented the degree to which the doctrines and practices of homeopathy were perceived to differ from mainstream medicine. This, explained Simpson, was no more or less than what Hahnemann had intended when he coined the term *allopathy* and acknowledged homeopathy as the only true medical doctrine. Hahnemann's sense of exclusiveness justified the actions of medical corporations to redefine the relationship between the two schools of practitioners. In effect, the resolutions by these medical bodies had "done nothing more than carry this opinion and dictum of Hahnemann . . . into virtual effect." As such, they were no more an act of injustice than for a Christian church to deny communion to those who practiced Muhammadanism or Buddhism.[56]

Meticulously referenced, Simpson's book presented a battery of arguments, challenges, and refutations. He took homeopaths at their word, which was to introduce a new practice of medicine and a sweeping reformation over the whole of therapeutics, joining issue with Old School medicine "on every inch of its possessions."[57] Using Hahnemann's own words, Simpson proceeded to build case upon case showing the inadequacies and inconsistencies of the founder, beginning with an exposition of mathematical models for Hahnemann's higher potencies, and moving to his theories on the itch, hospital statistics, vital force, spiritual tendencies, and shakings of drugs. By the end of the book, readers were ready to judge homeopathy guilty of outright dishonesty, cleverly concealing its quackery behind religious motifs. Homeopathy, according to Simpson, sought popularity among certain highbrow segments of society, particularly the clergy, and advocated the supersensibility of diseased organs to infinitesimal doses of drugs, including scents.

But Simpson went further by directly attacking Hahnemann's universal and infallible law of similars. In studying the evidence, he could find no degree of certainty or generality, much less a universal law. In fact, the alleged law broke down under testing since measles, for example, did not remove smallpox. Nor, for that matter, did Hahnemann's "unerring unchangeable law" have any characteristics of a law at all—only a pretension asserted by its believers.[58] Although Simpson agreed that cinchona cured ague, he challenged the homeopathic assertion that cinchona produced the symptoms of ague in a healthy person. That a few healthy individuals out of the thousands who took the drug might show the symptoms of ague could not be the foundation for a universal law in therapeutics, much less a law in any other of the sciences. A universal infallible law could not admit exceptions. Simpson's analysis brought him to one conclusion: "That cinchona does not produce ague or a disease analogous to ague; and that in relation to it, the 'infallible,' 'unerring' law of *similia similibus* does not hold good."[59]

It did not take long for homeopaths to respond to Simpson's critique. William Henderson, who had earlier offered a rebuttal to John Forbes, published a reply titled *Homeopathy Fairly Represented: A Reply to Professor Simpson's "Homeopathy" Misrepresented* (1854), with the American edition coming out three weeks after the English edition. Simpson's book might comfort "the weak and wavering" and perhaps gratify the "pugnacious feelings" of those desiring the downfall of homeopathy, but Henderson thought it failed to undermine the faith of believers.[60] He had sparred with Simpson many times in the course of their professional duties, so much so that their incessant wranglings had become a fixture in conversations at Edinburgh's coffee shops and social affairs. Henderson called Simpson "the parturient professor" (Simpson was professor of midwifery) who had written his book with defective information, destructive logic, and "vain confidence." He also referred to Simpson as "Haman," referring to the chief minister of the Persian king Ahasuerus, an enemy of the Jews, who was hanged on the same gallows he had prepared for Mordecai.[61] Henderson saw himself in the role of the proverbial David, championing New School reform and "launching his deadliest home-thrusts" against the Philistine giant Goliath (allopathy) with a smile and a good-humored laugh.[62]

But this time, David was no match. In fact, Henderson could not compete with Simpson's impact on the medical world. Unable to confront Simpson's criticisms in a clear and convincing manner, Henderson skirted issues and, like Neidhard's earlier rebuttal of Holmes, left a trail of compromising statements and unanswered questions in his wake. He admitted, for example, that Hahnemann never esteemed the curative powers of homeopathy to be effective in acute diseases. And although Henderson took exception to the criticisms of homeopathy's statistical triumphs, he admitted that "occasional mistakes" had sometimes happened in the use of numbers.[63] He conceded that Joseph Dietl's (1804-1878) expectant treatment in the New Vienna School, which proved so destructive of allopathic treatment, lowered materially the favorable influence of homeopathy on acute diseases such as pneumonia. He also concurred in the assessments of Holmes and Simpson that the greater proportion of incurable organic diseases found their way to the older allopathic hospitals rather than to the newer homeopathic hospitals. Still, he maintained that the schools were noticeably different. As for a direct comparison of statistics, "Let [Simpson] beware lest he provoke . . . a commission of inquiry into matters which had better remain as private as may be: Allopathy could ill stand such an investigation."[64]

Henderson defended Hahnemann, but only to a point. What Hahnemann said about psoric maladies was simply a hypothesis derived from what he supposed to be an analogy to syphilis. This, Henderson admitted, was the weakest part of homeopathy, but he had no doubt homeopaths would eventually come to terms with it. Similarly, Henderson felt Hahnemann's conception of infinitesimals had misled him into the dynamization hypothesis, and into believing medicines that were triturated or shaken acquired an increase of potency with each successive dilution. This doctrine, explained Henderson, was "inconsistent with the results" and had led Hahnemann's disciples to numerous and embarrassing contradictions.[65] Henderson refused to subscribe to the homeopathic belief that smaller doses resulted in a greater power of medicine. Nevertheless, he did recognize circumstances in which a smaller dose had a healing effect. The relationship, therefore, between medicinal substances and the living body was "very curious, very perplexing, and very little understood." In explaining this phenomena, Henderson suggested that some medicinal substances remained "inactive" until subdivided. For example, liquid mercury could be swallowed in ounces or pounds without any negative consequences, but a small amount, well triturated, could produce "violent effects."[66]

Finally, when Simpson questioned the accuracy of Hahnemann's claim of homeopathicity between drugs and diseases, Henderson responded laconically that even if the reported instances were fallacious, "the remedial virtues of cinchona would then stand merely as an exception to the law, or as an instance of the operation of some other law." No medicine produced all of its particular effects at all times and under all circumstances, and the failure of homeopathy to cure ague by cinchona proved nothing against its homeopathic relation to ague.[67]

SUMMARY

While the four horsemen of regular medicine predicted an apocalyptic end to homeopathy, William Tod Helmuth (1833-1902), chair of surgery and dean at New York Homeopathic Medical College and Hospital, thought differently. In his address before the Western Institute of Homeopathy meeting in St. Louis in 1865, Helmuth recounted the growth of homeopathy against the ridicule of its critics, arguing that until regular medicine could demonstrate more effective cures, homeopathy would continue to win the overwhelming confidence of the American people. All the so-called fatal blows meted out by allopathy had hit wide of the mark. The time would come, Helmuth predicted, when the numbers of publications, pharmacies, hospitals, dispensaries, and colleges, along with homeopathy's many influential patrons, would overwhelm the dissenters and New School medicine would become a coequal with regulars in every particular. Until that day, he urged his fellow homeopaths to stay clear of controversy "by sedulously cultivating a liberality of spirit" among themselves and extending that same spirit to those of the Old School.[68]

Chapter 8

Diversions, Spirits,
and Other Nonessentials

By midcentury, Hahnemann's practice of physic had incorporated a number of additional reform elements, most of which had come from outside homeopathy. For advocates, these additions made homeopathy that much more relevant to the patients it served; for skeptics, they were perceived as dilutions of Hahnemann's original principles and damaging to the future of New School reform. The dilutions included the use of lay doctors who practiced idiosyncratic forms of homeopathy; homeopaths who mixed their therapeutics with religion to create a subtle form of spiritualized homeopathy; and faddists who tinkered with such fringe systems as isopathy, Baunscheidtism, hydropathy, Mesmerism, movement-cure, and Grahamism. So common had these elements become within homeopathic ranks that in an address before the New York State Homeopathic Society in 1855, Dr. George W. Perine accused fellow homeopaths of frittering away the reputation of New School reform on "non-essentials," thereby humiliating themselves and diminishing the significance of homeopathy before the world.[1]

DOMESTIC MEDICINE

As Lamar Riley Murphy explained in *Enter the Physician; The Transformation of Domestic Medicine, 1760-1860*, traditional histories have "focused on the activities of doctors to explain changes in medicine" to the exclusion of a host of other nonprofessional healers, including the domestic and lay healer. Nevertheless, domestic, lay, and professional caregivers coexisted through the eighteenth and nineteenth centuries and even into the twentieth and twenty-first centuries. Indeed, the domestic and lay spheres of medical practice had been measurably assisted by the professional doctors as part of their desire "to induct the population into a learned medical ethos in which self-help occupied an integral but newly auxiliary role."[2] During the early years of homeopathy's diaspora, several of its more loquacious advocates wrote domestic or self-treatment texts intended for parents and lay practitioners. These were not unlike self-help texts authored by regular, eclectic, botanic, hydropathic, and Thomsonian doctors during the same period and designed to educate the population on matters of disease management. Some became immensely popular, rivaling John Wesley's *Primitive Physic* (1747; first American edition, 1764) which went through thirty-eight British and twenty-four American editions; William Buchan's *Domestic Medicine; Or Family Medicine* (1769) which, by 1843, had gone through twenty-two editions and been translated into several languages; and John C. Gunn's *Domestic Medicine* (1830), which went through its hundredth edition in 1870 and eventually replaced Buchan's as the domestic medical book of choice among Americans. Among the more successful homeopathic domestic texts were those by George E. Allshorn, Martin Freligh, Alvan E. Small, Ernest A. Lutze, Constantine Hering, Egbert Guernsey, Jonathan Adams Tarbell, John Epps, George Moore, and Joseph H. Pulte. Homeopathy also moved into veterinary practice where the popular *Homeopathic Veterinary Physician* (1854) by John Rush, F. A. Guenther, and Jacob F. Sheck served as a catalyst for a host of other writers of veterinary medicine, including Karl Boehm, Thomas Moore, and William Schwabe.[3]

These early domestic books, along with accompanying boxes of medicines (Epps's fifty-four remedies; Hering's forty-six remedies; and Laurie's fifty-nine remedies) provided by pharmacists, became the unofficial missionaries for New School reform. The purchasers of a domestic book and a box of pills were reminiscent of the buyers of Samuel Thomson's *Guide to Health* (1822) who, for $20, which covered the price of the book and patent right, could practice medicine on themselves and their families. Unlike Thomsonian instruction, which approached therapeutics with a six-step regimen of puking and sweating for almost every ailment, homeopathic instruction provided a specific remedy for specific symptoms. The popularity of these domestic texts among homeopathic users, especially women, reflected Hahnemann's early substitution of symptomatology for pa-

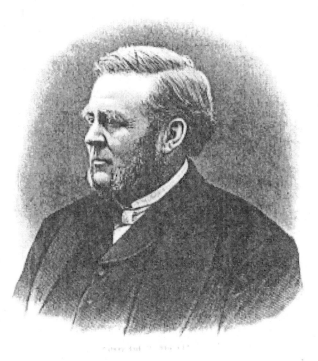

Egbert Guernsey, MD (1823-1904), author of *Homeopathic Domestic Practice*, 1856. (*Source:* Courtesy of the Lloyd Library and Museum, Cincinnati.)

thology. By refusing to countenance the existence of specific diseases and instructing followers to merely match the visible symptoms of an illness with the visible symptoms created by medicines taken in good health, Hahnemann had established a simplified therapeutic routine that amply suited the self-help rhetoric of the day. Self-help books and domestic practitioners did their best to serve families and friends in the absence or availability of licensed doctors.[4]

The first and most popular domestic homeopathic text published in the United States was Constantine Hering's *The Homeopathist, or Domestic Physician* (1835), translated from the fourth German edition. A mahogany box containing forty-six vials of medicines accompanied the text. Distributed by Jacob Behlert and J. N. Bauersachs at

260 Market Street in Philadelphia, the book sold for $2, or $5 with the box of vials.[5] Hering designed the book as a self-help guide for those living in remote areas and those who were traveling, or for self-treatment when it was too troublesome or expensive to call on a physician. The book described the most common causes of disease (affections of the mind, colds, overheating, disordered stomach, spirituous liquors, tobacco, and acids), and prescribed matching remedies. Hering urged patients with multiple complaints to note down all symptoms before deciding the proper remedy. If, for example, the reader suffered from a head cold, attended with headache and diarrhea, Hering directed the individual to investigate "colds," then "headache," and then "diarrhea," and identifying the remedy common to each of them. The book also provided directions for giving medicines, the regimen to be followed during treatment (including strict adherence to diet, clothing, baths, and physical and mental exercise), and an index referencing each of the forty-six medicines.[6]

Another popular text was Clemens Maria Franz von Bönninghausen's *Therapeutic Pocket-Book for Homeopathists; To Be Used at the Bedside of the Patient and in the Study of the Materia Medica* (1847). Like the German original, the English edition, edited by A. Howard Okie of Providence, Rhode Island, was published in a pocketbook format intended for country practitioners. Von Bönninghausen designed the book as an abridged substitute for the multivolume repertories that country practitioners found impossible to carry in their saddlebags or buggies. By providing a careful selection of the more common symptom complexes drawn from the *Materia Medica Pura* and other published works, the author made it easier for practitioners to select the proper remedy. The book was not intended to displace careful examination, but it did provide a shortened method for assessing symptoms. In effect, von Bönninghausen prejudged the value of each symptom and weighed its relative importance in the selection of remedies at the sickbed. Characteristic of von Bönninghausen's text was its reliance on the higher attenuations. "Convinced of the truth of this most important discovery [high dynamisations], I have scarcely given any other," he wrote.[7]

The American edition of Joseph Laurie's *Homeopathic Domestic Medicine* (London, 1842; American, 1843) relied heavily on information from Gottlieb H. G. Jahr's *Nouveau Manuel de Médecine Homeopathique* (1850), Franz Hartmann's *Therapie akuter Krank-*

heitsformen (1834), Samuel Hahnemann's *Materia Medica Pura,* and Constantine Hering's *The Homeopathist, or Domestic Physician.* Laurie, like von Bönninghausen, stood apart from most authors of domestic texts by recommending attenuations of the thirtieth potency and higher. Along with several other Europeans, he claimed to have obtained striking results with tinctures attenuated as high as the 1,800th power.[8] He further urged that medicines be taken while fasting; prohibited any excessive bodily or mental exertions; gave strict rules for diet when under treatment; and described the symptoms and characteristics of diseases. The text was especially popular with mothers looking for safe, gentle, and supportive treatments for infants and children. Sections addressing hygiene, clothing, organization of the sick room, and management of childhood diseases (sore throats, mumps, chicken pox, scarlet fever, etc.) made it particularly popular. Laurie's American editor and translator, A. Gerald Hull, MD (1810-1859), added his own advice to the text, suggesting that laypersons resort to the lower dilutions instead of those set down by the author for acute disease. Laurie prescribed the twenty-fourth or thirtieth attenuation of aconite, belladonna, or chamomile; Hull, on the other hand, recommended a drop or more of the tinctures mixed in a tumbler of water and given a tablespoon at a time. However, in chronic diseases, Hull agreed with the doses set forth in the text.[9]

During the cholera epidemic of 1848-1849, homeopaths claimed that Cincinnati had been spared the worst aspects of the disease due to the "skillful management" of Dr. Joseph H. Pulte, whose timely advice had enabled families to fight the early stages of the disease until a physician could be called to assist.[10] His subsequent book, *Homeopathic Domestic Physician* (1851), consisted of an explanation for the science of homeopathy; dietetic rules during treatment; specific descriptions and treatments for disease; a section on anatomy and physiology; and references on hygiene and hydropathy. Along with the text, Pulte provided a box of seventy-one medicines and four tinctures (arnica for bruises, contusions, fractures, and insect stings; calendula for lacerated wounds; ruta for chronic affections and contusions; and urtica urens for burns). Wisely, he refused to be drawn into the dispute between the high and low dilutionists except to say that all potencies were appropriate—whether a mother tincture, a first trituration, or a much higher dilution—depending on the judgment of the individual practitioner. For domestic family practice, however, he recommended the lower potencies: the third potency for vegetable medicines and the sixth for all mineral and animal medicines.[11]

Pulte considered Hahnemann the "father of scientific medicine" whose doctrines were "in beautiful harmony with all the other known laws of nature," demonstrating their practical superiority for all "self-thinking, independent minds." Compared with the physiological school of regular medicine, homeopathy represented the summum bonum of medical wisdom. Enlightened by the investigations of the microscope which had disclosed "new worlds" to the anatomist, physiologist, and pathologist, homeopaths were learning about the formative process of the cell in the living body and gaining new understanding concerning the dynamic nature of specific medication on the cell structure. In time, Pulte predicted, Old School medicine, hydropathy, and the movement-cure would unite into a single system with homeopathy at the head.[12]

Benjamin L. Hill's *An Epitome of the Homeopathic Healing Art, Containing the New Discoveries and Improvements to the Present Time; Designed for the Use of Families, for Travelers on Their Journey, and As a Pocket Companion for the Physician* (1859) was three inches by five inches in size and intended for the busy traveler. This abridged version enabled anyone with an ordinary capacity for observation to distinguish a particular complaint and ascertain its treatment. Hill, who began his career as an eclectic before turning to homeopathy, prescribed a list of twenty-seven mother tinctures, more or less dilute, in pellet or powder form, for the traveler's case; fourteen tinctures for special cholera cases; and forty-four tinctures for a full family case. The pellets and powders were placed dry on the tongue and allowed to dissolve before swallowing. Doses for an adult varied from four to seven pellets, less for children and infants.[13]

Another popular domestic text was *Family Homeopathy* (1864) written by John Ellis (1815-1896), a graduate of Berkshire Medical College in Pittsfield, Massachusetts. He later converted to homeopathy and taught at the Western Homeopathic Medical College in Cleveland before becoming professor of theory and practice at the New York Medical College for Women. To his discredit, Ellis used the book to market other works he had authored, particularly *The Avoidable Causes of Disease, Insanity, and Deformity* (1859). Even his own colleagues were embarrassed by the undignified manner in which he touted his writings. As Reuben Ludlam, co-editor of the

North American Journal of Homeopathy, explained, "We must be permitted to utter a protest against the value of such unprofessional . . . publications. Surely, it is time our literature [was] attaining something of dignity and influence."[14] In 1873, Ellis left medicine to find a new career in petroleum refining.[15]

A particularly interesting domestic text was *Robb and Company's Family Physician* (1880) which offered in plain language a trained physician's advice on the causes, symptoms, and cure of acute and chronic diseases; rules for preserving health; directions for the sick chamber; methods for preserving health and vigor; common rules in the treatment of women and children; the management of pregnancy and parturition; and observations on such areas as diet, proper clothing, and footwear. Although most other authors of domestic texts chose to account for the range of treatments within a single medical theory, *Robb and Company's Family Physician* gave patients the option of choosing among the different regimens of allopathy, hydropathy, and homeopathy.[16]

In all, more than thirty homeopathic domestic texts, along with scores of smaller monographs, were written for the American market and reflect the breadth of homeopathic popularity within the popular culture.[17] Parents were the most common purchasers of these books, buying them along with an accompanying box of medicines from a local pharmacy. The Cincinnati Homeopathic Pharmacy on 21st West Fourth Street was typical of stores that offered homeopathic tinctures, triturations, globules, pocket and family medicine cases, vials, sugar of milk, fresh cowpox virus, and books for domestic use.[18] Family medicine chests came in hard wood or leather, and cost from $2 to $10, depending on the number of vials included. The chests carried from fifteen to forty-five half-ounce or one-ounce vials of tinctures, dilutions, triturations, and medicated globules. Domestic texts and their medicine cases became the nucleus of a family's medical care.[19] William Radde, general agent for the Central Homeopathic Pharmacy of Leipzig, sold medicines in sets or by single vials of tinctures, dilutions and triturations; leather pocket cases that included a family guide and twenty-seven remedies; physician cases containing fifty to 400 vials of mother tinctures and triturations; isopathic remedies; refined sugar of milk; pure globules; and homeopathic chocolate.[20]

There is little doubt that domestic texts contributed to the popularity of homeopathy, attracting patients to the offices of their authors as

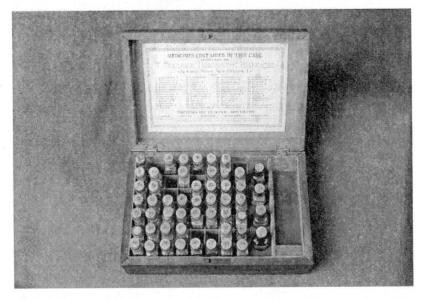

Homeopathic medicine chest from New Orleans. (*Source:* Photo courtesy of the Alabama Museum of the Health Sciences, Lister Hill Library, University of Alabama at Birmingham.)

well as to other practitioners. For that reason, most homeopaths were reluctant to publicly denigrate them. H. C. Allen, MD, for example, urged fellow homeopaths to disseminate their doctrines in every appropriate and justifiable manner. "If it is right for me to practice homeopathy," he explained, "it is my bounden duty to propagate its principles and further its advancement in every honorable manner."[21]

By midcentury, however, homeopathy's more academically trained physicians were in no mood to encourage the continued use of domestic texts. There were so many in circulation, complained one critic, that "their number has well nigh put a stop on the sale of 'shoe paper.'"[22] Another remarked that he hoped the utility of domestic treatises would soon end. These books, with their accompanying cases of medicine, had been "productive of vastly more injury than good," and it was time they be "discountenanced and discontinued." The use of pellets or globules in an attempt to popularize domestic homeopathy had degraded the true interests of the system. Physicians should encourage the publication of books for the professional rather than for the public. Otherwise, homeopathy should be listed among the purveyors of quackery.[23]

Part of the problem was that domestic text authors tended to steal from one another to fill their pages. According to critic J. W. Metcalf in the *North American Journal of Homeopathy,* Pulte had compiled his *Homeopathic Domestic Physician* (1850) a page at a time, cutting and pasting from the works of Christoph Wilhelm Hufeland and Henoch Schönlein. Offering readers a look at parallel columns of text that were strikingly similar in language and content, Metcalf thought it "sadly ridiculous" that Pulte would claim authorship of a work that was clearly not his. He accused Pulte of plagiarizing whole sections of Laurie's *Domestic Medicine* and Jahr's *Manual,* as well as Marcy's *Theory and Practice* (1850), Hering's *Domestic Physician* (1835), and Calvin Cutter's *Treatise on Anatomy, Physiology and Hygiene: Designed for Colleges, Academies and Families* (1850). About the only thing not stolen was Pulte's index, which was the work of his publisher. Metcalf concluded, "for the sake of Homeopathy, we regret that such a book should have ever seen the light."[24]

In writing about domestic texts, William H. Holcombe, MD, admitted that in numerous instances authors had actually supported antipathic, not homeopathic, treatment. For example, both Hering and Guernsey had recommended nauseating doses of tartar emetic, and Hering's recommendation of copaiba to the soles of the feet for gonorrhea was hardly a homeopathic recipe. Hering also resorted to using such terms as *vile trash, abominable medicines,* and *absolute poisons* to depict rival allopathic systems.[25]

Given the collapse of Thomsonism, the waning of Jacksonian fever, the growth of proprietary schools, and the more advanced state of medical science in the second half the nineteenth century, critics of domestic texts concluded that the writing of such works had become much more challenging, if not outright obsolete. This explains, in part, the mixed review given to the *Manual of Homeopathic Theory and Practice, with an Elementary Treatise on the Homeopathic Treatment of Surgical Diseases; Designed for Students, and Practitioners of Medicine, and As a Guide for Families, and an Intelligent Public Generally* (1858) written by Charles J. Hempel and Jacob Beakley. "We have had these domestic treatises used *ad nauseam,*" wrote reviewer J. R. Coxe Jr., of Philadelphia, and this particular volume was no exception in that it was written to serve the needs of practitioners, students, families, and the general public. The book's short-comings stemmed from the authors' attempt to serve too many different readers, each of whom had a different level of understanding.[26] Another reviewer, Edward P. Fowler, took a harsher view, concluding that the authors had no business teaching homeopathy, much less practicing it.[27]

In the late 1860s, the Cook County Medical Society in Illinois publicly rejected domestic texts, calling them detrimental to public health. The society objected to the books as a means of popularizing the practice of homeopathy, and condemned their accompanying medicine cases as "utterly worthless." Although once useful, they were now "superfluous."[28] Notwithstanding the society's official stance, before domestic texts moved to the backwaters of homeopathic practice, they served as midwife to a host of fads that grafted themselves to New School reform.

LAY DOCTORS

Parents may have been the intended audience for domestic texts, but they were not alone. Armed with a book, a box of medicines, good observation skills, and a keen intuition, so-called lay doctors (doctors de gratia) enjoyed favorable patronage among family, church, friends, and neighbors. Abraham Howard Okie considered them as important in homeopathy's struggle for recognition as the writings of German nobleman and humanist Ulrich von Hutten (1488-1523) had been in the defense of Lutheranism. "What would have become of the Reformation had not the laity taken part in it?" Okie asked rhetorically. Had the laity allowed theological controversies to be settled by theologians alone, Martin Luther and other church critics would have ended their days at the stake and the Reformation would have been a distant memory, nothing more.[29]

In some states, because of restrictive legislation, lay doctors had to dispense their medicines gratuitously and rely on the generosity of patients rather than the law to collect their fees. Nevertheless, the popularity of domestic texts and lay practitioners reflected the effects of democratization in medical licensing during the first half of the nineteenth century. With all manner of opposition to monopoly, elitism, orthodox intolerance, and restraint of trade, states repealed their regulatory laws on medical licensing. By the end of the 1840s, only

New Jersey, Louisiana, Michigan, and the District of Columbia retained any semblance of licensing control.[30]

Among lay doctors were many ministers who, caught between competing spiritual and physical functions, devoted their weekdays to the task of healing earthly bodies and their Sundays to saving souls. When the Reverend Dr. William Hunter was accused in 1855 of neglecting his ministerial duties by engaging in the practice of medicine, he denied the charge, explaining that he had done nothing more than follow in the footsteps of Methodism's founder, John Wesley (1703-1791). In an address before the Western Virginia Conference, Hunter explained that he had turned to homeopathy when living in Pittsburgh, Pennsylvania, before he became a Methodist preacher. When he moved to West Virginia to begin work as a minister, he soon found his medical expertise much needed in the region. Word of his success traveled quickly, and before long he was ministering to numerous families along his circuit. When regulars complained of his practice, Hunter referred them to scripture (Matthew 4:23; Mark 3:14; Luke 9:2), Wesley's *Journals* (5:187; 6:644, 689), and the preface to Wesley's *Primitive Physic* (1747). Hunter explained that he was performing work peculiar to the very character, office, and work of a Methodist minister and that he had done so without abusing his other duties. As it turned out, the conference "winked" at his alleged offenses and refused to censure him.[31]

In Maryland during the 1870s, at least nine Episcopal ministers practiced homeopathy on their congregations.[32] Other reverend doctors included W. A. Belding (Disciples of Christ), A. B. Palmer (Methodist), and John Ellis (New Church or Swedenborgian) in New York; Lancelot Younghusband (Baptist) and J. Y. Basset (Baptist) in Michigan; and William H. Holcombe (Swedenborgian) in Louisiana.[33] Ocasional itinerant minister-practitioners rented theaters and advertised sermons that they preached on Sabbath evenings, charging five cents per ticket to defray expenses. During the sermons, they would wander the fields of homeopathic medical theory and practice, using religious metaphors to cement homeopathy with Christianity, and referring curious or ailing listeners to their lodgings for further consultation. Not unexpectedly, Hahnemann's *Organon* became identified as the "bible" of homeopathy and, in this manner, many reverend healers maintained a comfortable livelihood.[34]

CHRISTIANITY AND SWEDENBORGIANISM

In the 1850s, James Y. Simpson (1811-1870), professor of midwifery at Edinburgh, noted a curious tendency among homeopaths to find their identity within a liberal Christian context. Not only did they describe themselves as converts from orthodox medicine but many—both academically trained and lay—were all too willing to combine Hahnemann's therapeutic principles with philosophical and religious theories to stress the unique spiritual forces in the healing process. Since homeopaths were already versed in refuting mechanistic and materialistic trends in eighteenth- and early nineteenth-century medicine, they converted to Christian perfectionism, sentimentalism, the emphasis on intuitive knowledge, the stirrings of the metaphysical imagination, and even strands of feminism. For many, homeopathy became a spiritual ministry touting a strong correlation with Hahnemann's natural laws and liberal theology's mood of optimism and perfectionist state of mind. Explained the English preacher Thomas R. Everest (1801-1855),

> When the old system [allopathy] shall have quite vanished from the earth, and the new one [homeopathy] shall be established, then will the Gospel of the kingdom of grace be preached as Jesus ordered it to be preached, and received as God intended it to be received.

To demonstrate the connection between the physical and spiritual orders of reality, Everest, who was treated by Hahnemann during the latter's years in Paris, established a homeopathic boardinghouse for young ladies in his parish at Wickwar where he taught that cleanliness, small doses of medicine, and good hygiene were the nearest thing to Godliness.[35]

One reason for the close affinity of homeopathy with Christianity stemmed from the direct relationship between symptomatology (including states of mind) and homeopathic provings. Homeopathic drugs were used to cure both bodily afflictions as well as certain moral and religious weaknesses. For example, Jahr's *Manual of Homeopathic Medicine* reported the feeling of "despair of eternal salvation" from the use of sulphur on the healthy body; a "despair of eternal happiness" with pulsatilla; the "absence of religious feeling" with lachesis; and an "irresistible desire to blaspheme and swear" with aconite. By applying these same medicines to patients harboring such tendencies, the homeopathist sought to cure them of these morally offensive feelings.[36]

For others, the basic doctrines of Hahnemann were nothing less than articles of faith. This meant ignoring the controversy over infinitesimals; emphasizing the spiritual (high dilution) aspects of homeopathy; and associating healing with evidence of divine purpose. It also meant recognizing medicine as a belief system rather than as a science; opposing strenuously the scientizing of medicine; suggesting a struggle of vitalism against materialism; preferring the use of religious metaphors to describe the healing processes; and stressing the simplicity of symptomatology and the power of each individual to become the instrument of his or her cure. In his *A Practical Appeal to the Public, Through a Series of Letters, in Defense of the New System of Physic by the Illustrious Hahnemann* (1833), John Gilchrist used such sobriquets as "Gospel of Medical Redemption" to describe Hahnemann's *Organon* and likened homeopathic dilutions to "the true Balm of Gilead."[37]

Among an inordinate number of sectarians, particularly those favoring the eclectic and homeopathic schools of thought, efforts to reconcile the competing interests of science and religion turned them first to the fluid forces in mesmerism, then to the discoveries of Franz Joseph Gall and the science of phrenology. This was soon replaced with the more speculative and esoteric sciences of *psychometry* (the influence of clairvoyance on the cerebral tissues of sensitive individuals) and *sarcognomy* (the correlation of soul, brain, and body to affect health and disease) founded by Joseph Rodes Buchanan (1814-1899), dean of the Eclectic Medical College of Cincinnati. From there, sectarians moved to the alluring world of Emanuel Swedenborg (1688-1772), a scientist and mystic whose interests included magnetic vision, clairvoyance, spirit seeing, and communications with spiritual essences above man. Those who were drawn to Swedenborg found a mind that was at home in both the spiritual and natural worlds, able to bridge them through the universality of God's providence.[38]

The relationship between homeopathy and the metaphysical thinking of Swedenborg was of particular interest to Professor Charles A. Lee who, writing in the *New Church Messenger* in 1854, expressed surprise that so many of the followers of Swedenborg were disciples of Hahnemann.[39] Edwin A. Lodge, general editor of the *American Homeopathic Observer,* asked: "Why are so many homeopathic physicians Swedenborgians? Who will tell us?" Since New Church (the popular name given to the Swedenborgian Church founded in 1784) thinking, like New School reform, appealed to many like-minded people searching for spiritual as well as physical uplifting, perhaps it was no accident that New Church and New School adherents were alike in their devotion to nature and optimistic in their meliorist and perfectionist tendencies. In reply to Lodge's inquiry, one respondent protested, arguing that a medical journal was not the appropriate medium to answer a religious question. Nevertheless, he went on to explain that all physicians should seek truth for its own sake, and since every truth should harmonize with all other truths, it followed that "theological truth must harmonize with scientific truth." To be true, theology must rest upon science, meaning that it should be confirmed by both reason and scripture. The facts of homeopathy, the respondent explained, were fully consistent with the spiritual and scientific writings of Swedenborg. For Swedenborgians, the word of God, which originally came to man through the prophets and the medium of the Old Testament, then again in the New Testament, came later through *correspondence,* Swedenborg's term used to describe the form of communication that bridged the natural and spiritual planes of reality. Swedenborg introduced this method of scriptural interpretation for mankind to discover, "somewhat as the angels do," the inner harmony and meaning of the Word. Here was the metaphysical imagination at its highest efficiency, guiding wisdom and energy to achieve both a spiritual and physical composure.[40]

To no great surprise, lay homeopaths sometimes chose the technique of clairvoyance to correlate symptoms and treatment, viewing New School reform as derivative of the theories set forth by Swedenborg.[41] Hahnemann's interest in vitalism, dynamization, and the theory of chronic diseases suggested a closer relationship between New School and New Church reform. Swedenborg's early works on matter and motion, along with his general conception of three planes of existence (the Divine, the Spiritual, and the Natural) had sufficient affinity with homeopathic physics and cosmology to provide the appearance of a genuine relationship. Moreover, Swedenborg's understanding of the soul as geometrical, mechanical, and finite blended as well with Hahnemann's concept of dynamization brought about by shaking, attenuation, and magnetization. Prominent American and English homeopaths who were Swedenborgians included John Ellis, Ernst A. Farrington, Hans Gram, Charles Hempel, Constantine Hering, William H. Holcombe, James T. Kent, William Wesselhoeft, and Garth Wilkinson. Wilkinson, an English physician and mystic, translated the works of Swedenborg in the 1840s, just prior to his conversion to New School medicine. Offended by the arrogance of the sciences, and especially of Old School medicine, he sought comfort in homeopathy, temperance, spiritualism, Fourierism, medical botany, and most importantly Swedenborgianism.[42]

Although many homeopaths chose to combine Hahnemann's principle of dynamization with Swedenborg's theory of correspondence, both Eduard von Grauvogl and Charles J. Hempel instead replaced Hahnemann's principle with what they believed was Swedenborg's more satisfactory explanation. "The day is fast approaching," Hempel predicted, "when the homeopathic profession will bow to Swedenborg as the great expounder of the philosophy of homeopathy." An active member of the Swedenborgian Church, Hempel drew from Swedenborg to explain the *harmonic* and *subversive* forces that operated within the body. Having characterized Hahnemann's theory as "vague, incomplete, and even erroneous," he suggested that the action of harmonic forces on matter produced substances that helped to support the healthy organism, while the action of subversive forces produced substances that restored the organism to its original condition of health after being disturbed.[43] Both were united in an indivisible bond and each endeavored to adapt the animal organism to its own particular nature. Disease represented the totality of the effects of subversive forces upon an organism. For example, the itch vesicle, the chancre, and the cauliflower excrescence were visible embodiments of internally active subversive forces and indicated "the degree of adaptation existing between the subversive forces and the organ."[44] Rather than use Old School measures to excite the contents or secretions of an organ, Hempel explained that the homeopathic physician chose a particular medicinal substance which, when raised to a spiritualized condition through trituration, embodied the "essence or spirit" of the subversive forces. When spiritualized, the subversive forces "converged" with the drug, and after a process of "materialization," left the organism. The challenge was in discovering the full range of homeopathic influence over the subversive forces in the organism.[45]

Among his many writings, Hempel sought to demonstrate how Swedenborgianism and the utopian socialist Charles Fourier constituted a union of science and religion such that Fourier's work unit, better known as a *Phalanx,* represented the practical expression of New Church theories. The Phalanx was the "tabernacle" in which all souls found a "holy and useful life" by transforming the "sublimest type of Christian Love" into living reality.[46]

William Holcombe of Natchez (and later New Orleans) was a Swedenborgian whose books *Our Children in Heaven* (1875) and *The Other Life* (1871) were intended to help parents adjust to the deaths of their children. Having lost two of his own by scarlet fever, and having fought for the Confederacy where he witnessed the deaths of numerous comrades, Holcombe reassured parents that their deceased sons and daughters were being cared for on the "other side." For Holcombe, the greatest manifestation of the human intellect was the emancipation of private judgment from the despotism of Church orthodoxy. Through the dissenting element that grew out of the Protestant Reformation and the compelling work of Swedenborg in illuminating rational understanding of the spiritual world, Holcomb explained the mystery of death, the universality of man, and the indestructible spiritual substances in which the soul lives.[47] Holcombe based his beliefs on Swedenborg's *True Christian Religion* (1853) and the idea that the Second Coming of Christ had already taken place.[48]

Holcombe also wrote *The Scientific Basis of Homeopathy* (1852) which welcomed New School reformers to the inner connections between the physical and spiritual realms. However, William A. Gardiner, editor of the *Philadelphia Journal of Homeopathy* (who was drawn to the less mystical side of homeopathy), pointed out that Holcombe's books were too obscure in their devotion to the sources of the soul's vitality and hoped he would eventually embrace the more advanced material side of homeopathic medicine.[49]

Other signs marked the affinity between homeopathy and Swedenborgianism. As an example, the publishers of the *American Homeopathic Observer* offered their journal at a discount if combined with a subscription to *The New Church Independent and Monthly Review,* edited by John S. Weller and published in LaPorte, Indiana.[50] Franz

E. Boericke and Adolph J. Tafel of Philadelphia, who began as homeopathic pharmacists in 1835, became one of the largest manufacturers of homeopathic remedies and food supplements as well as publishers of homeopathic and Swedenborgian books.[51]

In the latter decades of the nineteenth century, and leading into World War I, the ideas of Swedenborgian James Tyler Kent (1849-1916) formed a significant underpinning to what is today called "classical homeopathy." Kent matriculated at the Eclectic Medical Institute (EMI) of Cincinnati where, before graduating in 1870, he came under the influence of John M. Scudder (1829-1894), owner and manager of the school from 1862 to 1894. Scudder had authored numerous medical texts including *Specific Medication and Specific Medicines* (1870) and *Specific Diagnosis* (1874) which emphasized the importance of simplicity in prescribing therapeutic agents singly or in comparatively simple combinations. Like homeopaths, Scudder believed that a fixed relationship existed between the drug force and disease expression and recommended the use of a simple medication as a direct remedy for a specific pathological condition. Although he refused to recognize Hahnemann's "law" of cure, he did subscribe to symptomatic expression, or specific medication for specific conditions. Elements of Scudder's ideas could be found in the earlier writings of Charles J. Hempel and Gottlieb M. W. Ludwig Rau, but he diverged from homeopathic antecedents when he called his method *specific medication,* meaning "certain well-determined deviations from the healthy state will always be corrected by specific medications."[52] It is reasonable to conclude that Scudder's own Swedenborgian beliefs, as well as the New Church affiliations of other EMI faculty, influenced Kent's formative years. Later, Kent would delve into the metaphysical aspects of Hahnemann's writings to discover connections between Swedenborg and the ultrahigh potencies of homeopathy. Kent constructed a Swedenborgian foundation to Hahnemann's vitalistic principles by stressing the correlation between the principles of miasm and vitalism; rejecting modern scientific and pathological knowledge as a source or guide to diagnosis; emphasizing psychological (i.e., constitutional) symptoms in prescribing medicines; and prescribing only the higher potencies.[53] Thus, while mainstream homeopaths became increasingly linked to clinical laboratory science for pathology and diagnostic decision making, Kent and his followers roamed the fields of mental healing, the different

"states" of matter, the correspondence between disease and man's affections, and the vital force of the soul.[54]

Notwithstanding the fact that the majority of homeopaths in the United States were low-potency advocates, the mind-cure healing groups and therapies that flourished at the turn of the century gave added credence to homeopathy's high-potency purists. Loosely federated, these New Thought and metaphysical cults (Christian Science, Immanuel Movement, Swedenborgianism, etc.) shared common notions with homeopathy, including the power of mind over matter, an emphasis on vital force, a fascination with mental healing, and holistic therapies. The human body, which served as a temporary shelter for the soul, had a connection to the greater spiritual world that differentiated man from the rest of organic creation. Homeopathy's embracing of medicine's vitalistic traditions made it an attractive partner to Swedenborgianism and its transcendent view of the spiritual world.

One cannot read Kent's *The Art and Science of Homeopathic Medicine* (1900) without appreciating his strong and effective communication skills, reminiscent of Andrew Weil, the spokesman for the integration of Western medicine with the various mind/body aspects of alternative medical systems. For Hahnemannians, Kent's book constitutes much of what is present-day lay homeopathy. For historians of medicine, however, it fits into a broader context of philosophical works best represented in the writings of Hans Dreisch (1867-1941), Henry Louis Bergson (1859-1941), and J. Arthur Thomson (1861-1933) who advocated a form of "neo-vitalism" in opposition to the French materialism of the previous century.

FADS

Isopathy

Johann Joseph Wilhelm Lux (1773-1849), a veterinary surgeon in Leipzig who adopted homeopathy in 1820, grew increasingly disappointed with the early results of his newfound system and decided to counteract contagious diseases in animals with dilutions (up to the thirtieth potency) of body secretions contaminated with the same disease. Instead of the principle of *similia similibus curantur,* Lux chose *Æqualia Æqualibus curantur,* or *iidem iisdem curanture,* meaning the application of substances of the same nature and degree, not just similar, to the symptom complex. Although Hahnemann raised concerns with the practice, fearing that it had not been proven conclusively, numerous homeopaths were willing to test the method. Isopathy gained added meaning in 1848 when advocates announced that animal secretions possessed curative properties when applied to diseases of corresponding organs, i.e., a tincture made from the liver of the fox (hepatin) for diseases of the liver.[55]

Robert E. Dudgeon's *Lectures on the Theory and Practice of Homeopathy* (1854) took particular aim at isopathy, identifying it as a heresy that had originated in antiquity. It was strikingly similar to the doctrine of *signatures* that, for many nineteenth-century observers, had been a precursor to homeopathy. John Geary of the *Philadelphia Journal of Homeopathy* accused Constantine Hering of having introduced isopathic heresies into the homeopathic school when he proposed using *nosodes*, extracts from secretions taken during the course of a specific disease that were attenuated and used to cure the same disease in another patient. For example, Hering introduced lysin, prepared from the saliva of a mad dog, to treat hydrophobia, and recommended the watery excrements of cholera, the black vomit of yellow fever, and skin scrapings during malignant scarlet fever as proper homeopathic remedies. He also advocated the potentized fluids and solids of crushed insects to cure individuals of their bites.[56]

In 1852, the French Academy of Medicine condemned the work of doctors William Boeck and Casimiro Sperino, who had treated syphilis patients with attenuated amounts of syphilitic virus.[57] In 1867 the Michigan Institute of Homeopathy refused to countenance or approve isopathic remedies.[58] Regardless of official disdain, isopathy in various forms continued to find favor among lay practitioners well into the late nineteenth and twentieth centuries.

Vaccination

Although regulars considered cowpox vaccination the appropriate prophylactic against smallpox, for homeopaths, the implications were not so clear. "Could vaccination protect us from the small-pox otherwise than homeopathically?" asked Hahnemann rhetorically in his *Organon*. While Hahnemann was impressed with the "homeopathicity" of cowpox vaccination and believed that vaccinating an otherwise healthy individual by exciting an analogous disease proved efficacious in destroying smallpox on first appearance, others were not so inclined.[59] Reports in homeopathic journals recounted instances in which vaccination introduced other diseases along with it, including croup, diphtheria, pulmonary and mesenteric phthisis, typhoid fever, and even syphilis. Many of the reported cases came from arm-to-arm vaccination.[60] Some high dilutionists attributed gonorrhea and all of its consequences to vaccination. Assuming smallpox to be identical with gonorrhea, they concluded that cowpox was nothing but gonorrhea passed through a cow. These same critics also argued that syphilis and gonorrhea were associated diseases, the treatment of which called for a single globule of thuja—30, 300, or 1,000 tituration, according to the intensity of the disease.[61]

Convinced that doctors were inoculating innocent victims with "diseases and constitutional taints far worse and more permanent than small-pox," under the delusion of protecting the patient from an infection "to which nine-tenths of our patients will never be exposed," Henry C. Preston condemned vaccination as the "wholesale propagation of a filthy and destructive poison." In its present use, the virus passed not directly from the pure disease in the cow but through thousands of "vitiated constitutions" that were "charged with psoric and syphilitic miasm." Rather than use an unpotentized vaccine, Preston recommended the internal administration of the triturated virus known as vaccinin to deliver the prophylactic.[62] Pure vaccinin, dynamized by trituration, could be administered internally with specific prophylactic and dynamic effects.[63]

Preston's assumptions were not widely accepted by other homeopaths. In an article written in 1852 in the *Philadelphia Journal of Homeopathy*, Dr. J. Bryant warned doctors not to regard vaccination as an uncertain prophylactic or as an unnecessary and dangerous practice. Vaccination was an important prophylactic whose effects were real and long lasting. Bryant opposed vaccinin as a substitute for vaccination: "I do not believe that it can ever supersede the necessity of vaccination," he wrote, because like other medicines taken internally "its effects are transitory, and individuals will be protected by it no longer than they are under the influence of a recently-administered dose."[64]

Most mainstream homeopaths took issue with the eccentricities and practices of the antivaccinationists. "We lack words and energy sufficient to express our mortification that such theories and practice . . . have found a footing in our ranks," wrote the editor of the *North*

American Journal of Homeopathy in 1860.[65] The rational school of homeopaths, represented by P. W. L. Griesselich, Carl F. G. Trinks, and Alphonse Noack in Vienna; Johann Wilhelm Arnold, Daniel Roth, Jean-Paul Tessier in France; and William Henderson, John C. Peters, and William Holcombe in England and America, pointed to statistical evidence of the effectiveness of vaccination.[66] Indeed, health officer and homeopath Tullio S. Verdi, MD, of the District of Columbia found the benefits of vaccination clear and unmistakable. With so much written on the subject, he preferred to demonstrate with statistics taken by the city's board of health. More than 70,000 persons had been vaccinated against smallpox in the District of Columbia in 1872; and of the 925 reported cases of smallpox, 532, or 58 percent, had not been vaccinated. The mortality rate of this group was 209, or nearly 40 percent. Of those who had been vaccinated but who contracted the disease, the mortality rate was only 20 percent.[67]

By the 1870s, vaccination had become the cordon sanitaire between the more ideological high dilutionists and the eclectic or liberal wing of homeopathy. Those high dilutionists who rejected the practice considered it a crude procedure and vaccinated their patients only under protest, believing that the vaccine virus aroused "latent psoric or scrofulous taints" in the body, leading to a state of "vaccinosis," an impairment resulting in chronic disease. Their antipathy to the procedure continued into the twentieth century in the form of vitriolic statements and political action groups designed to halt the practice once and for all.[68]

Baunscheidtism

Lay homeopaths also rallied to the use of Baunscheidtism in the 1850s and 1860s. The treatment, known variously as the pyonex, or dermapathic regimen, originated from the invention in the 1840s of the vitalizer or resuscitator *(Lebenswecker)* by Carl Baunscheidt (1809-1873), a mechanic from Endenich, Germany, who studied medicine briefly before turning to invention. Popular in northern Germany and Prussia, the resuscitator was also fashionable in the German communities of Ohio, Pennsylvania, Missouri, and Illinois, and was copied by American imitators John Linden of Cleveland and Joseph Firmenich and L. Dodge of Buffalo. The device, which varied only slightly from one manufacturer to another, had all the properties of a medieval torture instrument. It consisted of a hammerlike handle attached by a spring to a circular piece of metal containing thirty or more gold-plated needles. When released, the spring drove the needles into the patient's skin. An irritative oil called oleum baunscheidtii (prussic acid), croton oil, or tartar emetic salve was then painted over the prick marks to produce an eruption. Within hours, the area of the rash became pustular and inflamed.[69]

Basic to this exanthematic method of cure was the belief that disease resulted from impure fluids retained too long in the system and subsequently deposited in various organs, corrupting the blood, and causing fever and pain. Although the body had its own built-in mechanisms to protect against the accumulation of harmful toxins, Baunscheidt users felt that the counterirritant and derivative powers of the artificially induced rash would hasten the body's natural healing power. Just as the healthy body eliminated toxins by means of exhalations from the lungs and the actions of the bowels, skin, and kidneys, so the resuscitator assisted in the elimination of toxins through an artificial eruption of the skin. The method corresponded to the use of blisters and setons placed on the skin to encourage pustular eruptions. By continuing the treatment over time, a physician could produce an ulcer and keep it open with the use of bread poultices and lint compresses. The ulcer then acted as a "vent" for the internal malady.[70]

Baunscheidtism differed from cupping, tartar emetic salve, Spanish-fly plasters, fomentations, and setons by promising to be less painful and messy and involving little nursing, yet achieving similar results. Like venesection or arteriotomy, which reduced the force of the blood on the diseased part by diminishing the general circulation, the counterirritative properties of Baunscheidtism created an artificial or secondary disease on the body's surface which drew the analogous internal action to the spot on the skin where it could be localized and treated more directly. It also caused a derivation or "local hyperemia" which brought more blood to the surface to relieve congestion at the diseased part.[71] Although contrary to Hahnemann's principle of *similia,* lay homeopaths used the device to treat diphtheria, pneumonia, and typhoid, explaining that its actions were "almost magical in restoring immediate warmth and circulation." The use and popularity of Baunscheidtism suggests that lay doctors carried in their medical handbags an assortment of conflicting regimens to treat patients.[72]

Grahamites

Food, drink, sleep, air, exercise, clothing, and occupation were all factors that homeopaths considered in their regimen for preserving health. On diet, they relied heavily on William Beaumont's *Experiments and Observations on the Gastric Juice and the Physiology of Digestion* (1833), on Justus von Leibig's *Chemistry in Its Application to Agriculture and Physiology* (1842), and on John A. Tarbell's *Sources of Health and the Prevention of Disease or, Mental and Physical Hygiene* (1850). The quality of air was equally important, i.e., the more air available to patients, the sooner they recovered. Homeopathy's only caution concerned drafts and damp evening air. Exercise was essential since it stimulated the appetite, invigorated the nerves, and gave vigor to the blood. Without it, the functions became torpid and sluggish. In choosing clothing, homeopaths recommended utility over "fancifulness" by urging the use of cotton, linen, and wool, according to the season, and the avoidance of tight waists, corsets, and poorly fitted shoes.[73] In general homeopaths identified several important rules for good health: rising early and dressing appropriately; washing the entire body daily; never sleeping in a warm room; avoiding damp clothes, sharp winds, and the damp evening air; eating meals at regular hours; and avoiding indigestible foods and stimulating drinks.[74]

Not surprisingly, America's academic homeopaths showed more than casual interest in the dietary preferences of food reformers, but on balance were unimpressed with their more visionary promises and platitudes. Lay homeopaths, on the other hand, fell in quickly with evangelical minister, lecturer, health reformer, and general agent of the Pennsylvania Temperance Society, Sylvester Graham (1794-1851), who challenged the American preference for hot breads and fried foods by urging temperance in eating, drinking, and other voluntary habits, including sex. A leader in the health movement, he recommended the use of whole, unbolted, and coarsely ground wheat as the most appropriate food staple for the new generation of Americans.[75]

By the 1830s, the eating and living preferences of the Grahamites, including those in Graham-based boarding houses in the Northeast, had acquired political agendas, most notably abolitionism and temperance. Graham also influenced other medical sectarians. There were efforts to build a coalition of Grahamites among the followers of botanic Samuel Thomson. The beliefs of the Grahamites were cited so frequently in Thomsonian magazines, and particularly among "New Light" or Independent Thomsonians such as Alva Curtis (1797-1881) of Cincinnati, that some advocated the alliance of Thomson's vegetable medicines with the vegetable diet of the Grahamites, creating a reform movement known as *Thomsonian Grahamism.* The effort, although fervent, never fully materialized since most Thomsonians refused to dilute their medical system with the politics and food habits of the more liberal vegetarians. A similar attitude prevailed among homeopaths. "I have met with a good many of these priests of starvation," recalled I. G. Rosenstein of Louisville. "Beans, roots, potatoes, and bran bread, is all they want." He preferred not to dictate diet. "In a country like ours, where every one is . . . his own judge in politics and religion," it was far better to preach nature's natural appetites and to refrain from unnatural desires and the detrimental consequences of intemperate appetites.[76]

Movement-Cure

Lay homeopaths and authors of domestic texts gave enthusiastic endorsement to the so-called movement-cure, practiced in Sweden and other European countries. This reform embraced gymnastics and the application of specific exercises to stimulate the healthy functioning of the body's organs. Along with diet and hygiene, it became a regular part of homeopathic literature.[77] The movement-cure was attributed to Peter Henry Ling (1766-1839) who, while studying fencing in Stockholm, Sweden, came to the conclusion that however valuable fencing was as an exercise, it could not accomplish the full and harmonious development of the body. Aiming at the reformation of health, strength, and beauty, he set out in 1805 to teach both fencing and gymnastic exercises. He studied anatomy, physiology, and the other natural sciences, viewing them as essential to the fullest development of human corporeal and mental nature. He sought to make gymnastics not only a branch of education for healthy individuals but also a remedy for disease.[78] To do this, he identified twenty-one different laws of physical development. Before long, his gymnastics were introduced into Sweden's military academies, town schools, colleges, universities, and orphan institutions.[79]

Although not intending to shake a patient's faith in "wise, prudent, conscientious, and learned physicians," movement-cure advocates such as George H. Taylor of New York City valued physical training far more than reliance on a doctor's skill. Taylor felt that individuals, properly taught, could take greater responsibility for their health, efficiency, and happiness.[80] Unfortunately, the medical profession and its science offered little besides dispensing old-style medication. Medicine's scope was too narrow to supply the pressing wants of society, and its therapeutic regimens had all but exhausted the vital energies of the body. As a specialty of medical practice, however, the movement-cure offered a physiological method to accomplish medicine's purposes. Taylor considered it "a means of enabling the natural tendencies of the system . . . to act more powerfully and effectually."[81] The moral and intellectual natures of man were capable of development, but physical training came first, fitting individuals for their destiny as intellectual beings.[82]

Hydropathy

The medicinal use of cold showers, wet sheets, compresses, douches, and other water techniques had many advocates over the centuries, but the disciples of Vincenz Priessnitz (1799-1851), a Silesian farmer, transformed the various techniques into a well-organized lay movement known as *hydropathy* in the first half of the nineteenth century. Founded on principles of humoral pathology and designed to remove offending fluids from the body, hydropathy quickly caught the attention of New School reformers. The *American Magazine* supported the legal rights of both homeopaths and hydropaths to practice, and claimed responsibility for officially encouraging a closer relationship between the two systems. In particular, the magazine encouraged a stronger relationship between hydropathy and the American Institute of Homeopathy, which formed in 1843.

Both academic and lay homeopaths viewed the systematic use of cold water internally and externally as a complementary, albeit auxiliary, branch of medicine and hygiene. The therapeutic use of cold water in combination with exercise and special diet strengthened the healing powers and often produced the crisis needed to throw off disease. For this alone, hydropathy was entitled serious consideration and praise. However, academic homeopaths were careful not to accept it as the only curative agent, superseding direct medication. According to J. H. Pulte of Cincinnati, when properly combined with homeopathy, the two systems formed "the most complete code of medical rule and action which has existed, as yet . . . each one supporting and strengthening the doings of the other." But Pulte was quick to denounce any pretensions of hydropathy to constitute by itself a perfect or complete medical system.[83]

Some elements within homeopathy looked with mixed feelings on the hydropathic movement, believing the therapeutical agent had much to commend itself, but only if the user adhered to the law of similars. As one of nature's most effective remedies, water had been employed as a prophylactic since the earliest days of humankind. Nevertheless, the "ultra water-doctors" of the 1850s assigned too much importance to the hydropathic art, deeming it more valuable than the vital principle itself. Conservative homeopaths were even stronger in their opposition, pointing out that mixing hydropathy with an attenuated medicine amounted to a compound prescription that violated one of the cardinal rules of their science, in other words, to use only one curative agent at a time. Moreover, as William A. Gardiner, editor of the *Philadelphia Journal of Homeopathy,* explained: "We are possessed of no physiological provings with a view of its [water] curative powers." He warned all followers of *similia similibus curantur* that they should not deviate from the "path of true science," preferring that the cold-water treatment be left to allopathy since empiricism seemed to be its only guide. By comparison with allopathy's doses of poisonous drugs, water could become the system's most benign treatment.[84] Over time, Gardiner did his utmost to convince believers that hydropathy was a bad idea which had no affinity with New School reform. Hydropathy was a form of treatment by *contrary,* not by *simile,* and was therefore to be viewed as an "adversary rather than a friend." Least hurtful among the various empirical practices, it was still incompatible with Hahnemann's method of cure.[85] While water had hygienic uses, hydropathy was no more essential to homeopathic practice than any other *non simile.*[86]

Gardiner's criticisms, although popular among the high dilutionists, lacked credibility among moderate elements in American homeopathy for whom water had both spiritual and physiological effects.

Besides, the early fortunes of both homeopathy and hydropathy were intricately tied to their combined appeal among the middle and upper classes, especially women. For a time, a climate of professional harmony existed between the two healing systems and their affluent clienteles. Both systems found secure niches in society and this contributed to their tolerance of each other. J. Davies, MD, of Chicago advocated the use of cold water as an "invaluable curative agent" when administered under hydropathic and homeopathic guidance.[87] In a paper read before the Massachusetts Homeopathic Medical Society in 1867, Samuel Gregg, MD, of Boston proposed the application of water to the skin as an "adjuvant for the removal of disease." Admitting that the beneficial effects of water could not be explained under the law of similars, he reminded his audience that the law of similars was not the *only* law of cure. In fact, there was no direct curative agent, only one that assisted or stimulated the organism to cure itself through the *vis medicatrix naturae*. To this end, the cold or wet water compress, sometimes applied with friction, proved especially helpful in inflammatory diseases where friction hastened suppuration. He also recommended a warm- or cold-water sitz or hip bath, hot- or cold-water douches, and wet sheets.[88]

Most water-cure establishments failed to survive the post–Civil War period. However, Kenosha, Wisconsin, laid claim to two homeopathic water-cure businesses in the 1870s.[89] Hydropathy also staged a comeback in the 1890s through the writings of Father Sebastian Kneipp (1821-1897) of Bavaria and the opening in 1903 of John Harvey Kellogg's Battle Creek Sanitarium which combined water cure with exercise, vegetarianism, massage, and electrotherapy for the nation's ailing neurasthenics. Stung by the need for a more valid ratiocination, academic homeopaths chose to distance themselves from lay homeopathy's sanative panaceas by vigorously emphasizing the more scientific side of medicine. Nevertheless, lay advocates continued to find fascination in the interplay of the body's physical, mental, and spiritual planes.

Electricity

In the 1840s and 1850s, both academic and lay homeopaths made much of electricity and electrical machines (frictional, galvanic, magnetic, and voltaic), suggesting in a vague manner the existence of an invisible physical force or fluid that bridged the spiritual and material worlds of man. This mind-body science lent to homeopthy an opportunity to affirm a close relationship between matter and spirit that, while mute on God, gave expression to a more imaginative universe. Hahnemann had shown great interest in animal magnetism and thought it valuable in healing certain disorders. With the early demise of mesmerism as a legitimate medical therapy in the 1850s, homeopathic attention shifted to general and localized faradization and galvanization. Homeopaths not only faradized the nerves, but offered to remove lead, gold, silver, mercury, and arsenic from patients diagnosed as "poisoned" by Old School doctors and their medicines. To alleviate this condition, patients would sit on a wooden chair with their feet immersed in a bath of hydrochloric acid. With the negative pole of the battery grounded in the bath, and the positive pole in the patient's hands, operators set in motion a electrolysis procedure designed to rid patients of the residual metals in their body as well as their connections with allopathic medicine.[90]

Before long, the editors of the *North American Journal of Homeopathy* suspected that the business of removing metallic poisons had fallen into the hands of "quacks and other incompetent persons" where it had become an "engine of mischief." The editors cautioned practitioners to be circumspect in their choice of patients, equipment, and treatments.[91] Similarly, Benjamin F. Joslin, author of *Principles of Homeopathy* (1850), warned fellow homeopaths against experimenting with the "delusive pretensions" of medical electricity. Homeopathic medicines, not electricity, were the only true regulators of the human organism.[92]

In 1851, homeopaths claimed to have developed an electrical machine that could demonstrate the truth of the law of similars, prove that the action of their remedies was totally independent of quantity, and verify the effect of remedies at the higher potencies. The basis for this claim was the magnetoscope, sometimes called the new magnetic indicator, invented by a Mr. Rutter at the Gas Works at Brighton, England, and used by Dr. Frederick H. F. Quin (1799-1878), Dr. E. M. Madden, and other leading members of the British Homeopathic Society. Quin claimed that even one globule of an 800th dilution of sulphur, when placed in the hand of the operator, produced a "reverse rotation of the pendulum of the magnetoscope." In fact, every remedy, no matter how diluted, affected the magnetic currents produced by the machine.[93] This, Quin proudly announced, proved that the effect of a homeopathic dose was independent of the quantity. Here, too, was proof of the increased medicinal action of drugs when triturated. Quin claimed that the magnetoscope had "all the certainty of a mathematical equation."[94]

Within months of these revelations, separate experiments by Madden and Quin produced strikingly different results. At first, Quin explained the differences on the basis of Madden's body not being "sufficiently free from lingering medicinal effects, originating before his conversion to homeopathy."[95] In other words, Madden's consumption of allopathic medicines in earlier years had adversely affected his body and therefore the accuracy of his magnetoscopic results. Then, in November 1851, Madden published a letter in the *Homeopathic Times* announcing that the instrument was of "no real value" and attributing the so-called evidence to "slight voluntary" as well as "unconscious movements" of the operator. After further experiments, Madden reported that the operator of the machine had produced all of the outcomes made by the instrument. "I have been constrained to conclude," he admitted in a letter to the *British Journal of Homeopathy*, "that in its present condition the Magnetoscope cannot be relied upon as a physical test of the action of our remedies." Following Madden's retraction, others discovered that inadvertent actions by the machine's operator had also affected results. Before long, England's leading homeopathic journal withdrew its support for the instrument.[96]

Electrotherapeutics remained on the fringe of academic homeopathy until the late 1870s and 1880s when the work of William A. Hammond (1828-1900), Julius Althaus (1833-1900), and Sir J. Russell Reynolds (1828-1896) gave it greater respectability. Early cases dealt with partial paralysis, numbness, and general stimulation of organs that were considered functionally deranged. From there, electrogalvanic treatment moved into many other areas and professors of electrotherapeutics were added to the faculty of a number of homeopathic medical schools.[97]

ECLECTIC SIRENS

The 1850s were a time of high anxiety for competing medical systems in the United States. This was certainly evident among the physiomedicals (New Light or Independent Thomsonians) who found themselves enamored by the more liberal eclectics and whose medical colleges gradually came under eclectic influence. The same was true within homeopathic circles where those favoring moderate interpretations of Hahnemann's principles struggled with their more orthodox colleagues. Until the eclectics became embroiled in their own internal feuds, they were the chief beneficiaries of these moderate swings within Thomsonism and homeopathy. Eclecticism was a system of medicine that ascribed to no single principle but willingly adopted any and all practices that benefited the patient. Generally the eclectics found much to admire in homeopathy and viewed it, along with hydropathy, allopathy, and physiomedicalism, as one of several systems dedicated to the cure of disease. The question for eclectics became whether to choose one "pathy" exclusively or choose the best from each of the systems on a case-by-case basis. Disposed early in their history to homeopathic ideas, and even adapting several homeopathic practices, the eclectics represented a plausible alternative to the rancor beginning to fester between the liberal and conservative wings of New School medicine. In fact, the eclectics had made homeopathy first among equals, preferring its small doses of specific medicine to the less precise claims of competing system builders. Anxious to make inroads, the eclectics advertised their medicines, books, and colleges in many of the homeopathic journals. But the very exclusivism that the eclectics despised was praised by the homeopaths. The eclectic, observed E. E. Marcy in 1853, was a "medical freebooter" who pinned his faith upon no law, had "no fixed rules of practice, but plunder[ed] from all sources regardless of consequences, sometimes sailing under an allopathic, and sometimes a homeopathic flag."[98]

The early adoption by more liberal Western homeopaths of indigenous herbs commonly used by botanic, Thomsonian, and eclectic doctors, caused them to be accused of "mixed practice" by their more conservative Eastern cousins.[99] These eclectico-homeopathists, as they were sometimes called, were harshly condemned. "The libel, so industriously circulated by this 'mixing' set," observed J. P. Dake, would eventually turn on itself. The faithful followers of Hahnemann would form no alliances that contradicted the principle of similars.[100]

For William Paine of Warren, Ohio, who had begun practice as an allopath before moving to eclecticism, "exclusivism in all its forms" was responsible for the high mortality of patients. The scientific eclectic practice of medicine offered the solution.[101] His *Treatise on the Principles and Practice of Medicine, and Pathology; Diseases of Women and Children, and Medical Surgery* (1867) sold in homeopathic pharmacies and was considered an important contribution to the liberal side of New School reform. But others found little to endorse in the book, believing that it represented the voyage of a "rudderless ship." "We do not wish to treat Prof. Paine's work hypercritically," cautioned the editors of the conservative *American Homeopathic Observer,* but "its faults are the faults of eclecticism."[102]

In 1873, there was talk of uniting the various medical schools under the term *medical union,* with the understanding that every qualified member of the medical profession should decide the proper methods to cure disease. This attitude was more common among eclectics than homeopaths, and even though union advocates published a journal called *Medical Union,* the contents of its pages were more eclectic than homeopathic.[103] Unionists looked to a time in the future when all the schools, including homeopathy and allopathy, were united under a single banner. For them, homeopathy had become a convenience, a "stepping-stone" in the direction of unity while eclecticism became the "guiding principle of their practice."[104]

The vision that the regular physician would eventually "lie down . . . with the homeopathic lamb" was one that appealed to some homeopaths, but it was anathema to others. Lying with the lion of allopathy, argued conservatives, would result in the "absolute surrender" of their principles. Nevertheless, a movement toward that end did emerge in New York City, based on the belief that "it is the right and duty of every qualified member of the medical profession to use his own judgment as to the proper methods to be adopted for the cure of his patients." Believing that homeopaths of the day were substantially different from Hahnemann's original followers, unionists emphasized the superior education provided in homeopathic schools; the tendency among homeopaths to prescribe doses in amounts similar to regulars; and the homeopathic practice of prescribing remedies suited to the disease at hand. The unionists also noted that regulars had modified their own practices by abandoning bleeding and heroic drugging. Indeed, the two systems now differed "in name rather than in fact"; and in almost every respect there was "little real difference between the practice of an accomplished regular physician, and that of the intelligent homeopathist who has abandoned the use of infinitesimal remedies."[105]

SUMMARY

As these "nonessentials" suggest, the form of medicine employed by homeopaths varied across the American landscape. Rather than relying on a single method, both academically trained and lay homeopaths took liberties with their system of healing by combining it with various supplemental remedies. This phenomenon, while more prominent among lay healers, was actually patterned along gender, class, religious, and even regional boundaries. Patients and their healers identified with what best suited their routine and their expectations. For some, healing seemed most effective when "mixed" with conventional medical techniques; for others, homeopathy was best approached through a more congenial metaphysical or quasireligious experience; and for still others, it was effective only to the degree that it was practiced according to its original principles.

Reflecting the spiritual and material restlessness of American society, nineteenth-century homeopaths were comfortable using a variety of therapeutic regimens. But, as critic Alfred Hughes explained in the pages of the *American Homeopathic Observer* in 1873, the public judged homeopathy on what they saw, read, or heard from its representatives. For better or worse, many of homeopathy's friends had supported a number of "absurd and foolish things." Hughes hoped that New School reformers would soon cleanse themselves of these errors. If not, they would face an increasingly hostile reception from the very individuals and social elite that had carried homeopathy into prominence.[106] Hughes' advice rang particularly true in the last quarter of the nineteenth century when homeopaths were forced to confront their identity in the light of the new scientific medicine. Would homeopathy look to the past? Would it stand with mesmerism, hydropathy, Grahamism, and other "nonessential" causes, seeking a rapport between the physical and metaphysical orders of reality?

Would it seek a home somewhere between protestant perfectionism and medical orthodoxy? Would it search for a universe governed by a single set of principles? Or would it make its future home in the laboratories of science?

Chapter 9

Biomedicine's Triumph

While proponents of New School reform fought over high and low dilutions, debated the merits of vitalism, and speculated on the etheric mediums for the transmission of their drug potencies, regular medicine enthusiastically joined the century's biomedical revolution and underwent a transformation in purpose and professional identity. Techniques and practices used for centuries fell out of fashion, discredited and abandoned. Bleeding, blistering, and purging, along with cauteries, setons, moxa, salivation, and heroic dosages of mercury, arsenic, tartar emetic, strychnine, opium, and other harsh drugs, disappeared from the medical handbag of those now attuned to the pronouncements from the medical capitals of Europe. True, orthodox doctors employed lame ratiocinations to explain the abandonment of their time-honored practices and did so without admitting errors of judgment; but the recognition of self-limited diseases, the clinical findings of the French and German schools, and the popular success of homeopathy—many of whose members came from orthodoxy's own ranks—had shaken regular medicine to its very core. The changes in medical practice had been so great in the aftermath of these catalysts that younger practitioners found it difficult to imagine the differences that once existed between the two schools. But as Naomi Rogers explained in *Culture, Knowledge, and Healing: Historical Perspectives of Homeopathic Medicine in Europe and North America* (1998), "American medicine was changing, but it had not necessarily drawn closer to the homeopathic ideal."[1]

MIGRATION

Homeopaths had their own interpretation of the unfolding events. According to editor Henry M. Smith in the *American Homeopathic Review* in 1858, the entire system of rational therapeutics underwent a transformation in response to the rise of homeopathy, changing what was formerly an art into a "positive science," and bringing "precision and certainty out of the doubts and empiricisms of former times." Dosages given in heroic amounts were now smaller, and bleeding to syncope, as well as salivation from mercury, were accidental or exceptional incidents rather than intentional practices. Many homeopathic remedies (e.g., arnica, rhus, nux vomica, and pulsatilla) were now popularly prescribed by allopathic doctors. Some regulars even used the law of similars in the application of caustic to ulcers. The homeopathic materia medica, including rhubarb and ipecac for dysentery; caustic and copper for dyspepsia; aconite in fever; and nitric and muriatic acid for chronic gastritis, had become routine. Smith enthusiastically reported that allopathy was "on the brink of Homeopathy."[2]

Marshall Hall's *Principles of the Theory and Practice of Medicine* (1839), Jacob Bigelow's *Nature in Disease* (1854), Sir John Forbes's *On Nature and Art in the Cure of Disease* (1858), and James Jackson's *Letters to a Young Physician Just Entering upon Practice* (1855), were praised by homeopaths for their simplicity and directness and for becoming effective instruments of change.[3] Hall (1790-1857), whose contributions to physiologic research marked him as a scientific leader of the age, warned of the evil effects of mercury. His views were frequently discussed in the sectarian journals. Homeopaths were also pleased with the third edition of John Hughes Bennett's *Clinical Lectures on the Principles and Practice of Medicine* (1859) because the author had taken note of the many changes in therapeutics due to knowledge gained from diagnosis and pathology. A professor of institutes and clinical medicine at the University of Edinburgh, Bennett was a pioneer in the use of the microscope in clinical pathology and a notably independent thinker who celebrated the diminished use of bloodletting and other antiphlogistic remedies in the treatment of acute inflammation. In response to those who reasoned that bloodletting had gone out of style because the modern constitution deteriorated after the 1832 cholera epidemic (thus medical men were simply adjusting their treatment, not their principles), Bennett asserted that human constitution had remained the same after 1832 and that bloodletting and other antiphlogistic remedies had actually been based on unsound principles of pathology. His popularity was so great among American eclectics that the Bennett College of Eclectic Medicine and Surgery (1868) in Chicago was named in his honor.[4]

John C. Peters, editor of the *North American Journal of Homeopathy,* explained that Bennett, a member of the expectant school within regular medicine, had sided with Louis in Paris and Joseph Skoda and Josef Dietl in Vienna in opposing bloodletting and tartar emetic. Peters recalled having personally observed the work of both Skoda and Dietl in 1841 and 1842, after which they abandoned heroic treatment for pneumonia and adopted the expectant system. "It would not do for them to adopt the homeopathic treatment," chided Peters, "but, as they were convinced that it was better than the ordinary method, and could not believe in infinitesimal doses, they concluded to try the do-nothing plan." Dietl had carried his expectant method from Vienna to Prague; from there it spread to Edinburgh where Bennett became its champion; and from there to New York, where Thon T. Metcalf touted its results. "Some of these men would hardly be willing to admit that homeopathy has led to their change of practice; but so it is," argued Peters.[5]

During the 1860s and 1870s, homeopaths noted with satisfaction the migration of New School remedies into allopathic texts, often without regulars suspecting their sectarian origins. This included nux vomica for constipation, neuralgia, and colic; aconite in rheumatic fevers and influenza; aconite and belladonna in erysipelas; belladonna in whooping cough and scarlet fever; arsenicum in asthma and diarrhea; gelseminum in neuralgia; and arnica for bruises.[6] "The time will come," predicted J. A. Cloud, MD, in *Homeopathy: Its Difficulties and Some of the Principal Errors Against It* (1869), "when the only difference between the schools will be in name."[7]

Similarly, it was apparent that homeopathy had begun moving toward allopathic practices by downplaying its exclusiveness and acknowledging the possibility of nonhomeopathic methods. In 1858, homeopath Lewis Dodge, MD, of Cleveland, Ohio, reported the beneficial results of bleeding followed by chloroform, in treating cases of puerperal convulsions, insisting that bleeding was strictly homeopathic and that members of the homeopathic school did an injustice by discarding it out of hand.[8] In 1859, James T. Alley, MD, of New York explained in the *North American Journal of Homeopathy* that measures such as bleeding, blistering, purgatives, and narcotics were not wrong in and of themselves. They formed an important and legitimate part of earlier treatments and in their day were "the most efficient method of giving the recuperative powers of nature a chance to remove disease." Their uncertainty, however, made them no longer a regimen of choice.[9]

Then, too, the doctrine of inifintesimals had lost much of its purchase following the devastating ridicule from Oliver Wendell Holmes, John Forbes, Worthington Hooker, and James Y. Simpson. Their repugnance of the high dilutionists and their call for a common-sense approach did much to force academic homeopaths to abandon, if not renounce, the transcendental and more mysterious aspects of their medicine and substitute a more laboratory-based system of biomedicine. Making this transition was more difficult for homeopaths than it had been for regular doctors, particularly those who had taken sides with the purists or Hahnemannians. For this latter group, the higher potencies, drug provings, and the extended time it took to build a complete medical history of each patient had become distinguishing characteristics of their medical practices. In renouncing these practices, which many did, homeopaths moved from a predominantly patient-oriented model to the very reductionist practice they had so vociferously opposed.

Reflective of this changing attitude, Louisianan William H. Holcombe admitted in the *North American Journal of Homeopathy* that homeopathy was "not a new and perfect science of medicine . . . no new gospel, no new revelation to the medical world." Instead it was a "grand reform" in only one of medicine's departments. Anatomy, chemistry, physiology, pathology, surgery, and obstetrics were left untouched by New School medicine. Far from rejecting the "accumulated experience of ages," large portions of allopathy, along with elements of hydropathy, electricity, galvanism, magnetism, mesmerism, and chronothermalism, contributed to the "grand collateral" of the healing art. Indeed, homeopathy did not negate the use of drugs for specific mechanical purposes, such as ergot to empty the uterus, belladonna to dilate the pupils, chloroform to relax the muscles, vermifuges to expel worms, purgatives to relieve obstruction, and even bloodletting. Nor did it deny the use of drugs for certain chemical objectives, such as vegetable acids to remedy scurvy; iron to correct impoverished blood; or chlorine, charcoal, lime, or creosote to arrest putridity—none of which were part of the materia medica of homeopathy.[10]

So where were the points of dispute between allopathy and homeopathy? asked Holcombe. Both schools, for example, held that drugs were poisons that cured by means of disease-producing attributes. The allopathist attempted to produce a state *opposite* the existing one, by vomiting, purging, sweating, stimulating, or depleting the patient. The homeopathist, in contrast, used medicines that produced *similar* diseases in the healthy person. The point of dispute between the two systems, Holcombe explained, was the vital or dynamic action of medicines and their application in disease: Where should the artificial disease be produced and to what extent?[11]

Holcombe reminded his readers that, for Hahnemann, the principle of similars was the *only* true basis of homeopathic practice and all other principles (e.g., size of dosage, pellets, granules, tinctures, dynamizations, diet) were ancillary to this basic law. Since Hahnemann himself had initially given large doses before reducing his amounts, any physician who prescribed an ounce of Epsom salts for diarrhea acted just as homeopathically as one who gave the same remedy in a hundred-millionth of a grain. Unfortunately, purists within homeopathy had "pushed the attenuating process . . . to an unnecessary and even absurd degree." Holcombe preferred to use "appreciable quantities" of medicines on his own patients, but he recognized that many of the operations of nature (e.g., heat, light, magnetism, electricity, sound) were performed by microscopic and even atomic and subatomic particles that transcended imagination. The same applied to the natural agents of diseases such as malaria, which were yet to be seen, weighed, or analyzed but which produced powerful effects on the living organism. Holcombe thought it reasonable to conclude that homeopathic medicines might operate in a similar manner, with "nothing being felt by the patient beyond the gradual removal of the disease." Nevertheless, dosage should be a matter of choice. "The whole scale . . . from the crude natural substance up to the highest infinitesimals, should be open to the choice and the practice of every candid and sensible man," he wrote.[12]

Unfortunately, explained Holcombe, allopaths had chosen to focus their attention on Hahnemann's "visionary theories" rather than on the therapeutic law itself. But *Hahnemannism* and *homeopathy* were two very different things. "If Hahnemannism were homeopathy," he wrote, "the system would have long ago been demolished." Instead, homeopathy had spread across Europe and the United States, giving impetus to the study of drug action by experimenting on a healthy organism and making pathology a practical branch of medical science. It also brought relief to those with chronic diseases and proved superior to allopathy against the great epidemics of cholera and yellow fever.[13]

Even Hahnemann's *Organon* became an object of criticism among homeopaths when J. C. Peterson, MD, challenged the founder's case reports as being "too miraculous" to be true. Hahnemann had once directed patients, particularly children, to smell a globule moistened with a thirtieth potency, and then only a single breathful. That a cure could be so effected strained credulity. Prescribing medicines only once every five to thirty days for fear of their power and dictating a certain number of shakes for each potentization were also fanciful notions. These actions, which bordered on the "transcendental and mysterious," were "unstable props" to support the structure of homeopathy.[14] Peterson found equally insupportable Hahnemann's *Materia Medica Pura,* which included page after page of symptoms produced by a magnet. As for the founder's condemnation of external applications, what physician had not used hot fomentations and mustard poultices? Or prescribed a brisk purge or emetic? For Peterson, the answer was obvious. Allopathy had "not labored in vain in three thousand years." The challenge was to bring back the ultrahomeopaths from the precipice of their highly attenuated position and, at the same time, drag "old fogy" regulars to common ground where physicians could replace "allopathy" and "homeopathy" with friendship and common sense.[15]

In an address before the Massachusetts Homeopathic Medical Society in 1865, Dr. H. B. Clarke admitted that, to its discredit, the homeopathic school had ignored allopathic advances in pathology and physiology. Praising their own triumphs, inflating their own value, and avoiding the imperfections of their own system, homeopaths had lost sight of allopathy's achievements in clinical therapeutics.[16] Professor Reuben Ludlam (1831-1899), in his remarks to the new class of matriculants at the Hahnemann Medical College of Philadelphia in 1868, agreed: "It is unreasonable to suppose that Hahnemann could have anticipated, much less perfected, all the various resources and applications of the law of cure," he told students. Hahnemann's range of vision, however strong, was still limited, and his "leaning to dogmatism" was a foible of human nature. Far better to "advocate and exercise the greatest liberty of thought," Ludlam advised, than to hide behind dogma. "We must have a creed, but, in the present imperfect state of medical science, that creed should be elastic and susceptible of amendment." In the present state of medicine, Ludlam realized that denominational differences were both necessary and salutary. He hoped, however, the day would come when reconstruction would be preferred to revolution and the motto, "not homeopathy less, but humanity more," would become reality.[17]

Further evidence of accommodation came from the editors of the homeopathic *U.S. Medical and Surgical Journal* in 1867 calling for new leadership as well as new scholarship among the rank and file.

> A leaden apathy has for a long time past been upon our homeopathic physicians. We want solid acquirements everywhere; we want in our schools more pathologists and learned physicians—as Bennett, Watson, and a score of others. Writers, for instance, upon female diseases, and their surgical and mechanical treatment; and writers on obstetrics, such as Bennett, of London, Sims, Simpson, and Barnes. When will issue from our ranks, writers of such worth as Rayer, Casenave, or Wilson on diseases of the skin? Louis Andral, and Skoda, on diseases of the chest—West on diseases of children—Ricord of syphilis; or such pathologists as Rokitansky, Virchow, or Rock? Homeopathy is here a *humiliated beggar* to allopathy. Produce—produce! Were it but the pitifulest infinitesimal fraction of a product, produce it, in God's name![18]

By the 1870s, a new trend became evident in more liberal (eclectic) homeopathic circles, one seeming intent on reducing the distinctions between the two schools and establishing instead a new professional identity. Not only were American homeopaths joining regulars in seeking specialized training in Germany but, increasingly, rifts were appearing within and among the organizations of homeopathic academicians. This included a marked similarity in the curriculum of both regular and homeopathic medical schools to the point that Dr. Thomas Nichol objected to the further use of the terms *homeopath, homeopathist,* and *homeopathician.* These "queer nicknames" concealed the fact that they were physicians. "We are not homeopaths, not homeopathists, least of all are we homeopathicians, but physicians practicing according to the homeopathic law," he reminded his colleagues. He wrote:

> We are true priests in the one Catholic Church of medicine. We are the true regular physicians for we practice according to a true *regula* or rule—a grand Law of Nature, and it is high time to discard all such nicknames.[19]

John C. Peters

John C. Peters (1819-1893) of New York, a leading American homeopath, served as editor of the *North American Journal of Homeopathy* from 1855 to 1861. During those years, readers and contributors alike noticed that the editorial staff refused to reduce all homeopathic practices to a single law or force them into a single "scientific enclosure." Perhaps, Peters speculated, there was an overarching law more general than the principle of similars to explain the healing process. Until that could be determined, he urged New School reformers to avoid endorsing homeopathy as the "whole, sole, and all inclusive truth in medicine." Better to tolerate all varieties of medicine.[20]

To complaints from readers that the journal was taking on allopathic tones, Peters and his staff responded by admitting to universal truths in both systems and suggesting that the two schools did "not differ so widely that there is no bond of union between them." Since homeopathic, allopathic, and even antipathic remedies acted specifically upon the disease, there was little reason to ignore all but the homeopathic. Even within homeopathy, there were two very distinct avenues of treatment: *rational* and *transcendental.* Rational treatment required a similarity of symptoms and disease, also that the remedial drug act specifically on the disease. To be effective, the dosage had to be large enough to "establish its peculiar influence and thus dislocate the disease, on the principle that two different actions cannot go on at the same time in the same place." By contrast, transcendental homeopathy claimed only one mode of cure and considered all others useless. Transcendental believers followed "too closely" the "bad example" of Hahnemann who had carried his theories into infinitesimal doses and condemned all nonhomeopathic remedies. Peters hoped

for a "fair compromise" between the two factions; unless this occurred, homeopathy would face an uncertain future.[21]

To no one's great surprise, Peters renounced homeopathy in 1861,
declaring his opposition to all medical exclusivity and urging the incorporation of homeopathic medicine into regular practice. In explaining his decision in the *American Medical Times,* he wrote that
the infinitesimal doses and even the principle of similars were no longer sustainable.[22] Thirteen years later, when Peters was a member of
the American Medical Association, the American Academy of Medicine, and president of the American Medical Library and Journal Association, he wrote *On Sects in Medicine* (1874). In it, he claimed that
although medical sects and systems had "flourished like parasites
around and upon medicine proper," regular medicine had never been
sectarian in thought or deed. What distinguished it from sectarian
medicine was its catholicity, its inclusiveness, and its willingness to
embrace "all rational systems and all useful discoveries."[23] Believing
that regular medicine was sufficiently broad to encompass the most
brilliant discoveries as well as the humblest additions, and believing
that it resisted nothing that was in accord with reason or "enlightened
experience," Peters insisted that regular medicine profited from even
its worst enemies. By contrast, sectarianism represented the ambi-
tions of a few bigoted individuals who were "so infatuated with the
discovery of some partial or apparent truth that they deceive[d] themselves and their followers into the belief that no greater truths have
ever been discovered, or ever will be again." Instead of adding to the
canon of medical science, sectarians endeavored to present their
"wonderfully narrow and contracted theories" as the only true medicine.[24]

According to Peters, no system, ancient or modern, had ever dominated the thinking of the profession. That was because the "church
of genuine physicians" had always witnessed a "continuous stream of
solid advancement" and therefore tolerated the discoveries made by
able anatomists, physiologists, surgeons, chemists, and practical physicians through the ages.[25] Their combined abilities gave great diversity to the healing art and represented the wisdom, experience, and
aspirations of the profession. Peters was fond of praising German reformer William Hufeland for having opened his *Journal of Practical
Medicine* to a multitude of ideas, including those of Samuel Hahnemann, and who believed that the true art of medicine was guided by

reason and experience through the ages, customs, and languages of humankind. Amid the early sects of dogmatics, pure empirics, methodists, pneumatics, episynthetics, and eclectics, medicine had never come under any single controlling influence. From Hippocrates to Aretaeus, Giorgio Baglivi, Thomas Sydenham, Albrecht von Haller, and Hermann Boerhaave, medicine welcomed every improvement, "but not to the exclusion of all others." Similarly, regular medicine made allowances for reasoned differences of opinion, "but not for the domineering preponderance of any one." This meant that true medicine welcomed each new and plausible remedy, regardless of form or size. Wrote Peters:

> While the principles of scientific and rational medicine are well fixed and founded they are so broad and catholic that no rational remedy or procedure for the cure of disease is excluded; so that it is exceedingly difficult for a generous-minded, reasonably unselfish, honorably ambitious, moderately prudent, and fairly learned and skillful physician to overstep the ethics and traditions of his profession.

Only by bigoted devotion to one truth, or by openly resorting to quackery, could a physician step out of the bounds of his profession.[26]

THE DIVIDE

With increasing numbers of homeopaths migrating to more liberal interpretations of Hahnemann's principles, both the "pure" and "eclectic" (sometimes called "mixer") wings of homeopathy struggled to work peaceably within the confines of their national organization, the American Institute of Homeopathy (AIH). In 1870, however, the status quo was disrupted when Dr. Carroll Dunham, former dean of New York Homeopathic Medical College and a self-proclaimed Hahnemannian, cast a pall over the annual meeting of the AIH in Chicago by openly recognizing the low-potency eclectic wing of the association and pleading for a greater liberty of opinion and practice within the school. To his credit, Dunham was merely reflecting New York homeopathy's openness to medical diversity within its own school, an attribute that other regions found less appealing. The once delicate balance between those attached to the ideals of homeopathic purity and those who hoped that homeopathy and allopathy might merge collapsed amid accusations that threatened schism within the association. In 1874, following several years of heated debate and simmering animosity over the nature of homeopathy, the liberal wing of the association managed to remove "homeopathy" as a requirement for membership in the AIH. The decision served as a direct challenge to conservatives, and when the AIH went further by denying the active medicinal efficacy of the higher potencies, the stalwarts of pure homeopathy broke with the institute and announced the establishment of a new organization, the International Hahnemannian Association, and adopted a set of defining resolutions, on June 26, 1880.

Whereas, We believe the *Organon of the Healing Art* as promulgated by Samuel Hahnemann to be the only reliable guide in therapeutics; and

Whereas, This clearly teaches that homeopathy consists in the law of similars, the single remedy, and the minimum dose of the dynamized drug, not singly, but collectively; and

Whereas, A number of professed homeopathists not only repudiate these tenets, but violate them in practice; and

Whereas, An effort has been made on the part of such physicians to unite the homeopathic with the allopathic school; therefore

Resolved, That the time has fully come when legitimate Hahnemannian homeopathy should free itself from all such innovations, hurtful alike to its reputation as a science and fatal to the best interests of the sick.

Resolved, That the mixing or alternating of two or more medicines displays on the part of the prescriber a lack of skill, besides being a species of empiricism, inexcusable and non-homeopathic.

Resolved, That in non-surgical cases we regard medicated topical appliances and mechanical appliances as relics of the defunct customs of past ages, unscientific, non-homeopathic and often injurious.

Resolved, That as "the best dose of medicine is ever the smallest," we cannot recognize as homeopathic the treatment of any physician who administers medicine in such quantities as to suppress symptoms by their primary or toxical action.

Resolved, That we have no sympathy in common with those physicians who would engraft on to homeopathy the crude ideas and doses of the eclectics, and we will not hold ourselves responsible for their "fatal errors" and failures in practice.

Resolved, That as some self-styled homeopathists have taken occasion to traduce Hahnemann as a "fanatic," "dishonest" and "visionary," and his teaching as "not being the standard of the homeopathy of to-day," that we denounce all such as being traitors to our cause and recreant to its best interests.[27]

These resolutions became a veritable declaration of principles of those calling themselves pure Hahnemannians. Its supporters included Adolphus Lippe, George F. Foote, Clement Pearson, Henry C. Allen, Oliver P. Baer, Phineas P. Wells, Edward W. Berridge, William H. Leonard, Thomas F. Pomeroy, J. P. Mills, Edward Rushmore, T. F. Smith, E. A. Ballard, T. P. Wilson, T. Wilhelm Poulson, and Edward Cranch. This same group organized Hering Medical College 1892 in Chicago devoted to the teaching of pure homeopathy.[28] They also formed the nucleus of the International Hahnemannian Association that carried the more restricted practices of the high dilutionists into the twentieth century. The association continued until 1959 when it merged back into the AIH, which has since turned to the advocacy of pure Hahnemannianism.[29]

Two distinct groups of homeopaths emerged within its colleges in the 1880s. One, a minority, believed in the universality of the law of similars; held that all other methods were in error; regarded high dosage, trituration, and succussion as integral parts of homeopathy; favored single doses of a remedy; and opposed alternation of remedies. The other, a clear majority, accepted the law of similars but recognized methods other than homeopathy; believed dosage to be secondary and not essential in treatment; honored Hahnemann as the founder of a distinct school of medicine but did not accept all of his ideas; held that the needs of the patient were more important than adherence to principle; and sought the best experiences from all schools.[30] This latter group, more liberal in their ideas and practices, described themselves as sectarian not by choice but through persecution by Old School doctors who forced homeopaths out of state and local societies, hospitals, and colleges. The resulting sectarianism had been "neither dishonorable nor disgraceful"; rather, it was "compatible with the highest degree of learning" and firm in the "preservation of its rights." If sectarianism had not been a part of medicine at this time, then the healing art would have become "an incongruous mass of poorly ascertained facts." Over the centuries, progress in medical science had been the work of illustrious leaders, many of whom were acknowledged sectarians—Draco who founded the dogmatists; Seraphion who originated the empirics; Thermison of the methodics; Aretaeus of the pneumatists; and Archigenes of the eclectics. These were followed by Friedrich Hoffmann, Jean Baptist Van Helmont, and Hermann Boerhave, and later William Cullen, John Brown, and Thomas Sydenham. Each man had founded a new school of medical thought or modified an older system to his own liking.[31]

William Tod Helmuth, president of the Homeopathic Medical Society of New York State, represented the liberal arm of homeopathy and, as such, preferred not to claim a monopoly on truth as had many other homeopaths. He explained in an address before his association:

> Do not understand me to imply that the homeopathic school is perfect, or that those who believe and practice according to the formula *similia similibus curantur* are by any means superior, as a class, to those who deny its verity.

Like other liberal homeopaths, he embraced a more catholic definition of homeopathic medicine, including a commitment to the demands of laboratory science. Only a judicious mixture of homeopathic and regular therapies would guarantee a respectful place for homeopathy in the modern age. Despite bigotry, intolerance, and outright jealousy, the differences between the two schools were not overwhelming, Helmuth added. While Old School medicine relied most often on the experiences of its great physicians, results were often variable and uncertain. New School medicine, on the other hand, professed to follow "whenever . . . practicable" the certain law of similars which rendered their practice "scientific."[32] As Helmuth remarked:

> Unity between the schools, as they exist today, can never be accomplished by legislation; it can never be brought about by controversy, and still less by the abnegation of a name; but it can be developed by that high degree of knowledge, that cultivation of the mental faculties, which, in its perfection, is able to eliminate self from science and can allow each school to freely and frankly acknowledge the good existing in the other.[33]

American Medical Association

While homeopaths were challenged by issues of professional identity, regular physicians in the 1870s and 1880s, particularly those in larger cities, experienced the phenomenal growth of the medical specialties and, in the process, began distancing themselves from the ideology of orthodoxy and with it the restrictive consultation clause of the American Medical Association's 1847 Code of Ethics. Liberal members of the Medical Society of the State of New York, including several national leaders and advocates of more rigorous scientific standards (ophthalmologists Cornelius R. Agnew and Daniel B. St. John Roosa, dermatologist Henry G. Pittard, and pediatrician Abraham Jacobi), rejected the code's exclusion clause and insisted on a physician's right to consult with any other licensed practitioner. For them, the mantle and ideology of laboratory science had become "the ultimate arbiter of propriety," eroding all theoretical distinctions and institutional boundaries between regulars and sectarians. But New York City's liberal medical community did not control the conservative political agenda of the AMA, and in 1882 the association's Judicial Council voted against seating New York's delegates at its annual meeting because of their decision to consult with all legally constituted medical bodies in the state, including homeopaths.[34]

Henry I. Bowditch, professor of clinical medicine at Harvard and former secretary, vice president, and president of the AMA, objected to the actions of the national association, accusing it of destroying "life-long friendships" and bringing dissension into its ranks. Like James Jackson in earlier years, Bowditch insisted on treating courteously and professionally all licensed practitioners. He urged state societies to follow the lead of New York and permit consultation "without loss of reputation"; permit members of all legally constituted medical societies to join in the state society "provided they agree to cease to call themselves by any peculiar name"; and annul the action of the Judicial Council which required every member to subscribe to a code of ethics—including the nonconsultation clause—or face expulsion.[35] Despite Bowditch's best efforts, the AMA's leadership (Austin Flint and Alfred Stillé) maintained the restrictions in the old code.

By the turn of the century changes across the medical landscape resulted in a gradual decline in homeopathy and a demonstrative change in the demeanor of allopathic practice. The impact of Pasteur's and Koch's bacteriology affected all aspects of medicine and forced the profession, including homeopaths, to focus their energies in new directions. Chairs of bacteriology proliferated as medical regimens once considered mainstays against disease were now rejected as useless and, in their place, new serum therapies were integrated into everyday practice. To be sure, there remained obvious differences in theory between high attenuationists and regulars; but in fact the same degree of difference existed within homeopathy between the high and low attenuationists. The high attenuationists largely ignored the introduction of serum therapies and antitoxins and continued to rely on bedside observation and the remedial powers of their favorite medicines. This ultimately caused them to be denounced as "unscientific" and out of touch with modern medicine. For homeopathy, German laboratory science was both a benefit and a threat. It gave homeopathy's stronger schools a place of importance in the scheme of medical education; but for most, German laboratory science threatened the very bedside authority that had made homeopathy distinctly popular in American culture. As Naomi Rogers explained, the new German laboratory science "neither unified homeopaths, nor provided them with stronger weapons to fight regular medicine." In effect, the tensions within homeopathy had become too fractious to allow for a healthy transition between New School reform and biomedicine. The defining elements of homeopathic practice remained unresolved and, with it, homeopathy's professional identity.[36]

It was evident, however, that regulars and homeopaths found it difficult to define themselves using their old terminology. Both applauded the advances taking place in medical science and both had strong ties to America's social and economic elites. Overwhelming evidence showed that New School doctors graduated from some of the best medical schools in the United States and Europe; founded colleges, hospitals, societies, dispensaries, clinics, and journals; recognized the benefits of microscopical pathology along with other new diagnostic techniques and practices; worked together with regulars to form integrated examining boards for the licensing of physicians; and shared with regulars a disdain for osteopathy, chiropractic, and Christian science. In their pursuit of a more laboratory-based medicine, homeopathy's more liberal low-potency wing sought to breach the barriers between themselves and regulars. In doing this, they became increasingly eclectic in their values and practices, leading to greater collaboration, especially among specialists and more affluent doctors. In fact, in Rochester, New York, in 1888, homeopaths and regulars squared off in a fund-raiser baseball game between the "blue pill" team and the "little pill" team—a sign that both schools had finally decided not to take themselves too seriously.[37]

In 1901, inspired by structural reforms undertaken by the British Medical Association and also by the reorganization of the American Institute of Homeopathy, the AMA revised its constitution and made membership in local societies the basis for affiliation. The strategist for this reorganization was George H. Simmons, MD, secretary for the AMA and editor of the *Journal of the American Medical Association*. Although a graduate of Hahnemann Medical College of Chicago, he had renounced homeopathy and, during his tenure with the AMA, membership increased to more than 80,000 licensed physicians in 1924, including irregulars. Key to this success in recruitment was the revision of the AMA's Code of Ethics in 1903, giving members greater freedom in matters of consultation, and admitting to membership eclectics and homeopaths provided they relinquish further use of those titles. Homeopathy and allopathy had at last come to an accommodation, due in part to the recognition among regulars that homeopaths were well educated and a recognition among homeopaths that they were now treating their own patients with a combination of both homeopathic and nonhomeopathic regimens.[38]

How well each would fare in their new relationship seemed evident on closer examination. The organized viciousness of past decades ended with the collapse of both old systems, replaced by the more rigorous standards of biomedically trained physicians. Both homeopathy and regular medicine were now fundamentally different from their forbears; with this, regular medicine's attitude toward homeopathy changed to one of indifference. Self-doubts that once had fed regular medicine's sensitivities, marshaled its vindictiveness, and framed its opposition were replaced by a confidence in science as the defining boundary between conventional and unconventional medicine. Regulars realized that the triumphs of medical science would push any unconventional practices to the fringes of respectability and that, in the drive to improve medical education, irregular colleges and inferior programs would ultimately be the losers in medical licensing examinations. The result was the relentless dilution of homeopathic identity even among its strongest supporters—America's social elite. Professional identity was now clearly tied to science. Only among hardcore Hahnemannians and lay practitioners did homeopathy continue to retain its distinctive stamp. For these believers, the familiar features that once defined homeopathy were still alive, although barely.

FIRE IN THE REAR

By the turn of the century, it was hard to find two homeopathic physicians with the same opinions on the subject of homeopathy. Many had found fault with their materia medica and thought it necessary to take all drugs through a reproving, especially of those potencies above the twelfth. Others had concluded that all practice should be carried out with high potencies, while similar hardliners recommended only the lower dilutions, alternating remedies, combination tablets, strong tinctures, and large doses. Some even advocated the use of patent medicines. Besides these differences, homeopaths were divided on whether to treat by way of the disease name or by individual symptoms and whether to use or abandon the repertory. According to William L. Morgan, MD, of Baltimore, fewer than 5 percent of the homeopathic physicians in the United States at that time really practiced according to the principles laid down by Hahnemann.[39] In attempting to understand these discrepancies, Morgan accused the colleges of being at the root of the problem in that very few students actually studied Hahnemann's *Organon* anymore. At best, it was mentioned only during faculty lectures. Searching the announcements of nine medical colleges, he found only two schools that offered lectures on the *Organon,* and only one of the two offered it through a full-time faculty member. Morgan concluded from this investigation that the only thing distinguishing homeopathic from allopathic colleges was the word *homeopathy* on their circulars.

Believing that the *Organon* stood in the same relation to therapeutics as arithmetic did for mathematics or as grammar did for language, Morgan insisted that it must once again become the anchor in all homeopathic instruction. Only when students had read and thoroughly studied the *Organon,* the system of chronic diseases, and the use of the repertory and materia medica, could they be considered capable of practicing homeopathy as it was intended. Only then would they be able to manage the life and health of their patients without resorting to the subterfuges of narcotics, coal oil derivatives, antitoxins, serum treatments, hypodermic treatment, and local treatments of any kind.[40] To accomplish this goal, Morgan urged the trustees of homeopathic colleges to provide greater oversight of their school's professors and teachers, ensuring that each was capable of teaching homeopathic philosophy and its applications in the various branches. Teachers should first understand what Hahnemann wrote and taught; they must be his faithful followers "before they undertake to reform on what Hahnemann did."[41]

Clearly a state of unrest existed within homeopathic colleges in the early 1900s. Critics were at variance as to both the cause and the remedy; but as to the facts there was little difference of opinion. Generally there was a consensus that courses were neither long enough nor thorough enough; that students and faculty were no longer loyal to the principles of Hahnemann; that the materia medica was not scientific enough; that provings lacked completeness; that clinical symptoms were recklessly unreliable; and that for an increasing number of practitioners, homeopathy did not mean much.[42]

Signs of uneasiness among conservatives occurred as early as 1893 when Michigan's homeopathic community learned that the dean of the Homeopathic College at the University of Michigan had called for a union of the two schools.[43] Several years later, the Inter-Collegiate Committee of the American Institute of Homeopathy denied recognition to the homeopathic medical department in the State University of Iowa for teaching isopathy and not pure homeopathy.[44] By 1902, this concern had spread among AIH members to the extent that the organization passed a series of resolutions intending to regulate the conduct of its colleges, including the following:

1. Resolved, That the teaching of the Principles of Homeopathy as enunciated in the *Organon,* the Homeopathic Pharmaceutics and Homeopathic Materia Medica be continued throughout the entire four year's course. The *Organon* and Homeopathic Pharmaceutics at least one year, the Homeopathic Materia Medica at least three years.
2. Resolved, That the clinical teaching in our schools should be brought into the greatest attainable harmony with the teachings of Materia Medica.
3. Resolved, That we disapprove of and discountenance all teaching which gives approval to what is known as the purely empiric use of medicine, or the use of proprietary medicine and combination tablets, believing that such teaching is productive of confusion in the minds of students, subversive of the principles of Homeopathy, and tends to retard the progress in the establishment of a Scientific Materia Medica and Therapeutics.[45]

The presence of "cloaked or sugar-coated" nonhomeopathic teaching was perceived as the ruin of the colleges. For the editor of the *Medical Advance,* it was time to end "the shabby, bastard colleges which parade a pretended homeopathy." For too long they had demonstrated their "shameful surrender" to the teachings of allopathy.

Wake up you other homeopathic colleges! In the name of homeopathy bestir yourselves! Purge yourselves of those whited hypocrites who are alienating homeopathic students, and are trailing the flag of Hahnemann in the mire. Get back to the homeopathy of the Fathers or else the skeleton of the late lamented Chicago Homeopathic College will not long remain the only college bones bleaching in the sun on the plains of Marathon.[46]

Flexner on Homeopathy

Abraham Flexner held few illusions concerning the future of medical sectarianism, believing sects that began with a set of preconceived notions, principles, laws, formulas, or dogmas had no role in scientific medicine. At the time of his study, which was backed by the power and prestige of the Carnegie Foundation for the Advancement of Teaching, 32 of the 155 schools he visited in 1909 and 1910 were sectarian (15 homeopathic, 8 eclectic, 8 osteopathic, and 1 physio-medical). According to Flexner, none of the fifteen homeopathic schools required more than a high school education for entrance and only five of them required even that.[47] In laboratory science, only Boston University School of Medicine showed any evidence of "progressive scientific work." In the homeopathic medical departments at Iowa and Michigan, where students received much of their science instruction from nonhomeopathic teachers, most were ill prepared because of admission standards lower than other university students. In this regard, the universities had inadvertently created a double standard within the student body that affected the program's reputation and its long-term integrity.[48]

When assessing hospital facilities, Flexner identified the University of Michigan Homeopathic Medical College, Boston University School of Medicine, and the New York Homeopathic Medical College and Flower Hospital as the only schools equal to the task of providing strong clinical teaching, in other words, learning by doing. The others were handicapped with inadequate space, insufficient beds, or lack of sufficient control over hospital staff. Just as any good medical school controlled its laboratory, so it must also control all teaching in the university hospital. The teaching of students was not to be relegated to part-time clinical teachers. However, many schools offered little more than amphitheater teaching because hospital rules prohibited students in the wards. In dispensaries, the problems were worse. Boston University alone had a commendable dispensary; the rest lacked sufficient equipment, facilities, diversity of patients, or appropriate organization. Finally, Flexner found that only the two state university departments in Iowa and Michigan and the New York Homeopathic Medical College and Flower Hospital had adequate funding, other than fee income. Most were dependent on tuition, a distinct liability when it came to replacing laboratory apparatuses and updating library and teaching materials. While some schools generated annual fees between $12,000 and $18,000, the clear majority were "hopelessly poor." Southwestern Homeopathic Medical College and Pulte Medical College, for example, each operated on less than $1,500 annually.[49]

Assessing the strengths and weaknesses of the country's homeopathic schools, Flexner concluded that only Boston University School of Medicine, the New York Homeopathic Medical College and Flower Hospital, and the Hahnemann Medical College of Philadelphia possessed the equipment needed to teach the fundamental branches of medicine. Even though they lacked full-time instructors, their laboratories in anatomy, pathology, bacteriology, and physiology were sufficient. The remaining schools were either deficient in laboratory facilities or, as with the school in San Francisco, refused to acknowledge their relevance. Of the fifteen homeopathic schools, Flexner considered six to be "utterly hopeless": Southwestern Homeopathic Medical College in Louisville, Pulte Medical College in Cincinnati, Southern Homeopathic Medical College in Baltimore, Hering Medical College in Chicago, the Detroit Homeopathic College, and the Kansas City Homeopathic Medical College.[50]

Over and over again, Flexner used such phrases as *poor record-keeping, blot on the state, scant and dirty, woe-begone, wretchedly dirty, without merit,* and *educational chaos* to describe weaker schools and departments—both regular and sectarian. Accused of being flippant and even arrogant in his choice of words, Flexner nonetheless found that he had the national press as well as the presidents of the most prestigious colleges and universities behind his broad social endictment of America's system of medical education. The commercially driven schools along with the "poor boy's" right to practice were liabilities that the country could no longer support. For Flexner, the signs were ominous. "The ebbing vitality of homeopathic schools is a striking demonstration of the incompatibility of science and dogma," he wrote.

One may begin with science and work through the entire medical curriculum consistently, exposing everything to the same sort of test; or one may begin with a dogmatic assertion and resolutely refuse to entertain anything at variance with it. But one cannot do both. One cannot simultaneously assert science and dogma; one cannot travel half the road under the former banner, in the hope of taking up the latter, too, at the middle of the march. Science, once embraced, will conquer the whole. Homeopathy has two options: one to withdraw into the isolation in which alone any peculiar tenet can maintain itself; the other to put that tenet into the melting pot. Historically it undoubtedly played an important part in discrediting empirical allopathy. But laboratories of physiology and pharmacology are now doing that work far more effectively than homeopathy; and they are at the same time performing a constructive task for which homeopathy, as such, is unfitted.[51]

Scientific medicine had rendered sectarianism obsolete, concluded Flexner. A new generation of practitioners had arisen, educated in the laboratories and clinics of modern medical schools and their teaching hospitals. For this new generation of medical doctors, there was no room for historical dogma; neither was there any further use for abstract propositions and discredited formula. Modern medicine required trained observers; a demand for the highest standards of evidence; a spirit of inquiry; a firm understanding of the natural sciences; a respect for the scientific method; a rejection of unproven assumptions; and an appreciation of trained teachers, specialized facilities, and state-of-the-art equipment. Only a reformation of medical education along more enlightened lines of structure and inquiry would remove the taint of inferiority so long endured by the United States among the nations of the Western world. If a school—regular or sectarian—taught pathology, bacteriology, and clinical microscopy, it committed itself to the scientific method. Therefore, its propositions would have to stand or fall on scientific evidence. Where once differences in theory and practice were the defining elements of professional identity, now, because of the influence of German scientific medicine, the laboratory became the symbol of professional identity.[52]

THE DILEMMA

Following the publication of Flexner's report, various state and county homeopathic societies passed resolutions challenging his claim that no homeopathic institution was doing any scientific work.[53] The editor of the *Journal of the American Institute of Homeopathy* remarked that "nothing during the past half century has done so much to place the medical profession in a bad light before the people as Bulletin No. 4 of the Carnegie Foundation Fund."[54] More pronounced was the resolution adopted by the faculty of the Detroit Homeopathic College.

Whereas, A certain non-medical person recently visited many of the educational institutions of the country, and afterwards put into public print his impressions and prejudices; and

Whereas, This person visited the Detroit Homeopathic College and after, at least, several minutes' conversation with the janitor or his assistant learned all the details of equipment and methods of conducting the college work; and

Whereas, The statements made by this individual were both untrue as to facts, and purposely distorted to such an extent that the Ananias Club would admit the author without any State Board examination; and

Whereas, The Trustees of the College have in the last few months spent several thousands of dollars in equipment and improvements; and

Whereas, The Michigan State Board of Registration in Medicine, with the Faculty, reviewed the methods of the College, its equipment and facilities for work, and found the equipment up to the demands of the Board, in some things beyond the demands, and made suggestions which were afterward adopted by the College for its betterment; and

Whereas, Our Faculty was never as complete or as efficient as at present, our clinical facilities as numerous or as good, or our class of students as industrious and well prepared.

Resolved, That the Faculty of this college declare such statements misleading and false and the conclusions not warranted by facts.

Resolved, That these resolutions be signed by the officers of the College and published in the homeopathic journals.[55]

Despite these reactions, by 1909 homeopaths had come full circle and, instead of hoping for a proliferation of medical colleges espousing the principles of New School reform, were mindful of the changes taking place in medical education and had concluded that it would be better if only a few well-established schools in urban areas were to continue. "If some such plan is not adopted now," wrote W. John Harris, MD, of St. Louis, "it will be only a question of a few years before some of the colleges now struggling along will die of marasmus."[56] The editor of the *Journal of the American Institute of Homeopathy* noted that Flexner had set an ideal standard for medical education. And although he had yet to realize that such a standard could not be reached at once, nevertheless the goal was important. "We, probably, are no worse treated than is the old school," commented the editor. Indeed, there had been more "fierce criticism" coming from allopathic schools than had come from homeopathic medical colleges. Believing that only a few colleges could ever reach the standard of a Johns Hopkins or a Harvard, nonetheless no school should be permitted to have low standards. "There is a mean which many a college can, and under the stimulus of the present discussion will, reach so that it will turn out well qualified men and women," he wrote. To be sure, the laboratory was not the whole of medical education. It was important surely, but "to make the laboratory the sine qua non of a medical education is distinctly elevating it to a level far above the requirements of . . . common sense."[57]

Symptomatic of this new attitude, at the opening of the 1910-1911 session of the Hahnemann Medical College of Philadelphia, the dean announced a radical change in the curriculum for junior and senior students. Following the plan of instructions in vogue at Johns Hopkins and Harvard, the didactic lectures were reduced to a minimum and advanced students were directed to devote large amounts of their time to practical clinical work in the hospital wards and in the outpatient department.[58] Boston University School of Medicine's dean was quite proud of the statements made by Flexner and used them to the school's advantage. In his opening address to the students, he made note of the report, the strength of the school's laboratory and clinical facilities, and noted that the entering class was the largest since 1900.[59]

For homeopaths, their reform movement seemed all but spent. Only fifteen homeopathic schools existed at the time of Flexner's visits in 1909 and 1910; ten in 1912; five in 1920; and only two in 1923. Similarly, eclectic schools declined from ten in 1909 to six in 1912, and the physiomedical schools went out of existence altogether. Of the ten homeopathic schools in 1912, four (Homeopathic Department of the State University of Iowa, Boston University School of Medicine, Homeopathic College of University of Michigan, and Hahnemann Medical College and Hospital in Philadelphia) had a failure rate of less than a 10 percent before state boards; one (New York Homeopathic Medical College and Hospital) had a 10 to 20 percent failure rate; and five (Hahnemann Medical College of the Pacific, Hahnemann Medical College and Hospital in Chicago, Hering Medical College in Chicago, Kansas City Hahnemann Medical College, and Cleveland-Pulte Medical College) reported failure rates in excess of 20 percent.[60] This resulted in the following rankings by the Council on Medical Education (see Exhibit 9.1).[61]

EXHIBIT 9.1.
Council on Medical Education: College Rankings

Class A Plus—Acceptable Medical Colleges

No homeopathic colleges

Class A—Colleges Lacking in Certain Respects but Otherwise Acceptable

1. Homeopathic College of the State University of Iowa, Iowa City
2. Boston University School of Medicine
3. Homeopathic College of the University of Michigan, Ann Arbor
4. New York Homeopathic Medical College and Flower Hospital, New York City
5. Hahnemann Medical College and Hospital, Philadelphia

Class B—Colleges Needing General Improvements to Be Made Acceptable

6. Hahnemann Medical College of the Pacific, San Francisco
7. Hahnemann Medical College and Hospital, Chicago

Class C—Colleges Requiring a Complete Reorganization to Make Them Acceptable

8. Hering Medical College, Chicago
9. Hahnemann Medical College, Kansas City, Missouri
10. Cleveland-Pulte Medical College, Cleveland

After an assessment by the Association of American Medical Colleges and the AMA's Council on Medical Education, 85 colleges closed or merged between 1904 and 1914, and 24 new colleges were organized, for a total of 101 medical colleges.[62] During the same period, homeopaths declined from a high of 1,909 students and 420 graduates in 1900, to 794 students and 154 graduates in 1914, a 63.3 percent fall off in the annual number of graduates. The eclectics faced a similar experience, dropping from a high of 1,014 students and 221 graduates in 1901, to 270 students and 70 graduates in 1914. This represented a decline of 68.3 percent in the annual number of graduates.[63]

Over the ensuing years, homeopaths saw a steady erosion of their colleges. By 1912, the Detroit Homeopathic had relinquished its charter, while in the College of Homeopathic Medicine in the State University of Iowa, all chairs except the two relating to homeopathic material medica and therapeutics were merged with those of the regular college.[64] A year later, Hering Medical College closed, as did the Kansas City Hahnemann Medical College of Kansas City University and the Homeopathic Medical College of Missouri.[65]

Accompanying the precipitous decline in homeopathic medical colleges was a corresponding demise of state and county medical societies. Formed first in Philadelphia and New York, their numbers had grown manyfold. During their prime, these societies secured legal rights and privileges for their practitioners, represented homeopathy in many public activities, and fended off propaganda and political activity directed at their members.[66] In the aftermath of the AMA's reorganization and revised Code of Ethics, a wholesale migration took place as sectarians took advantage of the opportunity to "mainstream" provided they relinquish their distinctive titles (i.e., homeopath, eclectic, botanic). Dr. C. A. L. Reed, known as the so-called politician of the AMA, went about the country inviting homeopaths to join regular state medical associations. The same invitation went out to eclectics. Homeopathy's national and state organizations continued a precarious existence, but those who had made the jump to regular medicine looked "with undisguised scorn upon the efforts of those of us who still endeavor to maintain the traditions of homeopathy and by their aloofness have given ample notice that the continued existence of homeopathy is of no concern of theirs," lamented R. F. Rabe, editor of the *Homeopathic Recorder*.[67]

In the aftermath of the Flexner report, the states passed licensing legislation that tightened standards through the establishment of examining boards. In the wake of these changes, all homeopathic colleges were placed under the supervision of the Intercollegiate Committee of the AIH, which provided oversight on entrance, curriculum, and graduation requirements. In 1914 the Intercollegiate Committee was transformed into a Council on Medical Education consisting of Dr. George Royal, professor of materia medica and therapeutics of the Homeopathic Medical College of Iowa State University; Dr. Willis A. Dewey, professor of materia medica and therapeutics of the Homeopathic Medical College of the University of Michigan; Dr. John P. Sutherland, professor of theory and practice at Boston University School of Medicine; Dr. John B. Garrison, laryngologist to the Laura Franklin Free Hospital for Children in New York; Dr. H. H. Baxter, former member of the Ohio State Board of Medical Examiners; and Dr. C. E. Sawyer, ex officio member from Marion, Ohio. Although the council made no attempt to grade teaching institutions using a classification system, it nonetheless supervised the entrance requirements, curricula, and general management of the ten remaining schools to see that they functioned within the laws of the states in which they were located. The council was also engaged in the work of hospital inspection and grading since it recognized that graduates would need to have at least one year of hospital experience for the diploma or a license to practice.[68] Subsequent reports to the AIH noted efforts by the schools to strengthen their laboratories, increase endowment, improve hospital accommodations, and systematize teaching.[69]

In effect, while individual homeopaths trained their guns on Flexner and the AMA for their intrusiveness into matters considered beyond their purview, individual schools as well as the AIH's own Council on Medical Education were taking seriously the actions of state examining boards and focusing on the fact that only Class A schools should be recognized and only their graduates should be permitted to take state board examinations. Although a few recalcitrant deans and trustees complained about the requirement of two years of college work preparatory to admission to a medical college, the fact was that the council considered the requirement "entirely reasonable" and by no means drastic. Already, sixty-five medical colleges and nineteen state licensing boards had adopted the standard.[70]

In 1918, eight homeopathic colleges were in place, five of which were coeducational and one exclusively for women. All met the requirements of the Federation of State Medical Boards of the United States and were on the accredited list of colleges of that organization. The Council on Medical Education of the AMA rated five of them as Class A, three as Class B, and one as Class C. Convinced that no discrimination had been levied against the homeopathic colleges, G. M. Cushing, MD, of Chicago read a paper before the AIH urging all colleges to seek Class A status or to close. "There is only one excuse for the existence of any medical college today, be it homeopathic or regular," he wrote, "and that is the production of a superior type of doctor." Unless that could be done,

> there is no excuse for our existence as a separate school and the money now used for carrying on our colleges can best be diverted into other channels and the students sent to institutions where they will be better trained.[71]

Ralph R. Mellon of Rochester, New York, spoke in similar language, noting that the AIH had to "face facts" regarding the future of homeopathy. The "day of grace" had passed some time ago, and he urged the AIH to establish a research institute that would demonstrate homeopathy's commitment to science. If this was not feasible, then "such a state of affairs forms a silent and ominous commentary on our degeneracy," he wrote.[72] The goal of such an institute would be to establish the law of similars in its "proper place" in modern medicine; establish the relation of drugs to immunity in infectious diseases; train persons for positions in materia medica; and to construct a materia medica intelligible for future doctors. The institute was not to "prove homeopathy" but rather to find successful applications to fight disease.[73]

Mellon's desire for a research institute was echoed by other homeopaths as well. Thomas J. Preston, dean of New York Homeopathic Medical College and Flower Hospital, felt that the seeds of homeopathy's educational malaise stemmed from the lack of research being carried out as part of the life of the colleges. Having research institutes separate from the colleges was not the answer. "We should have more research work done in our colleges because it helps to keep the spirit of the student alive," he wrote. Even if this meant fewer colleges, Preston favored the move provided the remaining schools achieved Class A status. The colleges were to teach the principles of homeopathy but not at the expense of scientific medicine. The time for "ultra-sectarianism" had passed.[74]

In reviewing the causes behind the disintegration of their education system and the closing of their schools, homeopaths identified several reasons—some obvious and others more obscure. According to R. F. Rabe, editor of the *Homeopathic Recorder,* the abolition of the preceptor system that had been in place years earlier and had been a time-honored custom with much to commend it was a contributing cause. The influence of a good preceptor meant that students were "born to homeopathy" before entering medical college and carried their enthusiasm for homeopathic principles into their student days. Now, students were dissipating valuable time in fraternity life. A second cause was due to the decision of state licensing board to exclude questions on the materia medica and therapeutics. From Rabe's point of view, homeopaths had made a fatal error when they permitted state legislators to abolish separate examining boards. Although homeopathic representation was permitted on the so-called unified boards, these token members had little practical value so far as the interests of homeopathy were concerned. Lastly, the editor noted that New School physicians were "ashamed" of their designation as homeopaths and avoided the title whenever possible. No longer did doctors routinely place the designation "homeopathist" or "homeopathic physician" on their shingles, preferring instead to use the more generic title of "doctor," "MD," or "physician."[75]

In the light of this reality, Rabe suggested three options. The first involved the abolition of homeopathy as a sectarian organization. If this were done, all homeopathic physicians would become members of the regular body of physicians and members as well of the American Medical Association. In surrendering the sectarian label, however, the homeopathic school would need to insist that its materia medica and therapeutics be included in the curriculum of regular medical colleges. In addition, provision would have to be made for "suitable clinical demonstration" in hospitals and clinics. Rabe considered the plan utopian but thought that in an ideal world it would "once and for all establish homeopathy as a therapeutic specialty, which in truth, it is."[76] The second option involved the closing of all but the strongest colleges. Perhaps three—located in New York, Philadelphia, and Chicago—would suffice. Each would be connected with a large free hospital, with ample opportunity to demonstrate its medical, surgical, and obstetrical capacity. In addition to volunteer and full-time instructors, a full-time materia medicalist and a full-time homeopathic pharmacologist to prepare all hospital and dispensary prescriptions would be available. This plan, if carried out, would ensure that proper instruction was given and that homeopathy would be sufficiently supported as well.[77] The third option involved the establishment of postgraduate schools of homeopathy attached to a hospital, dispensary, and laboratory, and staffed by paid teachers and clinicians. Those sincerely interested in homeopathy and desirous of becoming exponents of its principles would be attracted to their research and educational programs.[78]

Rabe was not alone in suggesting the establishment of postgraduate schools as the most effective means of furthering the interests of homeopathy. Increasingly, those who had been lamenting the condition of the colleges and the ever-dwindling numbers of practicing homeopaths found this the most acceptable route to the future. Having seen what happened with their educational institutions in the state universities of Ohio, Michigan, and Iowa, the Council on Medical Education of the AIH concluded in 1922 that the only salvation for homeopathy's educational institutions lay in the support of their two remaining independent colleges or in a genuine postgraduate program financed by the profession.[79]

Perhaps the best explanation for homeopathy's situation came from Stuart Close in an address before the faculty and students of the American Foundation for Homeopathy in 1925. He explained that colleges were going out of existence and older practitioners were dying off faster than they could be replaced. In addition, nearly all of the hospitals had passed into the hands of regulars or were under the control of persons who were only nominally homeopathic. The same was true of their societies. Few were still functioning. Close found it difficult to speak of the majority of the rank and file "without indignation and grief." Ignorant of homeopathy's history, its theories, and its principles, and given to accepting every new product of modern scientific medicine, they were no longer examples of true homeopathy. Instead, they were the product of "four generations of degenerating ancestors, each worse than the last."[80]

All things considered, Close argued for the need to separate the methods or principles of homeopathy from the remaining colleges in the same manner that it was once necessary to separate Christianity from the Catholic Church. Organizations are always dying, he observed, but truth, which is immortal, continually reembodies itself in new forms of organization. "It is always alive, always active, always in transition," he explained. Rather than be discouraged, he urged his fellow homeopaths to appreciate the broader context of the changes going on and the part they were playing in the new educational enterprise, in other words, building a new structure for the preservation of homeopathy's pure principles and the perfected methods of classical homeopathy. For Close, the American Foundation for Homeopathy, with its department of postgraduate teaching, was the embodiment of the new age. The postgraduate school idea was the solution to the educational challenges that had been around since the days of Hahnemann himself. These were to become the "tool factories" of homeopathy's future.[81]

The American Foundation for Homeopathy, organized by a group of physicians affiliated with the International Hahnemannian Association, was incorporated in the District of Columbia in 1924. In developing its educational program, the foundation maintained a postgraduate school, first in Washington and later in Boston, where classes were provided in the School of Fine Arts at 234 Beacon Street. Students came from Sweden, Switzerland, Yugoslavia, East Africa, India, and the United States. The six-week course required the reading of Hahnemann's *Organon,* Kent's *Lectures in Homeopathic Philosophy,* and Stuart Close's *Genius of Homeopath* as their textbooks. Discussions also included Alexis Carrell's *Man the Unknown.* The lectures covered such topics as vital force as expressed in health, disease, recovery, and cure; the relation of sickness to the patient; susceptibility; suppression; palliation; disease classification; and manifestations of latent disease. There was also a course of study in the materia medica; case taking and its relation to repertory study, particularly of Kent and Bönninghausen; and practical instruction in case management, including that of both acute and chronic patients. The course finally included clinical medicine and experience at the clinics of Dr. Ray W. Spalding at the Massachusetts Memorial Hospital and the Union Rescue Mission. Teachers for the program included Drs. H. A. Roberts, Julia M. Green, Ray W. Spalding, Eugene Underhill Jr., Elizabeth Wright Hubbard, C. A. Dixon, H. R. Edwards, and Miss Annie C. Wilson.[82]

American Foundation for Homoeopathy

POST-GRADUATE SCHOOL

The American Foundation for Homoeopathy has conducted for ten years a Post-Graduate School of Instruction in the Philosophy and Art of Homoeopathy. The eleventh summer session will open on the second Monday in July, 1932.

The School is open to graduates in medicine from any accredited medical school, irrespective of doctrinal distinctions. The instruction has been of value to physicians of all kinds whose practice has already been established, as well as to younger medical graduates who have completed their hospital training and are about to establish their practice. The Post-Graduate School offers courses in Homoeopathic Philosophy, Materia Medica, Use of Repertories, Case-Taking and Clinical Medicine. The work of the session embraces lectures and reading on the above-mentioned subjects and actual demonstration in the clinics. The work of the School is in charge of recognized masters in the art of prescribing, marked for their thoroughness, ability and experience in medicine. Applicants are required to present satisfactory evidence of the completion of a medical course of high standing.

The course of instruction is given at 234 Beacon Street, Boston, Mass., a wonderfully cool place overlooking the Charles River Basin. Living accommodations are provided at reasonable rates at the Stuart Club, 102 The Fenway, and here the professors and students mingle freely.

For particulars relating to the coming summer course address

Chairman
American Foundation for Homoeopathy

Box 4, Derby, Conn.

Advertisement for the American Foundation for Homeopathy Post-Graduate School, Boston, 1932. (*Source:* Courtesy of the Lloyd Library and Museum, Cincinnati.)

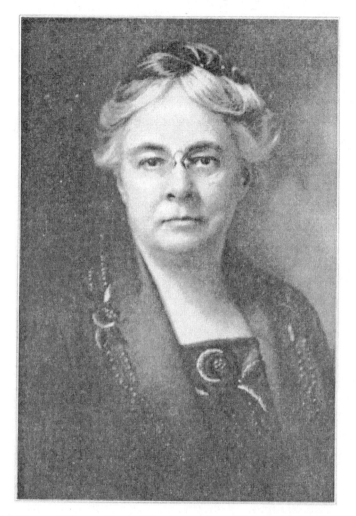

Julia M. Green, MD, president of the International Hahnemannian Association (1871-1963). (*Source:* Courtesy of the Lloyd Library and Museum, Cincinnati.)

Of the two remaining colleges, the Hahnemann Medical College of Philadelphia was in a better financial position than the New York Homeopathic Medical College and Flower Hospital, laying claim to a strong association of loyal alumni and a well-organized faculty who gave the level of teaching required of a Class A institution. Unfortunately, the college could not graduate a sufficient number of doctors to fill the dwindling ranks of homeopaths. The New York Homeopathic Medical College and Flower Hospital lacked essential funding and, in 1925, was rated B for not possessing the needed laboratory equipment. Recognizing that the cost of maintaining a medical college was more than students could support through tuition, and knowing as well that the college was handicapped by its Class B status (its graduates would therefore not be accepted for residency work in Class A hospitals and thirteen states would not permit its graduates to take their licensure examinations), the faculty and trustees knew that the future of the institution was in doubt. Also at question was whether Hahnemann Medical College of Philadelphia could survive once the New York Homeopathic Medical College was lost.[83]

By action of the AMA's Council on Medical Education and Hospitals on September 15, 1935, the teaching of homeopathy at the two remaining schools was placed in further jeopardy when it announced that after July 1, 1938, sectarian schools would no longer be included on its approved list.[84] The decision came as a mixed blessing to homeopaths. It caused some to ponder if it would not be better to let the expensive teaching of medicine be done by regular colleges and allow homeopaths to devote their time and energy to the study of homeopathy as a specialty in postgraduate studies. In this manner, training courses could be developed and a master's degree given in homeopathic practice. With sufficient support, endowment dollars could be used to preserve the active application of homeopathy in its pure form, following the example of homeopathic teaching in England and France.[85] By 1936, the New York Homeopathic Medical College and Flower Hospital and Hahnemann Medical College and Hospital of Philadelphia had relinquished their homeopathic status and become regular medical schools. By 1945, only five states had homeopathic examining boards and only one state, Arkansas, offered eclectics their own board, an empty gesture since the last eclectic school graduated its final class in June 1939.[86]

SUMMARY

Much of the criticism against homeopathy in the mid-1920s was not that it had failed to contribute to healing but that it remained a sect and, as such, fostered schism within the profession. In 1925, Morris

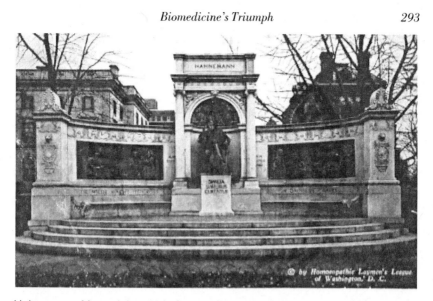

Hahnemann Memorial at 16th St. and Rhode Island Ave., N.W., Washington, DC. Note spelling of *Similia Similibus Curentur.* (*Source:* Courtesy of the National Library of Medicine.)

Fishbein, editor of the *Journal of the American Medical Association,* published a series of essays titled *The Medical Follies,* which provided a scathing criticism of medical sectarianism in the United States. Not surprisingly, homeopaths felt humiliated by the book, particularly since Hahnemann was classed with a dozen or more seductive quacks who had exploited society's more gullible elements. The result was a continuing decline in homeopathy's numbers and a corresponding phasing out of its societies.[87] In effect, homeopathy had come full circle, arriving in the early twentieth century at a point where it first started, in other words, attempting to become a medical specialization within regular medicine. But the failure of homeopathy to be recognized as a partner in scientific medicine sealed its fate. Viewed as an anachronism rather than as a legitimate medical specialty, homeopathy found few sympathizers among regulars. With its options restricted, academic homeopathy's once-impassioned plea for recognition and accommodation ended with its disappearance into regular medicine.[88]

Besides the sectarian label, homeopathy's insistence on fixed principles was an uncompromising position that, in the end, contributed significantly to its failure as an academic medicine. Having cast its lot with a vague metaphysical view of health and well-being, homeopathy became little more than a belief system set against the reductionist biomedical paradigm of the scientific age. To be sure, homeopathy retained a place in medicine as both a complementary and an alternative system, but its power base in the twentieth and twenty-first centuries shifted dramatically from academic to lay associations whose sensibilities were more aligned with holistic and herbal medicine, self-study groups, women's health advocacy, chiropractic, the vagaries of New Age culture, and persistent opposition to organized medicine. That, too, is a history worth telling.

Appendix A

Homeopathic Journals

Alumni News Letter

Date	1901
Location	Chicago
Editor	T.E. Constain
Description	Published three volumes.

American Climates and Resorts

Date	1893-1895
Location	Philadelphia
Publisher	W.A. Chatterton
Description	Monthly. Intended for laity.

American (The) Electro-Clinical Record

Date	1885
Location	Chicago
Editor	W.A. Chatterton
Description	Monthly journal of electricity. Succeeded by *The Medical Current*. Published but one year.

Sources include National Library of Medicine, *Index-Catalogue of the Library of the Surgeon-General's Office, United States Army, Series III* (10 volumes) (Washington DC: Government Printing Office, 1918-1952); Thomas Lindsley Bradford, *Homeopathic Bibliography of the United States, From the Year 1825 to the Year 1891, Inclusive* (Philadelphia: Boericke and Tafel, 1892); "American Homeopathic Periodicals," *The American Observer,* 9 (1872), 576-589; W.A. Dewey, "History of the Periodical Literature of the Homeopathic School," in William Harvey King, *History of Homeopathy and Its Institutions in America: Their Founders, Benefactors, Faculties, Officers, Hospitals, Alumni, etc., With a Record of Achievement of Its Representatives in the World of Medicine* (4 volumes) (New York: Lewis Publishing Company, 1905); Jay Yasgur, "Homeopathic Journals of the United States," *Pharmacy in History,* 40 (1998), 39-54; First Search Database; Google search engine.

American Health and Life

Date	1903
Location	New York
Description	Intended for laity.

American Homeopath

Date	1994
Location	Seattle, Washington
Publisher	North American Society of Homeopaths
Description	Annual.

American Homeopath

Date	1879-1884
Location	New York
Publisher	A.L. Chatterton Co.
Editor	E.C. Blumenthal
Description	Monthly. See *The American Homeopathist.*

American Homeopathic Journal of Gynaecology and Obstetrics

Date	1885-1895
Location	Ann Arbor; Chicago
Publisher	Advance Pub. Co.
Editor	Phil Porter
Description	Monthly. Changed in 1895 to *The Hahnemannian Advocate.*

American Homeopathic Observer; A Monthly Journal, Devoted to the Interests of Homeopathic Physicians

Date	1864-1885
Location	Detroit
Publisher	Edwin A. Lodge Homeopathic Pharmacy
Editor	Edwin A. Lodge; added Edwin M. Hale (1867); Bushrod W. James (1868); H.P. Gatchell, Thomas Nichol, L. Younghusband, E.W. Fish, and Carl Muller (1869); S. Lilienthal, Samuel A. Jones, and D.A. Colton (1870)
Description	A monthly journal devoted to the interests of homeopathic physicians. Praised for bringing before the profession new

provings, new remedies, and clinical cases illustrating the action of these medicines. Dr. L. Younghusband's name was dropped in 1870 following disclosure of his fraudulent degrees. The prefix *American* was added in April 1864 to distinguish the journal from the *Homeopathic Observer* of England. Known as "Lodge's Journal." Discontinued after the death of Lodge in 1885. Purchasers were also offered copies of *The Christian Unionist, The Christian at Work,* and *New Remedies.*

American Homeopathic Record

Date	1867
Location	New York
Publisher	J.T.S. Smith and Son
Editor	H.M. Smith
Description	Was to have been authorized by the American Institute of Homeopathy. Only one issue printed.

American (The) Homeopathic Review

Date	1858-1866
Location	New York
Publisher	John T.S. Smith and Sons
Editor	Henry M. Smith, Roger G. Perkins; P.P. Wells; C. Dunham
Description	Monthly; discontinued after six volumes. Contained many papers by Dr. Carroll Dunham. Opposed the *North American Journal of Homeopathy*. Contained many studies of the materia medica. Tried to find a middle ground between the high and low dilutionists.

American Homeopathist

Date	1864-1868
Location	Cincinnati
Publisher	Smith and Worthington
Editor	Charles Cropper; James G. Hunt
Description	Monthly; half professional and half nonprofessional journal. Adjunct to the Cleveland Homeopathic College. Miscellaneous monographs inserted in some volumes; includes proceedings of Indiana Homeopathic Institute for 1867. Published for four years. Merged in 1868 with the *Ohio Medical and Surgical Reporter.*

American (The) Homeopathist

Date	1877, 1885-1902
Location	Chicago; New York
Publisher	A.L. Chatterton and Co.
Editor	J.P. Mills; C.E. Blumenthal et al.
Description	Monthly. Changed name to *The American Homeopath* in 1879, and then back to *The American Homeopathist* in 1885, and then to *American Physician* in 1902.

American (The) Journal of Electrology and Neurology

Date	1879-1880
Location	New York
Publisher	Boericke and Tafel
Editor	J. Butler
Description	Quaterly. Continued in 1880 as *Medico-Chirurgical Quarterly.*

American (The) Journal of Homeopathia

Date	1834-1835
Location	New York
Publisher	Moore and Payne
Editor	John F. Gray; S.R. Kirby; A. Gerald Hull
Description	Bimonthly. Ambitious and devoted to upholding strict homeopathy. Suspended publication in 1835 after four issues and resumed in 1840 as *Homeopathic Examiner.* First American homeopathic journal. Intended for the profession and intelligent laypersons; not intended for dissemination to the public.

American Journal of Homeopathic Materia Medica

Date	1867-1871
Location	Philadelphia
Publisher	King and Baird
Editor	C. Hering; H.W. Martin
Description	Monthly. Organ of the Hahnemann Medical College of Philadelphia. Its object was to furnish the profession with a complete materia medica. Formerly called *The Journal of Homeopathic Clinics.* Published five volumes. Changed

name in 1871 to *The American Journal of Materia Medica and Record of Medical Science.*

American Journal of Homeopathic Materia Medica and Record of Medical Science

Date	1871-1876
Location	Philadelphia
Publisher	J.M. Stoddart
Editor	W.H. Bigler; A.R. Thomas (1871)
Description	Organ of the Hahnemann Medical College of Philadelphia. Its object was to furnish the profession with a complete materia medica. Nine volumes published.

American Journal of Homeopathic Medicine

Date	2002
Location	Alexandria, Virginia
Description	Quarterly. Formerly *Journal of the American Institute of Homeopathy.*

American (The) Journal of Homeopathy

Date	1838-1839
Location	Philadelphia
Publisher	W.L.J. Kiderlin and Co.
Editor	C. Hering; C. Lingen; C. Neidhard et. al.
Description	Bimonthly; there was but one volume published. Reissued in 1839 as *Miscellanies on Homeopathy.*

American (The) Journal of Homeopathy

Date	1846-1854
Location	New York
Publisher	C.G. Dean
Editor	S.R. Kirby; R.A. Snow
Description	Published semimonthly. On completion of second volume in April 1848, Snow resigned and Kirby continued alone as editor. Became a monthly.

American (The) Journal of Materia Medica

Date	1860-1861
Location	Chicago

Publisher   Halsey and King
Editor   George E. Shipman
Description   Only four numbers of the journal were published. Contained chiefly a record of provings.

American Magazine of Homeopathy

Date   1852
Location   Cleveland
Publisher   J.H. Pulte; H.P. Gatchell
Editor   J.H. Pulte; H.P. Gatchell
Description   Monthly. Formerly *American Magazine Devoted to Homeopathy and Hydropathy.* Contained articles on water cure, movement-cure, and health.

American Magazine Devoted to Homeopathy and Hydropathy

Date   1851-1854
Location   Cleveland; Cincinnati
Publisher   J.H. Pulte and H.P. Gatchell
Editor   J.H. Pulte; H.P. Gatchell; joined by C.D. Williams in 1854
Description   Monthly; contained popular articles on anatomy, physiology, hygiene, and dietetics. The second volume published under the title of *American Magazine of Homeopathy.* In 1854, it became a quarterly and was titled *Quarterly Homeopathic Magazine* and ceased to be a journal for popular reading.

American Medical Monthly

Date   1897-1904
Location   Baltimore
Editor   E.C. Price
Description   Previously titled *Southern Journal of Homeopathy.*

American Physician

Date   1902-1908
Location   Rahway, New York
Description   Formerly *The American Homeopathist.*

Amerikanische (Der) Deutsche

Date	1885
Location	Chicago
Editor	K. Puscheck
Description	A few volumes issued.

Amerikanische (Der) Hausartz

Date	1894-1895
Location	Essex, Iowa
Editor	Dr. Staads

Ann Arbor Alumnus

Date	1890
Location	Ann Arbor
Editor	R.S. Copeland; V.D. Garwood; W.H. Hodge
Description	Quarterly. Devoted to the interests of the students and alumni of the Homeopathic Medical College of the University of Michigan. Three numbers issued.

Ann Arbor Medical Advance

Date	1882-1884
Location	Ann Arbor
Editor	J.P. Geppert; T.P. Wilson
Description	Formerly *Cincinnati Medical Advance*. In 1884 became *Medical Advance*.

Annals of International Therapeutics

Date	1968-1975
Location	Vero Beach, Florida
Description	Quarterly.

Annual Announcement of the Central Michigan Homeopathic Medical Institute

Date	1872
Location	Lansing, Michigan
Publisher	Central Michigan Homeopathic Medical Institute
Editor	W.S. George
Description	Annual.

Annual Announcement of the Michigan Homeopathic College

Date	1873
Location	Jackson, Michigan
Publisher	Michigan Homeopathic College
Editor	P.H. Van Dyne
Description	Annual.

Annual Report of Homeopathic Literature

Date	1870-1875
Location	New York
Publisher	C.G. Pule
Editor	Raue
Description	Annual.

Annual Report of the Brooklyn Homeopathic Dispensary

Date	1869-1870
Location	Brooklyn
Publisher	Brooklyn Homeopathic Dispensary
Editor	George F. Nesbitt

Annual Report of the Brooklyn Homeopathic Hospital and Training School for Nurses

Date	1870s-1890s
Location	Brooklyn
Publisher	Brooklyn Homeopathic Hospital and Training School for Nurses
Description	Annual.

Argonaut (The)

Date	1890-1892
Location	Cleveland
Publisher	K.B. Waite
Editor	K.B. Waite
Description	Quarterly. Published in interest of the Cleveland Medical College.

Argus (The)

Date	1889
Location	Cleveland
Publisher	K.B. Waite
Editor	K.B. Waite
Description	Formerly *The College Argus.* Published by the Cleveland Homeopathic Hospital College.

Baltimore (The) Family Health Journal

Date	1889-1891
Location	Baltimore
Editor	Flora A. and Cora B. Brewster
Description	Name changed in 1891 to *The Homeopathic Advocate and Health Journal* (1891-1892). Intended for laity.

Big (The) Four

Date	1897
Location	Kansas City
Editor	C.W. Pyle
Description	Bimonthly.

Biomedical Therapy

Date	1983-1997
Location	Albuquerque, New Mexico
Publisher	Menaco Pub. Co.
Description	Quarterly. International journal of integrated medicine.

Body, Mind, Spirit

Date	1987-1998
Location	Johnston, Rhode Island
Publisher	Island Pub. Co.
Description	Bimonthly.

British Journal of Homeopathy

Date	1851
Location	New York
Publisher	William Radde

Editor	J.J. Drysdale; J.R. Russell; R.E. Dudgeon
Description	Quarterly. American reprint.

Brooklyn Homeopathic Hospital Bulletin

Date	1898
Location	Brooklyn

Bulletin

Date	1898
Location	Cleveland
Description	Published by the Cleveland Homeopathic College.

Bulletin

Date	1878
Location	St. Louis
Publisher	H.C.G. Luyties
Description	Publication of Luyties Homeopathic Pharmacy Company, with offices in St. Louis, Chicago, and New York.

Bulletin

Date	1904-1907
Location	Philadelphia
Publisher	Hahnemann Medical College and Hospital of Philadelphia

Bulletin of Medical Instruction

Date	1894-1896
Location	Boston
Editor	W.I. Talbot
Description	Represented the Boston University School of Medicine.

California (The) Homeopath

Date	1882-1893
Location	San Francisco
Publisher	Boericke and Schreck
Editor	W. Boericke; W.A. Dewey; C.L. Tisdale; H.R. Arndt et al.

Description   Bimonthly. Changed name in 1893 to *Pacific Coast Journal of Homeopathy,* and then to *Pacific Coast Homeopathic Bulletin.* The official organ of the state medical societies of California, Oregon, and Washington.

California (The) Medical Times

Date   1877-1878
Location   San Francisco
Editor   F. Hiller; S. Worth
Description   Quarterly. First homeopathic periodical on the West Coast. Four numbers issued.

Carlisle (The) Journal of Homeopathy

Date   1851
Location   Carlisle, Pennsylvania
Publisher   J.K. Smith
Editor   J.K. Smith
Description   Monthly; intended as a popular journal. Did not survive past inaugural issue.

Carnival (The) Record

Date   1887
Location   Philadelphia
Editor   C.F. McMichael; Miss L. Burling; Miss A. Mason
Description   A hospital fair paper for the Hahnemann Hospital Association of the Hahnemann Medical College of Philadelphia and the Lady Managers of the Children's Homeopathic Hospital of Philadelphia.

Central Journal of Homeopathy

Date   1920-1926
Location   Cleveland

Chicago Homeopath

Date   1854-1856
Location   Chicago
Publisher   D.S. Smith; S.W. Graves; R. Ludlam
Editor   Drs. D.S. Smith; S.W. Graves; R. Ludlam; D.A. Colton

Description   Bimonthly; designed for the nonprofessional reader and was the best of its kind. Three volumes issued.

Chicago Medical Review

Date   1880
Location   Chicago
Publisher   W.A. Chatterton
Editor   Chandler and Engelhard
Description   Bimonthly. Only two issues published.

Chironian (The)

Date   1884-1905
Location   New York
Publisher   Flower Hospital
Editor   E.H. Porter; P.W. Shedd; G.T. Hawley; E.R. Eaton et. al.
Description   Semimonthly. Published by the Alumni Association of New York Homeopathic Medical College and Flower Hospital.

Cincinnati Journal of Homeopathy

Date   1851-1852
Location   Cincinnati
Publisher   Society of Homeopathic Physicians of Cincinnati
Editor   B. Ehrmann; A. Miller; G.W. Bigler
Description   Monthly; published one year. Contained editorial articles, extracts from other journals, reviews of books, proceedings of societies, and items of news.

Cincinnati Medical Advance

Date   1873-1882
Location   Cincinnati
Publisher   J.P. Geppert; T.P. Wilson
Editor   T.P. Wilson; H.C. Allen et al.
Description   Monthly. Became *Ann Arbor Medical Advance* (1882), then *Medical Advance* (1884); changed name in 1895 to *The Hahnemannian Advocate*.

Cleveland Homeopathic Reporter

Date	1900-1902
Location	Cleveland
Publisher	J.R. Horner
Description	Devoted to the interests of the Cleveland Homeopathic Medical College. Changed name to *Cleveland Medical and Surgical Reporter* in 1902.

Cleveland Medical and Surgical Reporter

Date	1902-1912
Location	Cleveland
Description	Formerly *Cleveland Homeopathic Reporter.*

Climatologist (The)

Date	1891-1892
Location	Philadelphia
Publisher	Saunders
Description	Monthly.

Clinic (The)

Date	1875
Location	Cleveland
Description	Published by the faculty of the Cleveland Homeopathic College. Only a few numbers published.

Clinical (The) Record

Date	1889
Location	Chicago
Publisher	W.A. Chatterton
Editor	W.A. Chatterton
Description	Monthly record of clinical medicine, surgery, and materia medica. Published only a few issues.

Clinical (The) Reporter

Date	1888-1911
Location	St. Louis
Publisher	Schultz Pub. Co.; Foulon and Co.

Editor   I.D. Foulon; J.M. Kershaw; D.M. Gibson
Description   Monthly. Product of faculty of Homeopathic Medical
                 College of Missouri. United with *The St. Louis Journal of
                 Homeopathy* in 1895 and then the *St. Louis Journal of Ho-
                 meopathy and Clinical Reporter* (1895-1897). Then be-
                 came *The Clinical Reporter* (1897-1911).

Clinical (The) Review

Date   1885-1887
Location   Cleveland
Editor   C.L. Cleveland
Description   Monthly journal of medicine and surgery.

Clinique (The): A Monthly Abstract of the Clinics and of the Proceedings of the Clinical Society of the Hahnemann Hospital of Chicago

Date   1880-1927
Location   Chicago
Publisher   Hospital Board
Editor   R. Ludlam; Clifford Mitchell; H.V. Halbert; T. Bacmeis-
                 ter; C.A. Weirick; Rhoda Pike Barstow
Description   Monthly. The official organ of the Hahnemann Medical
                 College in Chicago and later amalgamated with Chicago
                 Homeopathic Medical College. Consolidated with *Medi-
                 cal Era* in 1904. Passed into the control of the Illinois Ho-
                 meopathic Medical Association in 1918 with T. Bacmeis-
                 ter as editor.

College (The) Argus

Date   1889
Location   Cleveland
Publisher   F.W. Roberts
Editor   K.B. Waite; F. Kraft
Description   Quarterly. Publication of the Cleveland Homeopathic
                 Hospital College. Became *The Argus* after two volumes.

College (The) Journal

Date   1860
Location   St. Louis

Publisher   St. Louis Homeopathic College
Description Bimonthly; published in the interest of the St. Louis Homeopathic College. Only two numbers published.

Compass (The)

Date   1890-1895
Location   Detroit
Publisher   Wilton and Wetherbee
Editor   S.H. Knight
Description Monthly. Became the *Grace Hospital Gazette* in 1895.

Correspondenzblatt der homoopathischen Aertze, herausgegeben durch die Nord Amerikanische Akademie der Homeopathischen Heilkunst zu Allentown an der Lecha

Date   1835-1837
Location   Allentown
Publisher   North American Academy of Homeopathic Healing Art
Editor   C. Hering
Description Fourteen numbers appeared. Issued by the North American Academy of the Homeopathic Healing Art, the first homeopathic school in the world.

Cresset (The)

Date   1887
Location   New York City
Editor   Edith H. Hamilton
Description Published for the New York Homeopathic Medical College and Hospital for Women.

Critique (The)

Date   1897-1909
Location   Denver
Editor   S.S. Kehr; J.W. Mastin
Description Formerly *Denver Journal of Homeopathy.* Claimed the largest circulation of a medical journal in the West. Ended when the Denver Homeopathic Medical College closed its doors.

Curopathist (The)

Date   1873-1874
Location   Indianapolis
Editor   J.T. Boyd
Description   Monthly. Intended for the laity and devoted to the interests of reform.

Dayton Herald of Health

Date   1851
Location   Dayton
Editor   H. Wigand
Description   Intended for the laity.

Denver Journal of Homeopathy

Date   1894-1897
Location   Denver
Editor   S.S. Smythe; S.S. Kehr; J.W. Mastin
Description   Changed name to *The Critique* (1897) at the end of third volume.

Deutsche (Der) Amerikanische Homeopatische Zeitschrift

Date   1885
Editor   K. Puscheck

Doctor (The)

Date   1876
Location   Baltimore
Description   Published during fair to support the Baltimore Homeopathic Free Dispensary. Only a few numbers issued.

Donation (The)

Date   1891
Location   Philadelphia
Editor   B.W. James
Description   Issued in aid of fair held for benefit of the Children's Homeopathic Hospital of Philadelphia. One number issued.

Dr. Ryan's Monthly Homeopathic Review

Date   18??

Duncan Brothers' Homeopathic Pharmacy Bulletin

Date   1881
Location   Chicago
Description   Issued irregularly as an adjunct to Duncan Brothers' Pharmacy.

Echo (The)

Date   1875
Location   New York
Editor   H. Sedley
Description   Published in thirteen numbers during the New York Homeopathic Hospital Fair.

Electro-Clinical Record

Date   1885
Location   Chicago
Editor   W.A. Chatterton

Faith's Record

Date   1871
Location   Chicago
Publisher   G.E. Shipman
Editor   G.E. Shipman
Description   Monthly. Served the Chicago Foundlings' Home.

Family Journal of Homeopathy

Date   1854
Location   St. Louis
Publisher   Association of Physicians
Editor   D. White; J.T. Temple
Description   Monthly; published for one year. Intended for the laity.

Family Medical Investigator

Date   1871
Location   Kansas City
Editor   J. Field
Description   Intended for the laity.

Fitchburg Homeopathic Hospital News

Date   1896
Location   Fitchburg, Massachusetts

Gentry's Record of Homeopathic Materia Medica

Date   1895
Location   Chicago

Globule (The)

Date   1869
Location   Philadelphia
Publisher   Young Folks
Description   In aid of the Homeopathic Hospital Fair. Three numbers
                issued.

Grace Hospital Gazette

Date   1895
Location   Detroit
Publisher   Grace Hospital
Description   Formerly *The Compass*.

Guilder (The)

Date   1900
Location   New York City
Description   Organ of the New York Medical College and Hospital for
                Women.

H.H.H. Record

Date   1883
Location   Pittsburgh

Description   Issued daily in aid of fair held by the Ladies' Association of the Pittsburgh Homeopathic Hospital.

Hahnemann Advocate

Date   1889
Location   Rochester, New York
Publisher   Pub. Committee of the Hospital
Description   Monthly organ of Hahnemann Homeopathic Hospital of Rochester.

Hahnemann (The) Monthly

Date   1866
Location   Cleveland
Publisher   Hahnemann Life Insurance Company
Description   Circulated gratuitously as an advertising medium of the Hahnemann Life Insurance Company. Only a few issues ever published.

Hahnemann Publishing House Circular

Date   1883
Location   Philadelphia
Editor   F.E. Boericke
Description   Published irregularly as an advertiser of new books.

Hahnemannian (The)

Date   1949-1990
Location   Lancaster, Pennsylvania
Description   Quarterly. Published by the Homeopathic Medical Society of the State of Pennsylvania.

Hahnemannian (The) Advocate

Date   1895-1902
Location   Chicago
Editor   H.W. Pierson; H.C. Allen
Description   Represented Hering Medical College and high potency homeopathy. Formerly *Medical Advance*.

Hahnemannian (The) Institute

Date	1850-1852
Location	Philadelphia
Publisher	Hahnemann Medical College of Philadelphia
Editor	Student editors

Hahnemannian (The) Monthly

Date	1865-1949
Location	Philadelphia
Publisher	King and Baird; Boericke and A.J. Tafel
Editor	J.H.P. Frost; Adolph Lippe; Robert J. McClatchey; W.H. Winslow; E.A. Farington; Pemberton Dudley; Clarence Bartlett; W.W. Van Baun
Description	Monthly. Intended to communicate the views of the faculty of the Homeopathic Medical College of Pennsylvania. Passed through numerous publishers and editors.

Hahnemannian (The) Periscope

Date	1901
Location	San Francisco
Description	Published by the Hahnemann Medical College of the Pacific.

Hahnemannian Pulse

Date	1892
Location	Chicago
Description	Issued by the Hahnemannian Medical College of Chicago.

Health and Life

Date	1880-1882
Location	Philadelphia
Editor	Starkey and Palen
Description	Quarterly. Emphasized the compound oxygen treatment process. Intended for the laity.

Health (The) Homeopathy

Date	1900
Location	Chicago
Editor	H.M. Pierson

Health (The) Record

Date	1885-1892
Location	Corning, New York
Editor	M.S. Purdy
Description	Quarterly. Intended for laity. First movement-cure journal published in America.

Herald (The) of Health and Homeopathy

Date	1890
Location	San Francisco
Publisher	Boericke and Runyon
Editor	W. Boericke
Description	Monthly. Intended for laity.

Herbal Update and Natural Healthcare Quarterly

Date	1990-1997
Location	Seattle, Washington
Description	Quarterly. Formerly *Quarterly Review of Natural Medicine.*

Home Papers

Date	1866
Location	Chicago
Publisher	C.S. Halsey
Editor	C.S. Halsey
Description	Monthly. Intended for laity. Published for only one year.

Homeopath (The)

Date	1858
Location	New York
Publisher	Charles T. Hurlburt
Editor	Charles E. Blumenthal

Description   Semimonthly intended to popularize the system. Published one year.

Homeopath (The)

Date   1858
Location   Philadelphia
Publisher   Boericke and Tafel
Editor   C. Hering; A. Lippe
Description   Devoted to pointing out mistakes in the *Symptomen Codex*. Generated controversy with the *Philadelphia Journal of Homeopathy*.

Homeopath (Der) und Diaetische Hausfreund

Date   1853-1854
Location   Buffalo, New York
Publisher   Lewis and Baar
Editor   Dioclesian Lewis
Description   Monthly. Intended for circulation among the German laity. Only a few numbers were published.

Homeopathic (The) Advocate and Guide to Health

Date   1851
Location   Keen, New Hampshire
Publisher   D. White
Editor   D. White
Description   Monthly; published as a paper for popular reading. Continued for a year.

Homeopathic Advocate and Health Journal

Date   1891-1892
Location   Baltimore
Publisher   Advocate Pub. Co.
Editor   Flora A. and Cora B. Brewster; E.C. Price et al.
Description   Monthly. Intended for laity. Formerly *The Baltimore Family Health Journal*. Published in the interest of the Maryland Homeopathic Hospital.

Homeopthic (The) Courier

Date	1881
Location	St. Louis
Publisher	H.L. Verdier
Editor	J.T. Boyd; J.T. Kent; W.C. Richardson; J.W. Thrasher
Description	Monthly. Two volumes issued.

Homeopathic Digest

Date	1976
Location	Ossining, New York

Homeopathic Envoy

Date	1890-1918
Location	Philadelphia; Lancaster, Pennsylvania
Publisher	E.P. Anshutz
Editor	E.P. Anshutz
Description	Monthly. Popular journal.

Homeopathic Examiner

Date	1840-1847
Location	New York
Publisher	Ludwig Felt and Co.; W. Dean; Radde
Editor	A. Gerald Hull; J.F. Gray; C.J. Hempel
Description	Monthly; Discontinued from December 1843 to August 1845 when a new series was commenced by Drs. John F. Gray and Charles J. Hempel. Formerly *The American Journal of Homeopathia.*

Homeopathic (The) Expositor

Date	1866-1867
Location	Milwaukee
Publisher	J.S. Douglas and Perrine
Editor	J.S. Douglas and Perrine
Description	Monthly; published for a few months only. Intended for laity.

Homeopathic (The) Expositor

Date	1879-1882
Location	Ithaca, New York
Publisher	E.J. Morgan Jr.
Editor	E.J. Morgan Jr.; A.M. Baldwin
Description	Quarterly. Intended for laity.

Homeopathic Eye, Ear and Throat Journal

Date	1895-1911
Location	Lancaster, Pennsylvania
Editor	A.B. Norton; J.L. Moffat; A.W. Palmer
Description	Monthly. Official organ of the Ophthalmological, Oto-logical and Laryngological Society (1911-1919). Became *The Journal of Opthalmology, Otology, and Laryngology* in 1911.

Homeopathic (The) Guide

Date	1895
Location	Louisville
Description	Intended for laity.

Homeopathic Heartbeat

Date	1978-1981
Location	Falls Church, Virginia
Description	Monthly. Published by the National Center for Homeopathy. Formerly the *Layman Speaks*. Succeeded by *Homeopathy Today*.

Homeopathic Hospital Envoy

Date	1896-1902
Location	Denver
Description	Supported by the ladies auxiliary of the Denver Homeopathic Hospital on Champa Street.

Homeopathic Hospital Reporter

Date	1868
Location	Cleveland
Publisher	Cleveland Homeopathic Hospital

Homeopathic Independent

Date	1868-1869
Location	St. Louis
Publisher	J. Conzelman
Editor	J. Conzelman; J.T. Temple; T.G. Comstock et al.
Description	Lasted for one year.

Homeopathic Journal of Materia Medica, Chemistry and Pharmacology

Date	1867
Location	Chicago
Publisher	Williams and Dwight
Description	Monthly. Lasted less than a year. Represented Williams and Dwight Homeopathic Pharmacists of Chicago.

Homeopathic Journal of Obstetrics and Diseases of Women and Children

Date	1879-1885
Location	New York City
Publisher	A.L. Chatterton Pub. Co.
Editor	H. Minton; L.L. Danforth; P. Porter; G.W. Winterburn; B.F. Underwood; G.F. Honan
Description	Quarterly. Name changed in 1886 to *Homeopathic Journal of Obstetrics, Gynaecology, and Paedology*. In 1905 it became *The Journal of Surgery, Gynecology and Obstetrics*.

Homeopathic Journal of Obstetrics, Gynaeocology, and Paedology

Date	1886-1904
Location	New York City
Publisher	A.L. Chatterton Pub. Co.
Editor	Phil Porter; G.W. Winterburn; B.F. Underwood; G.F. Honan
Description	Formerly *The Journal of Obstetrics and Diseases of Women and Children*. Became *The Journal of Surgery, Gynecology and Obstetrics* in 1905.

Homeopathic Journal of Surgery and Gynecology

Date	1898
Location	New York
Publisher	Medical Century Co.
Description	Became part of *Medical Century* magazine.

Homeopathic (The) Leader

Date	1883
Location	New York
Editor	W.Y. Cowl
Description	Two numbers issued.

Homeopathic Medical News Letter

Date	1851-1852
Location	St. Louis
Publisher	J. Granger, T.J. Vastine, and T.G. Comstock
Editor	J. Granger; T.J. Vastine; T.G. Comstock
Description	Monthly; intended for the patients of the editors. Published for one year.

Homeopathic News

Date	1854-1856
Location	Philadelphia
Publisher	Boericke & Tafel
Editor	Adolphus Lippe; Constantine Hering
Description	Published in eight pages and purported to be an independent advertising sheet. Published the errors of Jahr's *New Manual*.

Homeopathic News

Date	1871-1879
Location	St. Louis
Publisher	H.C.G. Luyties and Co.
Editor	C.H. Goodman; R.G.A. Meier; W.T. Helmuth et. al.
Description	Monthly. Name changed to *Monthly Homeopathic News* in 1879. Continued as trade journal until 1890 and then pirated other publications without credit.

Homeopathic News

Date	1876
Location	Kansas City
Publisher	Feld and Riley
Editor	J. Feld
Description	Monthly trade journal for the Kansas City Homeopathic Pharmacy.

Homeopathic Pioneer

Date	1845-1846
Location	Syracuse, New York
Publisher	H. Hull Cator and L.M. Tracy
Editor	H. Hull Cator; L.M. Tracy
Description	Monthly; published one year. Provided extracts from other journals, reviews of books, and case records.

Homeopathic Physician

Date	1881-1893
Location	Philadelphia
Publisher	Bedell and Bros. Pub.
Editor	E.J. Lee; Walter James
Description	Monthly. Devoted to high potency homeopathy. Designed to disseminate the popular views of homeopathic science.

Homeopathic Quarterly

Date	1869
Location	Buffalo, New York
Publisher	R. Gregg
Editor	R. Gregg
Description	Devoted to the elucidation of Gregg's theory of phthisis pulmonalis. Two volumes published.

Homeopathic Record

Date	1878
Location	Chicago
Publisher	W.F. Morrison
Editor	W.F. Morrison

Homeopathic (The) Recorder

Date	1885-1959
Location	Philadelphia; Brattleboro, Vermont
Publisher	Boericke & Tafel
Editor	J.T. O'Connor; C.F. Millspaugh; E.P. Anshutz et.al.
Description	Bimonthly, then became a monthly. Official organ of publisher. Merged with *Journal of the American Institute of Homeopathy* and in 1928 Boericke and Tafel announced they were passing control of magazine over to the American Institute of Homeopathy. High-class trade journal. Intent of new editor was to be "Simon-pure" in homeopathy.

Homeopathic Semi-Monthly Magazine

Date	1869
Location	St. Louis
Editor	J. Conzelman

Homeopathic (The) Student

Date	1895-1904
Location	Chicago
Publisher	Chicago Homeopathic College
Editor	C.W. Weirick
Description	Ceased publication with the consolidation of Chicago Homeopathic College and Hahnemann Medical College in 1904.

Homeopathic (The) Sun

Date	1868
Location	New York City
Publisher	William Radde
Editor	F.W. Hunt
Description	Monthly; devoted to popular homeopathic information, particularly life insurance. Published for just a few months.

Homeopathic Survey; A Journal for the Interests and Advancement of Homeopathy

Date	1926
Location	Washington, DC

Publisher	Foundation Press
Editor	Arthur and Julian Green; B.C. Woodbury Jr.
Description	Quarterly. Issued by the American Foundation for Homeopathy.

Homeopathic Times

Date	1875-1881
Location	New York City
Publisher	E. Guernsey, A.K. Hills, and J.B. Gilbert
Editor	E. Guernsey; A.K. Hills; J.B. Gilbert
Description	Monthly. Consolidation of *The Medical Union* and *New York Journal of Homeopathy*. Name changed to *New York Medical Times* in 1881 and continued until 1882.

Homeopathician (The)

Date	1914-1916
Location	Pittsburgh, Pennsylvania
Editor	Julia C. Loos; Wallace M. Loos
Description	Monthly.

Homeopathician; A Journal for Pure Homeopathy

Date	1912-1916
Location	Harrisburg, Pennsylvania
Publisher	Homeopathican Publishing Co.
Description	Monthly. Published six volumes.

Homeopatische (Der) Bote

Date	1886-1892
Location	St. Louis
Editor	W.F. Bockstruck
Description	Published irregularly.

Homeopatische (Der) Zeitschrift

Date	1883
Location	Newark, New Jersey

Homeopathischer (Der) Hausfreud

Date	1857
Location	Hermann, Missouri
Editor	J. Conzelman
Description	Published for only a short time.

Homeopathist (The)

Date	1850-1852
Location	Buffalo, New York
Publisher	D. Lewis
Editor	D. Lewis
Description	Semimonthly and later as monthly; lasted about two years and intended to spread the knowledge of homeopathy among the people. Lewis sold homeopathic medicines in Buffalo.

Homeopathist (The)

Date	1859
Location	Vermont, Illinois
Editor	J.M. Blaisdell
Description	Intended to diffuse knowledge of homeopathy among the people. Lasted only short time.

Homeopathist (The)

Date	1859
Location	Springfield, Massachusetts
Publisher	J.M. Buzzell
Editor	J.M. Buzzell; D. White
Description	Monthly; intended to be a popular sheet. Only three or four numbers were issued. Used to advertise Dr. Buzzell's private hospital in Springfield.

Homeopathist (The)

Date	1870-1874
Location	New York
Publisher	Homeopathic Mutual Life Insurance Co.
Editor	E.B. Holmes

Description   Issued in the interest of the Homeopathic Mutual Life Insurance Co. of New York.

Homeopathy Today

Date   1980
Location   Washington, DC; Alexandria, Virginia
Publisher   National Center for Homeopathy
Editor   Julian Winston
Description   Monthly newsletter of the National Center for Homeopathy. Formerly *Homeopathic Heartbeat*.

Homeotherapy

Date   1974-1980
Location   San Francisco
Editor   Robert Schore
Description   Bimonthly. Published by California State Homeopathic Medical Society. Formerly *Pacific Coast Homeopathic Bulletin*. Organ of the Homeopathic Physicians of the Pacific.

L'Homoion

Date   1861
Location   New Orleans
Editor   L. Caboche
Description   Monthly. Journal of the Societe Hahnemannienne de la Nouvelle Orleans.

L'Homoion

Date   1859-1860
Location   New Orleans
Editor   Dr. Taxil
Description   Monthly; published through December 1860.

Hospital Bazaar

Date   1874
Location   Chicago
Editor   Miss Kate N. Daggett

Description   Published in aid of the Hahnemann Hospital Charity Fair.
                Seven numbers issued.

Hospital Leaflet

Date   1889
Location   Rochester, New York
Publisher   Lady Supervisors of the Hospital
Description   Monthly. Published in interest of the Rochester Homeo-
                pathic Hospital.

Hospital Leaflet

Date   1895
Location   Buffalo, New York
Publisher   Board of Association Managers
Description   Monthly. Devoted to interests of the Buffalo Homeopathic
                Hospital.

Hospital Messenger

Date   1887
Location   Philadelphia
Publisher   Executive Bd.
Editor   Mrs. Charles Reese
Description   Published by the executive board of the Women's Homeo-
                pathic Association of Pennsylvania during the fair at St.
                George's Hall.

Hospital News

Date   1888
Location   Minneapolis
Description   One issue published under the auspices of the Homeo-
                pathic Hospital.

Hospital Tidings

Date   1895-1952
Location   Philadelphia
Description   Known also as *Hahnemann Hospital Tidings*.

Hospital (The) Visitant

Date	1894-1896
Location	Portland

Humphrey's Journal of Specific Homeopathy

Date	1855-1863
Location	Auburn, New York
Publisher	F. Humphreys
Editor	F. Humphreys
Description	Monthly. Intended for laity.

Indicator (The)

Date	1893
Location	Cleveland
Editor	B.B. Viets
Description	Organ of Cleveland Homeopathic Medical College.

Investigator (The)

Date	1879
Location	Richmond, Virginia
Description	Intended for laity.

Iowa Homeopathic Journal

Date	1907-19??
Location	Des Moines
Editor	J.G. Huntoon; John W. Cogswell
Description	Monthly journal of the Hahnemann Medical Association of Iowa.

Journal

Date	1941-1942
Location	Trenton, New Jersey
Description	Published by the New Jersey State Homeopathic Medical Society.

Journal of the American Institute of Homeopathy

Date	1909-present
Location	Cleveland; Denver
Publisher	Board of Trustees, AIH
Editor	W.A. Dewey; J.R. Horner; et al.
Description	Monthly. Later became quarterly. Superceded the *Medical Century*. Merged with *The Homeopathic Recorder* (1927). Journal includes bureaus of clinical medicine, homeopathy, materia medica, pedology, and sanitary science. Each article followed by a full discussion.

Journal (The) of Electro-Therapeutics

Date	1890-1892
Location	New York
Publisher	A.L. Chatterton and Co.
Editor	W.H. King
Description	Monthly.

Journal of Energy Medicine

Date	1980
Location	North Miami
Publisher	Energy Center Inc.
Description	Quarterly.

Journal of Homeopathic Clinics

Date	1867-1871
Location	Philadelphia
Editor	C. Hering; H.N. Martin
Description	Ceased after nine volumes. Title changed in 1871 to *American Journal of Homeopathic Materia Medica and Record of Medical Science*.

Journal of Homeopathic Practice

Date	1978
Location	Berkeley
Description	Quarterly.

Journal (The) of Homeopathics

Date	1889-1890
Location	New York
Publisher	H. Hitchcock
Editor	H. Hitchcock
Description	Monthly. Discontinued after two volumes. Devoted to the philosophy of homeopathy.

Journal (The) of Homeopathics

Date	1897-1903
Location	Philadelphia
Editor	J.T. Kent
Description	Merged with *Medical Advance* in 1903. Devoted to high-potency homeopathy.

Journal (The) of Ophthalmology, Otology, and Laryngology

Date	1889-1929
Location	New York City; Lancaster, Pennsylvania
Publisher	A.L. Chatterton and Co.
Editor	G.S. Norton; C. Deady; J.L. Moffat; M. Leal et al.
Description	Quarterly. Official organ of the Ophthalmological, Otological and Laryngological Society (1911-1929). Merged in 1911 with *Homeopathic Eye, Ear and Throat Journal.* In 1918 merged with the *Journal of the American Institute of Homeopathy.*

Journal of Orificial Surgery

Date	1892-1901
Location	Chicago
Publisher	Pratt and Holbrook
Editor	E.H. Pratt
Description	Monthly. Published nine volumes.

Journal of Pediatrics

Date	1902-1903
Location	Buffalo, New York
Editor	J.C. Chadwick

Journal of Surgery, Gynecology and Obstetrics

Date	1905-1910
Location	New York City
Publisher	A.L. Chatterton
Description	Bimonthly. Formerly *Homeopathic Journal of Obstetrics, Gynaecology, and Paedology.*

Journal of Ultramolecular Medicine

Date	1983
Location	Las Vegas, Nevada
Description	Published three times per year by Society of Ultra-molecular medicine.

Keystone (The)

Date	1889-1905
Location	Buffalo, New York
Publisher	Keystone Pub. Co.
Editor	J.T. Cooke; L.B. Lee; E. Hilliard; Jessie Shepard
Description	Monthly published under auspices of the Women's Aid Society of the Buffalo Homeopathic Hospital.

Layman Speaks

Date	1947-1978
Location	Falls Church, Virginia
Editor	Arthur Green
Description	Monthly. Published by the National Center for Homeopathy. Succeeding title *Homeopathic Heartbeat.*

Library of Homeopathic Classics

Date	1907
Location	New York
Editor	Shedd
Description	Supplement to the *New York Journal of Homeopathy.*

Madison Homeopathist

Date	1854
Location	Madison, Wisconsin

Publisher   Drs. Bowen and Giles
Editor   Drs. Bowen and Giles
Description   Monthly; lasted only a few months. Intended for laity.

Materia Medica Journal

Date   1896
Location   Chicago
Editor   H.C. Allen

Medical Advance

Date   1884-1903
Location   Ann Arbor
Editor   H.C. Allen
Description   Semimonthly. Formerly *Ann Arbor Medical Advance.* Became *Hahnemanian Advocate* in 1898. Merged in 1903 with *The Journal of Homeopathics* to develop true homeopathy into a science. Represented the tradition of Hering, Dunham, and Lippe.

Medical Arena

Date   1892-1903
Location   Kansas City
Editor   S.C. Delap
Description   Championed the Kansas City Homeopathic Medical College. Abandoned homeopathy in 1903 and became eclectic.

Medical Argus

Date   1890-1891
Location   Kansas City, Missouri
Publisher   F.F. Cassedy
Editor   F.F. Cassedy
Description   Monthly. Eight volumes issued. Devoted to homeopathy and the collateral sciences.

Medical (The) Call

Date   1881-1888
Location   Quincy, Illinois

Publisher   O.H. Crandall
Editor   W.D. Foster; O.H. Crandall
Description   Quarterly. Continued through three or four volumes.

Medical Century

Date   1893-1915
Location   Chicago; New York
Publisher   Medical Century Co.
Editor   C.E. Fisher; W.A. Dewey
Description   It first absorbed *The New Remedies* and then the *Northwestern Journal of Homeopathy*. In 1893 it acquired *Medical Era* and later combined with *Homeopathic Journal of Surgery and Gynecology*.

Medical Counselor

Date   1879-1886
Location   Chicago
Publisher   W.A. Chatterton
Editor   H.R. Arndt; N.B. Delamater; J.B. Mills
Description   Monthly. Changed with volume 11 in 1886 to *Medical Counselor and Michigan Journal of Homeopathy* and moved to Grand Rapids, Michigan. In 1889 it became *Medical Era,* and in 1893 it became *Medical Century.*

Medical Counselor and Michigan Journal of Homeopathy

Date   1886-1889
Location   Grand Rapids; Ann Arbor
Publisher   Medical Counselor Publishing Co.
Editor   H.R. Arndt; D.A. MacLachlan
Description   Semimonthly. See *Medical Counselor.* Merged with *Medical Era.*

Medical Counselor: A Twentieth Century Journal of the Medical and Collateral Sciences

Date   1896-1910
Location   Detroit
Description   Monthly.

Medical Current

Date	1886-1896
Location	Chicago
Publisher	W.A. Chatterton and Co.
Editor	H. Sherry; W.E. Reed; E.F. Storke; W.A. Smith
Description	Monthly. A continuation of *The American Electro-Clinical Record*.

Medical Debates

Date	1899
Location	New York

Medical Era

Date	1883-1903
Location	Chicago
Publisher	Gross and Delbridge
Editor	C. Gatchell; C.E. Fisher; R.N. Tooker; J.E. Gross; T.D. Williams
Description	Became *Medical Century* in 1893, and then returned back to *Medical Era*. Became the official organ of the Illinois Homeopathic State Medical Association. Became *The Clinique* in 1902.

Medical Era

Date	1896-1902
Location	Detroit
Description	Merged with *Medical Counselor and Michigan Journal of Homeopathy*.

Medical Forum

Date	1904-1907
Location	Kansas City
Editor	W.E. Cramer; C. Ott
Description	Monthly.

Medical Herald

Date	1881
Location	St. Louis

Editor   C.H. Goodman; C.W. Taylor
Description   Monthly. One copy issued.

Medical (The) Institute of Philadelphia

Date   1886-1905
Location   Philadelphia
Publisher   Hahnemann Institute
Editor   J.W. LeSeur; W.S. Morris et al.
Description   Monthly. The student publication of the Hahnemann Col-
                lege.

Medical Investigator

Date   1856
Location   St. Louis
Editor   D. White
Description   Intended as a weekly homeopathic newspaper. Published
                for a few months.

Medical Investigator

Date   1861-1874
Location   Chicago
Publisher   C.S. Halsey
Editor   T.C. Duncan; E.M. Hale; R. Ludlam; G.E. Shipman
Description   Bimonthly; intended as newspaper for the profession and
                advertising sheet for the publishers. Eleven volumes is-
                sued. Changed name to *Medical Investigator and Busi-
                ness Advertiser.* In 1875 became *The United States Medi-
                cal Investigator.*

Medical Investigator and Business Advertiser

Date   1863
Location   Chicago
Publisher   C.F. Halsey
Description   Formerly *Medical Investigator.*

Medical Magazine

Date   1901-1903
Location   Milwaukee
Editor   H.B. Dale

Medical (The) Mission Herald

Date	1895
Location	Chicago
Description	Intended for laity.

Medical (The) News

Date	1889
Location	Orrville, Ohio; Elkhart, Indiana
Editor	H.A. Mumaw
Description	Quarterly.

Medical News and Bulletin

Date	1888-1889
Location	Orrville, Ohio
Description	Formerly *The Medical News*. Became *The Semi-Monthly Bulletin of the Western Exchange*.

Medical (The) and Scientific News

Date	1896-1898
Location	Elkhart, Indiana
Description	Formerly *National Medical Exchange Monthly Bulletin*.

Medical (The) Student

Date	1888-1905
Location	Boston
Description	Monthly. Undergraduate publication of Boston University. Editor chosen by students.

Medical (The) and Surgical Record

Date	1889-1892
Location	Omaha
Editor	D.A. Foote; E.F. Allen
Description	Continuation of *The Surgical Record* (1888-1889).

Medical Topics

Date	1890
Location	Chicago
Publisher	W.A. Chatterton
Description	Quarterly. Two numbers published.

Medical (The) Union

Date	1873-1875
Location	New York
Publisher	C.T. Hurlburt
Editor	E. Guernsey; J.C. Minor; C.E. Blumenthal et al.
Description	Merged with *New York Journal of Homeopathy* to become *Homeopathic Times* in 1875. Two volumes published.

Medical (The) Visitor

Date	1885-1905
Location	Chicago
Publisher	T.S. Hoyne
Editor	W.A. Smith; H.B. Dale
Description	Monthly. Directory of homeopathic physicians. Passed into the hands of Halsey Brothers, Homeopathic pharmacists of Chicago.

Medical (The) World

Date	1881
Editor	C.H. Goodman; C.W. Taylor

Medico-Chirurgical Quarterly

Date	1880
Location	New York
Editor	J. Butler; G.M. Dillow
Description	Published single volume. Formerly *The American Journal of Electrology and Neurology*.

Michigan Journal of Homeopathy

Date	1848-1854
Location	Detroit

Publisher	G.W. Pattison
Editor	John Ellis; E.H. Drake
Description	Monthly. Published irregularly; contained articles addressed more to the laity than the profession. Two volumes issued.

Michigan Journal of Homeopathy

Date	1872
Location	Detroit
Publisher	E.R. Ellis
Editor	E.R. Ellis
Description	Quarterly. The second rendition was the product of the faculty of the Detroit Homeopathic College. Contained the announcement of the Detroit College and matters of interest to the medical profession. Four issues published.

Midwest Homeopathic News Journal

Date	1927

Milwaukee Homeopathic Medical Reporter

Date	1848
Location	Milwaukee
Publisher	L.M. Tracy and J. Douglas
Editor	L.M. Tracy; J. Douglas
Description	Monthly. Criticized for advertising the journal's two editors.

Minneapolis Homeopathic Magazine

Date	1892-1903
Location	Minneapolis
Publisher	Minneapolis Pharm. Co.
Editor	H.C. Aldrich
Description	Monthly. Published ten volumes.

Minnesota (The) Homeopath

Date	1854
Location	St. Paul
Editor	G. Hatfield
Description	Bimonthly. Published only a few numbers.

Minnesota Medical Monthly

Date	1886-1888
Location	Minneapolis
Publisher	T. Gardiner
Editor	W.E. Leonard; P.M. Hall; R.D. Matchan et al.
Description	Monthly. Published two volumes.

Miscellanies on Homeopathy

Date	1838-1839
Location	Philadelphia
Publisher	L.J. Kiderlin and Co.
Editor	C. Hering; C. Lingen; C. Neidhard et al.
Description	Thought to be one of the best books for physicians and laymen on homeopathy. Formerly *The American Journal of Homeopathy*.

Mistletoe (The)

Date	1891-1892
Location	Philadelphia
Editor	Mrs. R.S. Pencer; Mr. G. A. Barrows et al.
Description	Published for the benefit of the Hahnemann Hospital of Philadelphia.

Monthly Homeopathic News

Date	1871-1903
Location	St. Louis
Publisher	H.C.G. Luyties; R.G.A. Meier
Editor	H.C.G. Luyties; W.T. Helmuth; C.H. Goodman
Description	Monthly. Formerly *Homeopathic News*.

Monthly Record

Date	1857-1909
Location	New York
Publisher	Five Points House
Description	Published in connection with the Five Points House of Industry that was under homeopathic control.

Munson's Homeopathic Bulletin

Date	1872-1892
Location	St. Louis
Publisher	Munson Homeopathic Pharmacy
Editor	J.W. Munson
Description	Monthly. A gratuitous advertising journal.

National Medical Exchange Monthly Bulletin

Date	1888-1900
Location	Elkhart, Indiana
Description	Formerly *The National Medical News*. Later became *The Medical and Scientific News*.

National (The) Medical News

Date	1891
Location	Orrville, Ohio
Description	Formerly *The Semi-Monthly Bulletin of the Western Exchange*. Later became *The National Medical Exchange Monthly Bulletin* (1891).

Natural Medicine Law

Date	1997
Location	Rockville, Maryland
Publisher	Muscatatuck Pub. Co.
Description	Bimonthly.

Nature Cure Magazine

Date	1907-1909
Location	Chicago
Publisher	Nature Cure Publishing Co.
Description	Monthly.

New England Journal of Homeopathy

Date	1992-2001
Location	Amhurst, Massachusetts
Publisher	New England School of Homeopathy Press
Description	Quarterly. Published primarily clinical material.

New England Medical Gazette. A Monthly Journal of Homeopathic Medicine, Surgery, and the Collateral Sciences

Date	1866-1905
Location	Boston
Publisher	S. Whitney; Otis Clapp and Sons
Editor	H.C. Angell; I.T. Talbot; H.C. Clapp; C.F. Nichols; W. Wesselhoeft; C.A. Chase; J.L. Coffin et al.
Description	Monthly; devoted to the progress of homeopathy in New England. Considered "progressive" in character and viewed high and low attenuations as "open questions" to be treated fairly. Represented the interests of the Boston University School of Medicine.

New (The) Remedies

Date	1889-1892
Location	Chicago
Publisher	Gross and Delbridge
Editor	J.E. Gross; E.M. Hale et al.
Description	Bimonthly. Merged in 1892 with *Medical Century*.

New York Amusement Gazette

Date	1888
Location	New York City
Description	Daily bulletin of the fair for the benefit of the Homeopathic Free Hospital.

New York Journal of Homeopathy

Date	1846-1854
Location	New York City
Publisher	S.R. Kirby and R.A. Snow
Editor	S.R. Kirby; R.A. Snow
Description	Biweekly; monthly after 1848. Discontinued after 1854.

New York Journal of Homeopathy

Date	1873-1875
Location	New York City
Publisher	Carle and Grener
Editor	W.T. Helmuth; T.F. Allen; S.A. Jones et al.

Description   Monthly. Merged with *The Medical Union* to become *Homeopathic Times* in 1875. Two volumes published. Prepared under auspices of the New York Homeopathic Medical College. Became *New York Medical Times.*

New York Medical Times

Date   1881-1896
Location   New York
Publisher   E.P. Coby and Co.
Description   Monthly. Formerly *The Homeopathic Times.* Went over to allopathy.

North American Homeopathic Journal

Date   1851-1855
Location   New York City
Publisher   William Radde
Editor   Constantine Hering; E.E. Marcy; J.W. Metcalf
Description   Quarterly. Suspended operations in November 1853 following the resignation of Hering and the poor health of Metcalf; resumed in August 1856 as *The North American Journal of Homeopathy.* Prominent feature was report of provings and clinical cases.

North American Journal of Homeopathy, a Quarterly Magazine of Medicine and the Auxiliary Sciences

Date   1856-1923
Location   New York City
Publisher   William Radde
Editor   John C. Peters (New York); E.E. Marcy (New York); William H. Holcombe (Nachez, Mississippi); Henry C. Preston (Providence, Rhode Island). In 1860, the editorial board changed; and again in 1861, bringing in a broader range of regional editors.
Description   Quarterly. Took public issue with the editorial policies of the *Philadelphia Journal of Homeopathy.* Was accused of being in league with eclecticism and "other empirical schools," and with contributing "to render our house fearfully divided against itself." John C. Peters of New York was the chief editor until 1861 when F.G. Snelling took over. With the tenth volume, the journal dropped the

words *A Quarterly Magazine of Medicine and the Auxiliary Sciences* from its title. In 1870, the journal began a new series under editors F.W. Hunt and Samuel Lilienthal. Quarterly changed to monthly in 1885. Editorship changed in 1885 to G.M. Dillow and in 1892 to Eugene H. Porter. Formerly *North American Homeopathic Journal*.

Northwestern (The) Annalist

Date	1876-1877
Location	Dubuque, Iowa
Editor	E.A. Guilbert
Description	Quarterly. Dedicated to introducing homeopathy into the University of Iowa. Only four numbers issued.

North-Western Journal of Homeopathia

Date	1848-1852
Location	Chicago
Publisher	George E. Shipman
Editor	George E. Shipman
Description	Monthly; continued for four years. Contributions from the best writers on homeopathy. Extracts and reports from foreign periodicals.

Northwestern Journal of Homeopathy

Date	1889-1891
Location	Cedar Rapids, Iowa
Publisher	Medical Pub. Co.
Editor	A.C. Cowperthwaite
Description	Monthly. Merged in 1893 with *Medical Century*.

North Western Journal of Homeopathy

Date	1858
Location	Chicago
Publisher	Association of Homeopathic Physicians
Editor	Cowell and Halsey
Description	Quarterly; claimed to be a new series of the journal conducted by Shipman. Purported to be a quarterly magazine of medicine and the auxiliary sciences and edited by an as-

sociation of homeopathic physicians. Lasted only one issue.

North (The) Western Sanitarian

Date	1894
Location	Kenosh, Wisconsin
Description	Intended for laity.

Northern Ohio Medical and Scientific Examiner

Date	1848-1849
Location	Cleveland; Columbus
Publisher	Oliver and Gilmen
Editor	A.W. Oliver; J. Wheeler; C.D. Williams; J. Gilman; W.B. Waterman
Description	Name changed to *Ohio Medical Examiner* after four issues.

Occidental (The)

Date	1869
Location	St. Louis
Publisher	J.V. Hogan
Editor	G.S. Walker; T.G. Comstock
Description	Monthly. Organ of the Homeopathic Mutual Life Insurance Company. Published less than a year.

Ohio Medical Examiner

Date	1848
Location	Columbus, Ohio
Publisher	A.W. Oliver; John Gilman
Editor	A.W. Oliver; John Gilman
Description	First journal whose title did not bear the distinguishing name "homeopath" or "homeopathy."

Ohio Medical and Surgical Reporter

Date	1867-1877
Location	Cleveland
Publisher	Beckwith and Co.; Witte and Co. (1868)
Editor	T.P. Wilson; G.W. Barnes; H.H. Baxter (1870) et al.

Description   Bimonthly; organ of the Cleveland Homeopathic Hospital
                College and the profession of Ohio. Formerly *American
                Homeopathist.*

Pacific Coast Homeopathic Bulletin

Date   1943-1974
Location   Glendale, California
Description   Issued by the California State Homeopathic Medical Soci-
                ety. Published thirty-two volumes. Became *Homeother-
                apy* in 1974.

Pacific Coast Journal of Homeopathy

Date   1893-1940
Location   San Francisco
Publisher   Journal Pub. Co.
Editor   William Boericke
Description   Quarterly.

Pan-Therapist

Date   1923-1924
Location   New York
Publisher   Auto-Hemic Therapy Foundation Society
Description   Monthly. Formerly *North American Journal of Homeopa-
                thy.*

Pellet (The)

Date   1872
Location   Boston
Editor   J.B. Aldrich; J.M. Bugbee
Description   A record of the Massachusetts Homeopathic Hospital
                Fair.

Pellet (The)

Date   1876
Location   Brooklyn
Description   Published in the interest of the Brooklyn Homeopathic
                Hospital Fair. One number was issued yearly.

Pellet (The)

Date	1884
Location	Cincinnati
Editor	Mrs. W. Owens; Miss F.E. Worthington; Stella Hunt
Description	Published during fair held in aid of the Ohio Hospital for Women and Children.

Pellet (The)

Date	1886
Location	Chelsa, Massachusetts
Editor	Mrs. C.A. Richardson; Mrs H. Sawyer
Description	Published by the Chelsa, Massachusetts, Hospital Aid Association.

People's (The) Health Journal of Chicago

Date	1885-1892
Location	Chicago
Publisher	People's Health Journal Co.
Editor	L.D. Rogers; S. Ida Wright Rogers
Description	Monthly. Intended for laity. Devoted to health, hygiene, and preventive medicine.

Periscope (The)

Date	1878
Location	Dubuque, Iowa
Publisher	Remedial Instrument Co.
Editor	R.S. Gee
Description	Bimonthly. Organ of the Remedial Instrument Company. Devoted to physical, mental, and moral culture.

Pharmacy Bulletin

Date	1881
Location	Chicago
Publisher	Duncan Brothers

Phi Alpha Gamma Quarterly

Date	1901
Description	National fraternity.

Phials

Date	1900-1905
Location	Ann Arbor
Publisher	Parker and Snyder
Description	Annual.

Philadelphia Homeopathic Journal

Date	1838
Location	Philadelphia
Publisher	Association of Homeopathic Physicians
Editor	Constantine Hering, Lingen, and Neidhard
Description	Six numbers of thirty-six pages each issued; subsequently published under title *Miscellanies on Homeopathy.*

Philadelphia Journal of Homeopathy

Date	1852-1856
Location	Philadelphia
Publisher	Rademacher and Jacob F. Sheek
Editor	William A. Gardiner; Alvan E. Small (1854); John F. Geary (1855)
Description	Monthly; originally intended to uphold strict Hahnemannian view of homeopathy. Contained clinical records, monographs on special diseases, studies of the materia medica, provings of remedies, editorial articles, etc. Considered strong reference source.

Physician's and Surgeon's Investigator

Date	1880-1889
Location	Buffalo, New York
Publisher	Physicians and Surgeons' Association
Editor	S.W. Wetmore; A.A. Hubbell; S.N. Brayton; A.S. Couch; F.P. Lewis; G.W. Lewis; L.A. Bull; J.M. Lee
Description	Monthly. Issued ten volumes. Edited by the faculty of the College of Physicians and Surgeons of Buffalo.

Polychrest (The)

Date	1915-1920
Location	Columbus, Ohio

Publisher   College of Homeopathic Medicine
Editor   A.E. Hinsdale; J.A. Ferree
Description   Quarterly. Later became *The Central Journal of Homeopathy.*

Popular Homeopathic Journal

Date   1866
Location   Elgin, Illinois
Publisher   Smith and Lee
Editor   C.A. Jaeger
Description   Monthly. Devoted to promote the cause of homeopathy and to enlighten the public on its theories and its superiority in practice over other systems of medicine. Six numbers issued.

Popular (The) Medical Examiner

Date   1885
Location   New York
Publisher   N.Y. Medical Examiner Co.
Editor   W.M. Cate
Description   Monthly. Intended for laity.

Post Graduate Bulletin

Date   1897
Location   Chicago

Practicien (Le) Homeopathique

Date   1857-1858
Location   New Orleans
Publisher   L. Caboche
Editor   L. Caboche
Description   Monthly; continued a little more than a year.

Proceedings of the American Institute of Homeopathy

Date   1800s-1866
Location   New York City
Publisher   American Institute of Homeopathy
Description   Annual.

Progress; A Monthly Journal Devoted to Medicine and Surgery

Date	1903-1909
Location	Denver
Editor	D.A. Strickler
Description	Monthly. Resulted from split among Colorado homeo-paths in 1903. Claimed to represent the interests of the Denver Homeopathic Medical College.

Publishers (The) Record

Date	1883
Location	Chicago
Publisher	W.A. Chatterton
Editor	C.H. Evans
Description	Monthly. Journal of information concerning books and periodicals on medical and related subjects.

Pulte (The) Quarterly

Date	1890-1893
Location	Cincinnati
Publisher	Pulte Medical College
Editor	T.M. Stewart et al.
Description	Quarterly. Published in the interests of the Pulte Medical College, its alumni, and the profession.

Quarterly Bulletin

Date	1904
Location	Philadelphia
Description	Organ of Hahnemann Medical College of Philadelphia.

Quarterly Bulletin of Homeopathic Literature

Date	1871-1885
Location	Philadelphia; New York
Publisher	Boericke and Tafel
Description	Quarterly. Succeeded by *The Homeopathic Recorder.*

Quarterly Homeopathic Journal

Date	1849-1854
Location	Boston

Publisher   Otis Clapp
Editor   A.C. Becker; J.E. Birnstill; B. De Gersdoff; J.A. Tarbell
Description   Mainly devoted to the translation and republication of homeopthic news gathered from Germany, France, and England. Recognized two groups of homeopaths: those who accepted the theories of psora and infinitesimals and those who did not.

Quarterly Homeopathic Magazine

Date   1854
Location   Cleveland
Editor   Drs. J.H. Pulte; H.P. Gatchel; C.D. Williams
Description   The editors made frequent use of European homeopathic literature. Formerly *The American Magazine Devoted to Homeopathy and Hydropathy*. One volume issued.

Record (The)

Date   1873
Location   Boston
Publisher   Otis Clapp and Son
Description   Issued irregularly by the Homeopathic Association of Boston University.

Regular (The) Physician

Date   1884
Location   Havanna, New York
Editor   A.P. Hollett
Description   Quarterly. Organ of the Southern Tier Homeopathic Medical Society.

Resonance

Date   1979
Location   Seattle, Washington
Publisher   The Foundation
Editor   Melanie Grimes
Description   Bimonthly. Newsletter of the International Foundation for Homeopathy.

St. Louis Clinical Review

Date	1878-1884
Location	St. Louis
Publisher	Maynard and Co.
Editor	P.G. Valentine; W.B. Edmonds; S.B. Parsons; F. Kraft; J.M. Kershaw
Description	Monthly. United with *The St. Louis Periscope and Homeopathic Medicine and Surgery* to form *The St. Louis Periscope and Clinical Review.*

St. Louis Journal of Homeopathy

Date	1895
Location	St. Louis
Publisher	Schultz Pub. Co.
Description	Joined with *The Clinical Reporter.* Became *St. Louis Journal of Homeopathy and Clinical Reporter* (1895).

St. Louis Journal of Homeopathy and Clinical Reporter

Date	1895-1897
Location	St. Louis
Publisher	Schultz Pub. Co.
Description	Formerly *St. Louis Journal of Homeopathy.* Became *The Clinical Reporter* in 1897.

St. Louis (The) Periscope and Clinical Review

Date	1884-1886
Location	St. Louis
Publisher	F.W. Nixon
Editor	W.B. Edmonds; S.B. Parsons; F. Kraft et al.
Description	Formed by the merger of *The St. Louis Periscope of Homeopathic Medicine and Surgery* and *St. Louis Clinical Review.*

St. Louis (The) Periscope of Homeopathic Medicine and Surgery

Date	1884
Location	St. Louis
Editor	E.C. Franklin

Description Monthly. United with *St. Louis Clinical Review* to become *The St. Louis Periscope and Clinical Review.*

Sanitary Gleanings

Date   1884-1885
Location   Philadelphia
Publisher   Shermon and Co.
Editor   B.W. James
Description Intended for laity. Only twelve numbers published.

Semi-Monthly (The) Bulletin of the Western Exchange

Date   1889
Location   Orrville, Ohio
Description Formerly *Medical News and Bulletin.* Later became *The National Medical News.*

Similibus (The)

Date   1872
Location   New York
Editor   Mrs. Carroll Dunham; Mrs. Henry D. Paine
Description Published for the benefit of the Homeopathic Surgical Hospital. Complete in ten numbers.

Simillimum

Date   199?
Location   Portland, Oregon
Description Quarterly. Organ of the Homeopathic Academy of Naturopathic Physicians.

Small Remedies and Interesting Cases

Date   1990
Location   Seattle, Washington; Dubuque, Iowa
Publisher   International Foundation of Homeopathy
Description Annual. Proceedings of the professional case conference.

Southern Homeopathic Pellet

Date   1884-1885
Location   Austin, Texas
Description Renamed *Southern Journal of Homeopathy.*

Southern (The) Journal of Health

Date   1885
Location   Atlanta; Ashville, North Carolina
Editor   H.P. Gatchell
Description Intended for laity.

Southern Journal of Homeopathy

Date   1885-1897
Location   Austin, Texas; New Orleans
Publisher   C.E. Fisher
Editor   C.E. Fisher
Description Monthly. Formerly *Southern Homeopathic Pellet.* In 1897
             it became *American Medical Monthly.*

South-Western (The) Homeopathic Journal and Review

Date   1847-1850
Location   St. Louis
Editor   John J. Temple; Thomas Houghton
Description Monthly; extended through three volumes. First homeo-
             pathic periodical published in the West.

Student Newsletter and Hospital Tidings

Date   1895
Location   Chicago
Description Published by the Chicago Homeopathic Medical College.

Sugar Pills

Date   1874
Location   Cincinnati
Description In aid of the Homeopathic Free Dispensary at Seventh and
             Mound Streets. Six numbers issued.

Surgical (The) Record

Date	1889
Location	Omaha
Publisher	A.L. Stonecypher
Editor	E.F. Allen; D.A. Foote
Description	Bimonthly. Name changed to *The Medical and Surgical Record* in 1889.

Syracuse Clinic

Date	1898-1900
Location	Syracuse, New York
Publisher	Clinic Pub. Co.
Editor	E.E. Keeler
Description	Also called *Good Health Clinic*.

Syracuse Homeopathic Hospital Record

Date	1899
Location	Syracuse, New York

Texas (The) Homeopathic Pellet

Date	1883-1884
Location	Austin, Texas
Publisher	C.E. Fisher
Editor	C.E. Fisher
Description	Monthly. Medical journal devoted to the missionary interests of homeopathy. In 1884 changed name to *Southern Homeopathic Pellet,* then to *Southern Journal of Homeopathy* in 1885. In 1897, it became the *American Medical Monthly.*

Theory and Practice of Medicine

Date	1893
Location	Chicago
Publisher	Medical Advance Co.
Editor	H.W. Pierson

Transactions of the American Institute of Homeopathy

Date	1867-1909
Location	Boston
Publisher	American Institute of Homeopathy
Description	Annual. Transactions of the sessions of the American In-stitute of Homeopathy. Some sessions were held in con-junction with international congresses.

Transactions of the Homeopathic Medical Society of the State of New York

Date	1862-1919
Location	New York
Publisher	Homeopathic Medical Society of the State of New York
Description	Annual. Published total of fifty-four volumes.

Transactions of the Homeopathic Medical Society of the State of Pennsylvania

Date	1867
Location	West Chester, Pennsylvania
Publisher	Homeopathic Medical Society
Editor	Taylor and Hickman
Description	Annual.

Transactions of the Illinois Homeopathic Medical Association

Date	1800s
Location	New York
Publisher	Illinois Homeopathic Medical Association
Description	Annual.

Transactions of the New Jersey State Homeopathic Medical Society

Date	1854
Location	Caldwell, New York
Publisher	Homeopathic Medical Society
Description	Annual.

Transactions of the Southern Homeopathic Medical Association

Date	1800s
Location	Baltimore

Publisher   Southern Homeopathic Medical Association
Description   Annual.

Transformation Times

Date   1982
Location   Portland, Oregon
Publisher   Swift Communications
Description   Monthly.

United States Journal of Homeopathy

Date   1860-1863
Location   New York
Publisher   C.T. Hurlburt
Editor   E.E. Marcy; Henry C. Preston et al.
Description   Quarterly. Marcy and Preston withdrew from the *North American Journal of Homeopathy* and associated with fifty-two other homeopathic physicians to publish this journal. It continued for two years and then merged into the *North American Journal of Homeopathy* in 1863. The editors recognized only one therapeutic law, that of *similia similibus curantur,* and under no circumstances would admit that it was one of several laws of cure. Such admissions were for the eclectic and ultraallopathist but not the homeopath.

United (The) States Medical Investigator

Date   1875-1892
Location   Chicago
Publisher   Duncan Brothers; W.E. Reed; W.A. Chatterton
Editor   C.H. Evans; T.C. Duncan
Description   Semimonthly. See *Medical Investigator.*

United States Medical and Surgical Journal; A Quarterly Magazine of the Homeopathic Practice of Medicine and Medical Science in General

Date   1865-1875
Location   Chicago
Publisher   C.S. Halsey
Editor   George E. Shipman; A.E. Small et al.

Description   Quarterly. First published under the auspices of the West-
                       ern Institute of Homeopathy. Later issued by Professors
                       A.E. Small, R. Ludlam, W. Danforth, and R.N. Foster, all
                       of the Hahnemann Medical College of Chicago. Merged
                       in 1875 into *The United States Medical Investigator.*

University (The) Homeopathic Observer

Date   1903-1905
Location   Ann Arbor, Michigan
Publisher   University of Michigan
Editor   W.B. Hinsdale
Description   Quarterly. Organ of the medical department of the Univer-
                       sity of Michigan, Ann Arbor.

Wayside (The)

Date   1888
Location   Nappanee, Illinois
Editor   H.W. Mumaw
Description   Quarterly. Intended for laity and devoted to physical and
                       social culture. Four numbers issued.

Western (The) Homeopathic Observer

Date   1863-1871
Location   St. Louis
Publisher   H.G.C. Luyties
Editor   William Tod Helmuth; G.S. Walker; E.C. Franklin
Description   Monthly; contained short and interesting articles for the
                       profession. Discontinued at close of seventh volume.

Western (The) Journal of Homeopathy

Date   1859
Location   St. Louis
Publisher   Strong and Co.
Editor   E.C. Franklin
Description   Monthly; intended for the homeopathic profession in the
                       Mississippi Valley as a means of communication among
                       them.

Western New York Journal of Homeopathy

Date   1846-1854
Location   New York
Publisher   Drs. Kirby and Snow
Editor   Drs. S.R. Kirby; R.A. Snow
Description   Only one number was published and this was reprinted under the title of *American Journal of Homeopathy.*

Wisconsin (The) Medical Record

Date   1885
Location   Wisconsin
Editor   E.F. Storke
Description   Issued only one number. Represented interests of Wisconsin Homeopathic Medical Society.

Your Health; A National Health Magazine

Date   1927-1930
Location   Chardon, Ohio
Publisher   American Institute of Homeopathy
Description   Monthly. Official organ of the Women's Homeopathic League. Formerly *Your Health and the Central Journal of Homeopathy.* Became *Your Health Magazine.*

Your Health Magazine

Date   1930-1931
Location   Camden, New York
Publisher   Your Health Pub.
Description   Monthly. Family magazine of good health.

Your Health and the Central Journal of Homeopathy

Date   1926-1927
Location   Chardon, Ohio
Publisher   Homeopathic Medical Society of Ohio
Description   Monthly.

Appendix B

Homeopathic Colleges

Alumni Association of Homeopathic Colleges of Missouri

Location   St. Louis
Date   1876-1880
Comments   In 1880 a portion of faculty seceded and revived the St. Louis College of Homeopathic Physicians and Surgeons which held only two sessions. (See corresponding entry.)

American College of Medical Science

Location   New York
Date   1858
Comments   No information available.

Boston University School of Medicine

Location   Boston
Date   1869-1918
Comments   Incorporated in 1869 and lectures commenced in 1873. First class graduated in 1874. Merged with the New England Female Medical College in 1874. (See corresponding entry.) Became nonsectarian in 1918.

Buffalo College of Rational Medicine

Location   Buffalo, New York
Date   1879
Comments   Extinct. Fraudulent.

Central Michigan Homeopathic Medical College

Location   Lansing
Date   1871-1873

Comments   Incorporated in 1871 and opened the same year. Also called Michigan Homeopathic College. Held only one session. Became extinct 1873.

Chicago Homeopathic Medical College

Location   Chicago
Date   18,76-1904
Comments   First class graduated in 1877. Consolidated with Hahnemann Medical College and Hospital in 1904. (See corresponding entry.)

Cleveland Homeopathic Hospital College

Location   Cleveland
Date   1867-1870
Comments   School remained small and eventually merged with the Western College of Homeopathic Medicine, which became known as Cleveland Homeopathic Medical College.

Cleveland Homeopathic Medical College

Location   Cleveland
Date   1898-1910
Comments   Formed by union of Cleveland University of Medicine and Surgery and Cleveland Medical College. Merged in 1910 with Pulte Medical College to form Cleveland-Pulte Medical College. (See corresponding entries.)

Cleveland Medical College

Location   Cleveland
Date   1890-1898
Comments   Incorporated in 1890 and commenced lectures same year. First class graduated in 1892. Joined Cleveland University of Medicine and Surgery to form Cleveland Homeopathic Medical College in 1898. (See corresponding entries.)

Cleveland University of Medicine and Surgery

Location   Cleveland
Date   1894-1898

Comments   Formerly Cleveland Homeopathic Hospital College. (See corresponding entry.)

Cleveland-Pulte Medical College

Location   Cleveland
Date   1910-1914
Comments   Formerly Cleveland Homeopathic Medical College. In 1910 it absorbed Pulte Medical College. Property transferred to Ohio State University in 1914 to form Ohio State University College of Homeopathic Medicine. (See corresponding entries.)

College of Homeopathic Medicine and Surgery of the Kansas City University

Location   Kansas City
Date   1896-1900
Comments   First class graduated in 1897. Name changed to Hahnemann Medical College of the Kansas City University in 1901. United in 1902 with Kansas City Homeopathic Medical College to form Kansas City Hahnemann Medical College. (See corresponding entries.)

College of Homeopathic Medicine and Surgery of the University of Minnesota

Location   Minneapolis
Date   1888-1909
Comments   Absorbed Minnesota Homeopathic Medical College (see corresponding entry) in 1888. First class graduated in 1889. Abolished by Board of Regents in 1909 and absorbed by University of Minnesota College of Medicine and Surgery.

College of Physicians and Surgeons

Location   Buffalo, New York
Date   1879-1884
Comments   Illegally organized. First class graduated 1881. Charter revoked in 1884.

Denver Homeopathic Medical College

Location	Denver
Date	1894-1907
Comments	First class graduated in 1896. In 1907 it became nonsectarian as the Westminster University College of Medicine. Changed name in 1908 to Denver College of Physicians and Surgeons. Extinct in 1909.

Detroit Homeopathic College

Location	Detroit
Date	1899-1912
Comments	Formerly Homeopathic Medical College of Detroit. (See corresponding entry.) First class graduated in 1900. Extinct 1912.

Dunham Medical College and Hospital

Location	Chicago
Date	1895-1903
Comments	First class graduated in 1896. Merged with Hering Medical College (see corresponding entry) in 1903.

German Homeopathic Medical College

Location	Chicago
Date	1891-1900
Comments	Located at 512-14 Noble Street near Milwaukee Avenue. Lectures commenced in 1891 and given in both English and German. Extinct. Chartered by Johann Malok. Not recognized.

German-American Homeopathic Medical College

Location	Chicago
Date	1892
Comments	Extinct. Chartered by Johann Malok. Fraudulent.

Hahnemann Hospital College of San Francisco

Location	San Francisco
Date	1888-1902

Comments   Formerly Hahnemann Medical College. Name changed in 1902 to Hahnemann Medical College of the Pacific. (See corresponding entries.)

Hahnemann Medical College

Location   San Franscisco
Date   1881-1888
Comments   Incorporated in 1881 and lectures commenced in 1884. First class graduated in 1884. Name changed in 1888 to Hahnemann Hospital College of San Francisco. In 1902 name changed again to Hahnemann Medical College of the Pacific. Merged with University of California Medical School in 1915. (See corresponding entries.)

Hahnemann Medical College and Hospital

Location   Chicago
Date   1855-1922
Comments   First class graduated in 1860. In 1904 college absorbed Chicago Homeopathic Medical College. (See corresponding entry.)

Hahnemann Medical College and Hospital of Philadelphia

Location   Philadelphia
Date   1885-present
Comments   Formerly Hahnemann Medical College of Philadelphia. Commenced lectures in 1886. Coeducation since 1941. Dropped required courses in homeopathy in 1945 and discontinued last elective class in 1959. (See corresponding entry.)

Hahnemann Medical College of the Kansas City University

Location   Kansas City
Date   1901-1902
Comments   Formerly College of Homeopathic Medicine and Surgery of the Kansas City University. United in 1902 with Kansas City Homeopathic Medical College to form Kansas City Hahnemann Medical College. (See corresponding entries.)

Hahnemann Medical College of the Pacific

Location   San Francisco
Date   1902-1915
Comments   Formerly Hahnemann Hospital College of San Francisco. Merged with University of California Medical School in 1915. (See corresponding entries.)

Hahnemmann Medical College of Philadelphia

Location   Philadelphia
Date   1867-1885
Comments   Incorporated in 1867 and lectures commenced same year. Classes graduated in 1868 and 1869. Merged with the Homeopathic Medical College of Pennsylvania in 1869 and kept name. Became Hahnemann Medical College and Hospital of Philadelphia in 1885. (See corresponding entries.)

Hering Medical College

Location   St. Louis
Date   1880-1882
Comments   Organized in 1880 and held two sessions. In 1882 united with the Homeopathic Medical College of Missouri. (See corresponding entry.)

Hering Medical College and Hospital and Postgraduate School of Homeopathy

Location   Chicago
Date   1892-1913
Comments   First class graduated in 1893. Absorbed Dunham Medical College and Hospital (see corresponding entry) in 1903. Closed in 1913.

Homeopathic College

Location   Buffalo, New York
Date   18??-1874
Comments   Extinct prior to 1874.

Homeopathic College of Physicians and Surgeons

Location	Buffalo, New York
Date	1879-1880
Comments	First and only class graduated 1880.

Homeopathic College of Vermont

Location	Vermont
Date	1854
Comments	Never organized by the Vermont State Society.

Homeopathic Department of the University of Nebraska College of Medicine

Location	Lincoln, Nebraska
Date	1883-1887
Comments	Lectures commenced in 1883. First class graduated in 1884. Extinct 1887.

Homeopathic Hospital College

Location	Cleveland
Date	1870-1894
Comments	Merged with Homeopathic Medical College for Women in 1870. (See corresponding entry.) First class graduated in 1871.

Homeopathic Medical College for Women

Location	Cleveland
Date	1868-1870
Comments	Incorporated in 1868 and opened the same year. Only one session held. Merged with the Homeopathic Hospital-College in 1870. (See corresponding entry.)

Homeopathic Medical College of Detroit

Location	Detroit
Date	1872-1899
Comments	Suspended in 1876. Reorganized in 1899 as Detroit Homeopathic College. (See corresponding entry.) Extinct 1912.

Homeopathic Medical College of Missouri

Location   St. Louis
Date   1864-1909
Comments   Reorganized in 1882 and absorbed Hering Medical College and St. Louis College of Homeopathic Physicians and Surgeons. (See corresponding entries.) Became extinct in 1909.

Homeopathic Medical College of Pennsylvania

Location   Philadelphia
Date   1848-1869
Comments   Incorporated in 1848 and lectures commenced same year. First class graduated in 1849. In 1869 it united with Hahnemann Medical College of Philadelphia and took the latter title. Became Hahnemann Medical College and Hospital of Philadelphia in 1885. (See corresponding entries.)

Homeopathic Medical College of St. Louis

Location   St. Louis
Date   1873-1883
Comments   Suspended after 1875. Extinct since 1883. Fraudulent.

Homeopathic Medical College of the State of New York

Location   New York City
Date   1860-1869
Comments   Incorporated in 1860 and lectures commenced same year. First class graduated in 1861. Assumed titled of New York Homeopathic Medical College in 1869; New York Homeopathic Medical College and Hospital in 1887; New York Homeopathic Medical College and Flower Hospital in 1909; and New York Medical College and Flower Hospital in 1936. (See corresponding entries.)

Independent Medical School of Philadelphia

Location   Philadelphia
Date   1854

Comments   Chartered in 1854 and prospectus provided by Constantine Hering and Adolph Lippe. Never organized.

Kansas City Hahnemann Medical College

Location   Kansas City
Date   1902-1915
Comments   First class graduated 1903. Formed by the union of the Kansas City Homeopathic Medical College and the Hahnemann Medical College of the Kansas City University. In 1915 name changed to Southwest School of Medicine and Hospital. (See corresponding entries.) Held one session under new name. Extinct in 1916.

Kansas City Homeopathic Medical College

Location   Kansas City
Date   1888-1902
Comments   Incorporated in 1888 and commenced lectures same year. First class graduated in 1889. United in 1902 with Hahnemann Medical College of the Kansas City University to form Kansas City Hahnemann Medical College. (See corresponding entries.)

Michigan School of Homeopathy and Surgery

Location   Detroit
Date   1863
Comments   Extinct.

Minnesota Homeopathic Medical College

Location   Minneapolis
Date   1886-1888
Comments   Incorporated in 1886 and commenced lectures the same year. Ceased to exist in 1888 and became the College of Homeopathic Medicine and Surgery of the University of Minnesota. (See corresponding entry.) Supported by the state.

National Homeopathic Medical College

Location   Chicago
Date   1891-1895

Comments   Opened at 541 North Halstead Street in 1891. Coeducational. Offered a three-year course of study, each session being six months. First class graduated 1892.

National Homeopathic Medical College

Location   Washington, DC
Date   1893-1896
Comments   First class graduated in 1894. Merged into the Washington Homeopathic Medical College (see corresponding entry) in 1896.

New England Female Medical College

Location   Boston
Date   1848-1874
Comments   First class graduated in 1849. Gravitated to homeopathy. Merged in 1874 with Boston University School of Medicine. (See corresponding entry.)

New York Homeopathic Medical College

Location   New York City
Date   1869-1887
Comments   First class graduated 1870. Formerly Homeopathic Medical College of the State of New York. Became New York Homeopathic Medical College and Hospital in 1887. (See corresponding entries.)

New York Homeopathic Medical College and Flower Hospital

Location   New York City
Date   1909-1936
Comments   Formerly New York Homeopathic Medical College and Hospital (see corresponding entry). Renamed New York Medical College and Flower Hospital in 1936.

New York Homeopathic Medical College and Hospital

Location   New York City
Date   1887-1909

Comments   Formerly New York Homeopathic Medical College. Later named New York Homeopathic Medical College and Flower Hospital in 1909. (See corresponding entries.)

New York Medical College and Hospital for Women

Location   New York City
Date   1866-1918
Comments   Formerly New York Medical College for Women. (See corresponding entry.)

New York Medical College for Women

Location   New York City
Date   1863-1866
Comments   Incorporated in 1863. First class graduated 1864. Assumed title New York Medical College and Hospital for Women in 1866. (See corresponding entry.) Became extinct 1918.

North American Academy of the Homeopathic Healing Art

Location   Allentown, Pennsylvania
Date   1835-1841
Comments   Founded in 1835 and incorporated in 1836. Teaching was entirely in German. Extinct around 1841. Last meeting of the directors was in 1842.

Ohio State University College of Homeopathic Medicine

Location   Columbus
Date   1914-1922
Comments   Organized when the property of the Cleveland-Pulte Medical College of Cleveland (see corresponding entry) was transferred to the Ohio State University. Classes graduated from 1915 to 1922. College abolished in 1922 by the Board of Trustees.

Penn Medical University

Location   Philadelphia
Date   1853-1880

Comments   Incorporated in 1853 and lectures commenced same year. Suspended lectures in 1863 and reorganized in 1873. An independent school teaching both homeopathy and eclecticism. Provided a graded course of study. Closed in 1880.

Post-Graduate School of Homeopathics

Location   Philadelphia
Date   1890-1900
Comments   Incorporated in 1890 and commenced lectures same year. Founded by James Tylor Kent and funded by John Pitcairn, founder of Pittsburgh Plate Glass and a leader in the Swedenborgian Church. The school trained thirty physicians over the course of its history and its free clinic treated more than forty thousand patients. In 1900, Kent moved the school to Chicago where he became dean of the Dunham Medical College and Hospital. In 1903, Dunham merged with Hering Medical College. (See corresponding entries.)

Pulte Medical College

Location   Cincinnati
Date   1872-1910
Comments   Incorporated in 1872 and lectures commenced same year. First class graduated in 1873. Merged in 1910 with the Cleveland Homeopathic Medical College to form the Cleveland-Pulte Medical College. (See corresponding entries.)

St. Louis College of Homeopathic Physicians and Surgeons

Location   St. Louis
Date   1869-1882
Comments   Formed in 1869 from faculty of the Alumni Association of Homeopathic Colleges of Missouri. Held two sessions. Suspended in 1871 and revived in 1880. Consolidated with Hering Medical College and the Homeopathic Medical College of Missouri in 1882. (See corresponding entries.)

St. Louis Hahnemann Medical College

Location	St. Louis
Date	1873-1874
Comments	Graduated one class of four students. Extinct 1874.

Southern Homeopathic Medical College

Location	Baltimore
Date	1907-1910
Comments	Formerly Southern Homeopathic Medical College and Hospital (see corresponding entry). Extinct 1910.

Southern Homeopathic Medical College and Hospital

Location	Baltimore
Date	1890-1907
Comments	Incorporated in 1890. First class graduated in 1892. Co-education established in 1902. Name changed in 1907 to Southern Homeopathic Medical College (see corresponding entry). Extinct in 1910.

Southwest School of Medicine and Hospital

Location	Kansas City
Date	1915-1916 ·
Comments	Formerly Kansas City Hahnemann Medical College (see corresponding entry). Held one session. Extinct in 1916.

Southwestern Homeopathic Medical College

Location	Louisville
Date	1893-1910
Comments	First class graduated in 1894. Extinct in 1910.

State University of Iowa, College of Homeopathic Medicine

Location	Iowa City
Date	1877-1919
Comments	Incorporated in 1877 and lectures commenced in same year. First class graduated in 1878. Supported by the state. Offered a three-year graded course of study. Abolished in 1919.

University of Michigan Homeopathic Medical College

Location   Ann Arbor
Date   1873-1922
Comments   Created by special appropriation of Michigan legislature
             in 1873-1874. Lectures commenced in 1875 and first class
             graduated in 1877. Abolished by Board of Regents in
             1922.

Washington Homeopathic Medical College

Location   Washington, DC
Date   1896
Comments   Closed for failure to meet legal requirements.

Western College of Homeopathic Medicine

Location   Cleveland
Date   1849-1857
Comments   Incorporated in 1849 and lectures commenced in 1850.
             First class graduated in 1850. Name changed in 1857 to
             Western Homeopathic College; in 1870 to Homeopathic
             Hospital-College and absorbed the Homeopathic Medical
             College for Women. In 1894 became Cleveland Univer-
             sity of Medicine and Surgery. In 1898 it joined Cleveland
             Medical College to form Cleveland Homeopathic Medical
             College. (See corresponding entries.)

Western Homeopathic College

Location   Cleveland
Date   1857-1870
Comments   Formerly Western College of Homeopathic Medicine. Be-
             came the Homeopathic Hospital-College in 1870. (See
             corresponding entries.)

Western Homeopathic Medical College

Location   St. Louis
Date   1857-1864
Comments   Incorporated in 1857 and lectures commenced in 1859.
             First class graduated in 1860. No sessions held between

1861 and 1864. Reopened in 1864 as Homeopathic Medical College of Missouri.

Women's Medical College of St. Louis

Location   St. Louis
Date   1883-1884
Comments   Organized in 1883 and held only one course of lectures. Extinct 1884.

Notes

Introduction

1. John F. Gray, "Early History of Homeopathy in New York," *North American Journal of Homeopathy,* 12 (1864), 322.

2. E. E. Marcy, *Homeopathy and Allopathy: Reply to an Examination of the Doctrines and Evidences of Homeopathy, by Worthington Hooker, M.D.* (New York: William Radde, 1852), pp. 124-125.

3. J. C. Reeve, "Some of the Latest Systems in Medicine," *Transactions of the Annual Meeting of the Ohio State Medical Society,* (1885), 31-35.

4. Motzi Eklöf, "Doctor or Quack: Legal and Lexical Definitions in Twentieth-Century Sweden," in Robert Jütte, Motzi Eklöf, and Marie C. Nelson (eds.), *Historical Aspects of Unconventional Medicine: Approaches, Concepts, Case Studies* (Sheffield: European Association for the History of Medicine and Health Publications, 2001), p. 104.

5. Guenter B. Risse, "Introduction," in Robert Jütte, Guenter B. Risse, and John Woodward (eds.), *Culture, Knowledge, and Healing: Historical Perspectives of Homeopathic Medicine in Europe and North America* (Sheffield: European Association for the History of Medicine and Health Publications, 1998), p. 1.

Chapter 1

1. "Concise Review of Dr. R. E. Dudgeon's Lectures on the Theory and Practice of Homeopathy, Delivered at the Hahnemann Hospital School of Homeopathy," *Philadelphia Journal of Homeopathy,* 3 (1854), 102; Paul F. Curie, *Principles of Homeopathy* (London: Thomas Hurst, 1837), p. 40.

2. Stephen Simpson, *A Practical View of Homeopathy, Being an Address to British Practitioners on the General Applicability and Superior Efficacy of the Homeopathic Method in the Treatment of Disease. With Cases* (London: J. B. Baillière, 1836), p. 319.

3. Quoted in Joseph Hooper, "Sketch of the Life of Hahnemann," *American Homeopathic Observer,* 3 (1836), 180.

4. Simpson, *A Practical View of Homeopathy,* p. 320.

5. Quoted in Hooper, "Sketch of the Life of Hahnemann," p. 183; Samuel Hahnemann, "On the Great Necessity of a Regeneration of Medicine," in Robert E. Dudgeon (ed.), *The Lesser Writings of Samuel Hahnemann* (New York: William Radde, 1852), pp. 511-512.

6. Samuel Hahnemann, "Instructions for Surgeons Respecting Venereal Diseases, Together with a New Mercurial Preparation," in Dudgeon, *The Lesser Writings of Samuel Hahnemann,* pp. 136-153; Hahnemann, "On the Great Necessity of a

Regeneration of Medicine," p. 512; Hooper, "Sketch of the Life of Hahnemann," p. 183; Worthington Hooker, *Homeopathy: An Examination of Its Doctrines and Evidences* (New York: Charles Scribner, 1851), p. 13; Iris Ritzmann, "Children As Patients in Early Homeopathy," in Martin Dinges (ed.), *Patients in the History of Homeopathy* (Sheffield: European Association for the History of Medicine and Health, 2002), pp. 118-140. In a strongly written article titled "Hahnemann and Homeopathy," John C. Peters, president of the Medical Society of the County of New York, president of the New York Neurological Society, and former editor of the *North American Journal of Homeopathy,* reviewed Hahnemann's claims for the discovery of belladonna as a preservative against scarlet fever. When Hahnemann first announced his prophylactic, he refused to divulge the name of the medicine, and only promised to do so after 300 individuals had subscribed the equivalent of $3.50 to receive the contents of his secret medicine: a 24th millionth part of a grain of dry belladonna juice. According to Peters, few physicians agreed to the "black-mail" and most considered Hahnemann's practice as "selfish, avaricious and quackish." For those who purchased the medicine by subscription but found it ineffective, Hahnemann responded that the medicine could have lost its power due to the distance it had been sent and the long period it may have been kept; neglect by the patient to take the right precautions in preparing and administering the medicine; the effects of weather; and the potential effects of other epidemics. Hahnemann later claimed that belladonna was only to be used against "mild" scarlet fever. Numerous physicians tested his claim and found it wanting. These included H. C. Wood Jr., Jonathan Pereira, George B. Wood, Thomas Waring, Alfred Stillé, Charles D. Meigs, and William Pepper.

7. Samuel Hahnemann (trans.), *William Cullen's Abhandlung über die Materia medica* (2 volumes) (Leipzig: Schwickert, 1790).

8. Hooper, "Sketch of the Life of Hahnemann," pp. 184-185; J. Rutherfurd Russell, "Sketch of the Origin and Progress of Homeopathy," *British Journal of Homeopathy,* 1 (1843), 3; "Hahnemann in the Cradle," *Philadelphia Journal of Homeopathy,* 4 (1855), 41; Benjamin C. Woodbury Jr., "The Homeopathic School of Medicine," Lloyd Library and Museum, Eclectic Medical College, Box 37, folder 1,076, p. 297. According to William Leo-Wolf writing in 1835, Hahnemann's recommendation of drug trials on healthy persons had nothing to do with Haller's recommended trials with simple drugs. Instead, Haller had recommended them to show the particular effects of drugs that might lead, indirectly, to results valuable for the cure of disease "as many would try some newly discovered plant or other substance to learn whether it contains wholesome nourishment, or some medical property which may be successfully used in extraordinary cases." See William Leo-Wolf, *Remarks on the Abracadabra of the Nineteenth Century; Or on Dr. Samuel Hahnemann's Homeopathic Medicine, with Particular Reference to Dr. Constantine Hering's Concise View of the Rise and Progress of Homeopathic Medicine* (New York: Carey, Lea and Blanchard, 1835), p. 88.

9. Hooper, "Sketch of the Life of Hahnemann," pp. 184-185; Russell, "Sketch of the Origin and Progress of Homeopathy," p. 3; "Hahnemann in the Cradle," p. 41; Woodbury, "The Homeopathic School of Medicine," p. 297.

10. Max Neuburger, "The Doctrine of the Healing Power of Nature Throughout the Course of Time," *Journal of the American Institute of Homeopathy,* 25 (1932), 1427-1428.

11. Hahnemann quoted in Neuburger, "The Doctrine of the Healing Power of Nature Throughout the Course of Time," p. 1428.

12. Simpson, *A Practical View of Homeopathy*, p. 59.

13. Dr. Perine, "Address Before the New York State Homeopathic Society," *North American Journal of Homeopathy*, 4 (1855), 174.

14. Doctor Lacombe, *Homeopathia Explained, Being an Exposition of the Doctrine of Hahnemann, According to the Opinions Published by the Principal Physicians of the Faculty of Paris* (New York: James E. Betts, 1835), p. 10. See also Glynis Rankin, "Professional Organization and the Development of Medical Knowledge: Two Interpretations of Homeopathy," in Roger Cooter (ed.), *Studies in the History of Alternative Medicine* (New York: St. Martin's Press, 1988), pp. 51-52.

15. Quoted in Russell, "Sketch of the Origin and Progress of Homeopathy," pp. 5, 8.

16. Edward Bayard, "Discoveries of Hahnemann—With a View of the Past and Present State of Medical Science," *Philadelphia Journal of Homeopathy*, 4 (1855), 46.

17. Quoted in Russell, "Sketch of the Origin and Progress of Homeopathy," pp. 9-10.

18. Quoted in Russell, "Sketch of the Origin and Progress of Homeopathy," p. 11; Samuel Hahnemann, "Essay on a New Principle for Ascertaining the Curative Powers of Drugs, with a Few Glances at Those Higherto Employed," in Dudgeon, *The Lesser Writings of Samuel Hahnemann*, pp. 259-261.

19. Hahnemann, "Essay on a New Principle for Ascertaining the Curative Powers of Drugs, with a Few Glances at Those Higherto Employed," pp. 265, 267.

20. Quoted in Russell, "Sketch of the Origin and Progress of Homeopathy," p. 12.

21. Hahnemann, "Essay on a New Principle for Ascertaining the Curative Powers of Drugs, with a Few Glances at Those Higherto Employed," p. 262.

22. Perine, "Address Before the New York State Homeopathic Society," pp. 164-165.

23. William Coleman, *Biology in the Nineteenth Century: Problems of Form, Function and Transformation* (New York: John Wiley and Sons, Inc., 1971), pp. 24-26, 48-53, 150-151.

24. Quoted in Russell, "Sketch of the Origin and Progress of Homeopathy," p. 14.

25. Samuel Hahnemann, "Are the Obstacles to Certainty and Simplicity in Practical Medicine Insurmountable?" in Dudgeon, *The Lesser Writings of Samuel Hahnemann*, p. 310.

26. Samuel Hahnemann, "A Preface," in Dudgeon, *The Lesser Writings of Samuel Hahnemann*, p. 348.

27. Samuel Hahnemann, "Fragmentary Observations on Brown's Elements of Medicine," in Dudgeon, *The Lesser Writings of Samuel Hahnemann*, pp. 350, 355, 359, 361.

28. Hufeland quoted in Dudgeon, *The Lesser Writings of Samuel Hahnemann*, p. 350.

29. Samuel Hahnemann, "Aesculapius in the Balance," in Dudgeon, *The Lesser Writings of Samuel Hahnemann*, pp. 410-411.

30. Ibid., p. 412.

31. Ibid., pp. 419-420.

32. Thomas Lindsley Bradford, *Life and Letters of Dr. Samuel Hahnemann* (Philadelphia: Boericke & Tafel, 1895), p. 72.

33. Samuel Hahnemann, "The Medicine of Experience," in Dudgeon, *The Lesser Writings of Samuel Hahnemann,* pp. 440, 447-448; Robert E. Dudgeon, "A Century of Homeopathy," Lloyd Library and Museum, Eclectic Medical College, Box 37, Folder 1,082, p. 18.

34. Samuel Hahnemann, "Spirit of Homeopathic Doctrine of Medicine," in Dudgeon, *The Lesser Writings of Samuel Hahnemann,* pp. 617-621.

35. Samuel Hahnemann, "On the Great Necessity of a Regeneration of Medicine," in Dudgeon, *The Lesser Writings of Samuel Hahnemann,* p. 517.

36. Samuel Hahnemann, "On the Present Want of Foreign Medicines," in Dudgeon, *The Lesser Writings of Samuel Hahnemann,* p. 486.

37. In this book I will be using several English editions of the *Organon* to explain Hahnemann's theories. The original 1810 edition was not translated into English until 1913 by C. E. Wheeler. It was published as a historical document for Everyman's Library by J. M. Dent and Sons in London and E. P. Dutton and Company in New York. This translation will be used to explain Hahnemann's earliest thinking. But the first American edition was published in 1836, translated by Robert F. Dudgeon and prepared from the 1833 British translation of the fourth German edition. Other editions will include the eighth American edition (1923) translated from the fifth edition by Dudgeon, and the sixth edition translated into English in 1922 by William Boericke, MD.

38. Samuel Hahnemann, *Organon of Homeopathic Medicine* (Allentown, Pennsylvania: Academical Bookstore, 1836), pp. 10-11.

39. Ibid., pp. 15-17, 19.

40. Ibid., pp. 107-109, 110, 115-116. See also Charles J. Hempel, *Homeopathy, a Principle in Nature: Its Scientific Universality Unfolded; Its Development and Philosophy Explained; and Its Applicability to the Treatment of Diseases Shown* (New York: C. T. Hurlburt, 1860), p. 44.

41. Hahnemann, *Organon of Homeopathic Medicine* (1836), pp. 24-25.

42. Ibid., pp. 30-31, 33.

43. Ibid., pp. 34-35.

44. Quoted in Hahnemann, *Organon of Homeopathic Medicine* (1836), pp. xiii, 76-77.

45. Hahnemann also distinguished between *homeopathic,* meaning "similar," and *homopathic,* meaning "common, identical, or the same." See Samuel Hahnemann, "Nota Benne for My Reviewers," in Dudgeon, *The Lesser Writings of Samuel Hahnemann,* p. 659; Puhlman, "The History of Homeopathy in Germany," p. 11.

46. Hahnemann, *Organon of Homeopathic Medicine* (1836), pp. 80-81; Samuel Hahnemann, *Organon of the Rational Art of Healing* (London: J.M. Dent and Sons, 1913 [1810]), p. 2.

47. Hahnemann, *Organon of Homeopathic Medicine* (1836), pp. 84, 91; Hahnemann, *Organon of the Rational Art of Healing* (1810), pp. 4-6, 9.

48. Hahnemann, *Organon of Homeopathic Medicine* (1836), 191; Hahnemann, *Organon of the Rational Art of Healing* (1810), pp. 18-19, 83.

49. Hahnemann, *Organon of the Rational Art of Healing* (1810), pp. 50-51.

50. Ibid., p. 56.

51. Hahnemann, *Organon of Homeopathic Medicine* (1836), pp. 143-145; Joseph H. Pulte, *Homeopathic Domestic Physician: Containing the Treatment of Diseases; with Popular Explanations of Anatomy, Physiology, Hygiene and Hydropathy: Also an Abridged Materia Medica* (Cincinnati: H.W. Derby and Co., 1851), pp. 39-42; Dinges, *Patients in the History of Homeopathy,* p. 4.

52. Samuel Hahnemann, "On the Effects of Coffee, from Original Observations," in Dudgeon, *The Lesser Writings of Samuel Hahnemann,* pp. 391-392.

53. Ibid., pp. 402, 404-405.

54. I. G. Rosenstein, *Theory and Practice of Homeopathy. First Part, Containing a Theory of Homeopathy, with Dietetic Rules, Etc.* (Louisville: Henkle and Logan, 1840), p. 136. In the United States, homeopathists tended to allow patients to drink black tea, having decided that it had become, like coffee, a common drink for most constitutions. See James McNaughton, "Annual Address Delivered Before the Medical Society of the State of New York, February 6, 1838," *Transactions of the Medical Society of the State of New York,* 4 (1838), p. 13.

55. Hahnemann, *Organon of the Rational Art of Healing* (1810), pp. 62-65, 85-86, 90.

56. Ibid., pp. 99, 101.

57. Russell, "Sketch of the Origin and Progress of Homeopathy," p. 21.

58. Hooper, "Sketch of the Life of Hahnemann," p. 188.

59. Gustav Puhlman, "The History of Homeopathy in Germany," *Transactions of the World's Homeopathic Convention, Held at Philadelphia, Under the Auspices of the American Institute of Homeopathy, at Its Twenty-Ninth Session, June 26-July 1, 1876* (2 volumes) (Philadelphia: Sherman and Company, 1880), pp. 14-15.

60. Samuel Hahnemann, *Materia Medica Pura* (4 volumes) (New York: Radde, 1846), Vol. II, pp. iv-v.

61. Hahnemann, *Materia Medica Pura,* Vol. I, pp. ix-xi.

62. Ibid., p. 21.

63. Ibid., p. 36.

64. Ibid., pp. 144-147.

65. Hahnemann, *Materia Medica Pura,* Vol. II, p. 102.

66. Hahnemann, *Materia Medica Pura,* Vol. III, pp. 22-23.

67. Hahnemann, *Materia Medica Pura,* Vol. III, pp. 27-41; Martin Dinges, "Men's Bodies 'Explained' on a Daily Basis in Letters from Patients to Samuel Hahnemann (1830-35)," in Dinges, *Patients in the History of Homeopathy,* pp. 101-105.

68. Hooper, "Sketch of the Life of Hahnemann," pp. 188-189; Dudgeon, "A Century of Homeopathy," p. 19.

69. Thomas Lindsay Bradford, *The Life and Letters of Dr. Samuel Hahnemann* (Philadelphia: Boericke & Tafel, 1895), pp. 128-129; see also Martin Dinges (ed.), *Patients in the History of Homeopathy* (Sheffield: European Association for the History of Medicine and Health, 2002).

70. John F. Gray, "Early History of Homeopathy in New York," *North American Journal of Homeopathy,* 12 (1864), 324.

71. Bradford, *Life and Letters,* p. 131.

72. Gustav Puhlman, "The History of Homeopathy in Germany," *Transactions of the World's Homeopathic Convention, Held at Philadelphia, Under the Auspices of the American Institute of Homeopathy, at Its Twenty-Ninth Session, June 26-July*

1, 1876, Volume II: *History of Homeopathy* (2 volumes) (Philadelphia: Sherman and Company, 1880), p. 16. Hahnemann's only son, Friedreich (b. 1786), seems to have been among the early provers of his father's medicines. After taking his degree at Leipzig, he married a widow, thereby giving offense to his father and causing an estrangement between the two. The son established a practice in Wolkenstein and when his success led to jealousy among professional colleagues, the Medical College of Saxony forbade him from practicing. Little is known of his whereabouts after his move although he was thought to have lived in Dublin, Ireland, before moving to New York. In 1830, an individual by the name of Frederick Hahnemann reportedly traveled through Pennsylvania curing people with various small powders. He was described as a hunchback who dressed strangely and spoke with a heavy German accent. See Robert E. Dudgeon (ed.), *The Lesser Writings of Samuel Hahnemann* (New York: William Radde, 1852), p. 235.

73. Samuel Hahnemann, *Organon of Homeopathic Medicine* (Allentown, PA: Academical Bookstore, 1836), pp. 143-145; Bernhardt Fincke, "Improved Process of Preparing Homeopathic Medicines," *American Homeopathic Observer,* 9 (1872), 10-11. The decimal potency was introduced after Hahnemann's death.

74. Hahnemann, *Organon of Homeopathic Medicine* (1836), pp. 200-201, 205; B. F. Joslin, *Principles of Homeopathy. In a Series of Lectures* (New York: William Radde, 1850), pp. 40-41. See also Renate Wittern, "The Origins of Homeopathy in Germany," *Clio medica,* 2 (1991), 55.

75. Hahnemann, *Organon of Homeopathic Medicine* (1836), p. 205.

76. Ibid., p. 208.

77. Benjamin C. Woodbury Jr., "The Homeopathic School of Medicine," in the Lloyd Library and Museum, Eclectic Medical College, Box 37, Folder 1,076, p. 302.

78. "Teachings of Common Sense," *Philadelphia Journal of Homeopathy,* 3 (1854), 91-93.

79. Joslin, *Principles of Homeopathy. In a Series of Lectures,* pp. 40-41.

80. Hahnemann, *Organon of Homeopathic Medicine* (1836), pp. 143-145.

81. Samuel Hahnemann, *The Chronic Diseases: Their Specific Nature and Homeopathic Treatment* (5 volumes) (New York: William Radde, 1845-46), Vol. V, pp. v-vi.

82. Puhlman, "The History of Homeopathy in Germany," pp. 18-19.

83. Bradford, *Life and Letters,* pp. 164-165.

84. Ibid., p. 166.

85. Hahnemann, *The Chronic Diseases,* Vol. I, p. 23.

86. Ibid., pp. 27-28.

87. Ibid., p. 111.

88. For Charles Hempel, these treatments failed due to their making no direct impression upon the vital principle but only upon the disease. Only by treating the sycosis with appropriate internal, and not external, antipsorics would a cure be possible. See Hahnemann, *The Chronic Diseases,* Vol. I, pp. 113-114.

89. Hahnemann, *Organon of Homeopathic Medicine* (1836), pp. 153, 191.

90. Bradford, *Life and Letters,* pp. 171-172.

91. Worthington Hooker, *Homeopathy: An Examination of Its Doctrines and Evidences* (New York: C. Scribner, 1851), p. 51.

92. Puhlman, "The History of Homeopathy in Germany," p. 25.

93. Wittern, "The Origins of Homeopathy in Germany," pp. 55-56.

94. Joseph Hooper, "Sketch of the Life of Hahnemann," *American Homeo-pathic Observer,* 3 (1866), 191.

95. Quoted in Bradford, *Life and Letters,* p. 304.

96. Ibid., p. 301.

97. Quoted in Puhlman, "The History of Homeopathy in Germany," p. 23.

98. Ibid., p. 29.

99. Bradford, *Life and Letters,* pp. 327-329.

100. Ibid., p. 406.

101. Hooper, "Sketch of the Life of Hahnemann," p. 190.

102. Bradford, *Life and Letters,* pp. 350-351, 357; Robert Jütte, "The Paradox of Professionalisation: Homeopathy and Hydropathy As Unorthodoxy in Germany in the 19th and 20th Century," in Robert Jütte, Guenter B. Risse, and John Woodward (eds.), *Culture, Knowledge, and Healing: Historical Perspectives of Homeopathic Medicine in Europe and North America* (Sheffield: European Association for the History of Medicine and Health Publications, 1998), p. 74.

103. Bradford, *Life and Letters,* pp. 376-377, 412, 472. See also Anna Cora Mowatt, *Autobiography of an Actress* (Boston: Ticknor, Reed, and Fields, 1854).

104. T. W. Gordon, "Beauties of Homeopathy Exemplified," *Weekly Medical Gazette,* 1 (1855), 417-423.

105. Samuel Hahnemann, "How Can Small Doses of Such Very Attenuated Medicine As Homeopathy Employs Still Possess Great Power?" in Dudgeon, *The Lesser Writings of Samuel Hahnemann,* pp. 728-729.

106. Bradford, *Life and Letters,* p. 424; William Harvey King, *History of Home-opathy and Its Institutions in America* (4 volumes) (New York: Lewis Publishing Company, 1905), Vol. I, p. 38.

107. Hooper, "Sketch of the Life of Hahnemann," p. 191; "Hahnemann," *British Journal of Homeopathy,* 1 (1843), 329.

108. Bradford, *Life and Letters,* pp. 468-472, 476; Jütte, "The Paradox of Professionalisation," p. 74.

109. A. R. Thomas, "Homeopathic Medical College of Pennsylvania," *Transac-tions of the World's Homeopathic Convention, Held at Philadelphia,* Volume II: History of Homeopathy, p. 798.

110. Prof. Neidhard, "Hahnemann," *American Homeopathic Observer,* 7 (1870), 206. Two years later, in 1872, the French government officially recognized Mélanie's American diploma and granted her the right to practice homeopathy. See Rima Handley, *A Homeopathic Love Story: The Story of Samuel and Mélanie Hahnemann* (Berkeley: North Atlantic Books, 1990), p. 208; Julian Winston, *Faces of Homeopathy* (Tawa, New Zealand: Great Auk Publishing, 1999), p. 43.

111. Erwin H. Ackerknecht, "Elisha Bartlett and the Philosophy of the Paris Clinical School," *Bulletin of the History of Medicine,* 24 (1950), 42-60; Erwin H. Ackerknecht, *Medicine at the Paris Hospital, 1794-1848* (Baltimore: Johns Hopkins University Press, 1967); Michel Foucault, *The Birth of the Clinic: An Ar-chaeology of Medical Perceptions* (New York: Pantheon Books, 1973); Caroline Hannaway and Ann La Berge (eds.), *Constructing Paris Medicine* (Atlanta: Rodopi, 1999); W. F. Bynum, *Science and the Practice of Medicine in the Nineteenth Cen-tury* (Cambridge: Cambridge University Press, 1994).

Chapter 2

1. Robert C. Fuller, *Alternative Medicine and American Religious Life* (New York: Oxford University Press, 1989), Chapter 2 (pp. 12-37).

2. Henry M. Smith, "Homeopathy in New York," *Transactions of the World's Homeopathic Convention, Held at Philadelphia, Under the Auspices of the American Institute of Homeopathy, at Its Twenty-Ninth Session, June 26-July 1, 1876,* Volume II: *History of Homeopathy* (Philadelphia: Sherman and Company, 1880), pp. 440-441; John F. Gray, "Early History of Homeopathy in New York," *North American Journal of Homeopathy,* 12 (1864), 326.

3. H. W. Felter, "Pathfinders," Lloyd Library and Museum, Eclectic Medical College, Box 37, folder 1,070, pp. 17-18; "Homeopathy in the United States," *Transactions of the World's Homeopathic Convention,* Volume II: *History of Homeopathy,* pp. 440-441.

4. Felter, "Pathfinders," p. 18; Gray, "Early History of Homeopathy in New York," pp. 326-327.

5. "Homeopathy in the United States," p. 441.

6. Smith, "Homeopathy in New York," p. 444; "Homeopathy in the United States," pp. 441-443. By this time, Hahnemann's *Organon* had gone through three German editions and had been translated into French. In addition, his six-volume *Materia Medica Pura* was in its second edition.

7. Felter, "Pathfinders," p. 19; Smith, "Homeopathy in New York," pp. 442-445.

8. Gray, "Early History of Homeopathy in New York," pp. 335-336.

9. Felter, "Pathfinders," p. 19; "Homeopathy in the United States," pp. 445-446.

10. Smith, "Homeopathy in New York," pp. 445-447; "Homeopathy in the United States," p. 447.

11. Smith, "Homeopathy in New York," pp. 448-449; Gray, "Early History of Homeopathy in New York," pp. 332-333; "Homeopathy in the United States," pp. 448-449.

12. Smith, "Homeopathy in New York," pp. 447-448; "Homeopathy in the United States," p. 447.

13. Smith, "Homeopathy in New York," p. 448.

14. Smith, "Homeopathy in New York," pp. 449-450; "Homeopathy in the United States," p. 450.

15. "Concerning the American Institute," *American Homeopathic Observer,* 2 (1865), 255; "Homeopathy in the United States," p. 451; Smith, "Homeopathy in New York," pp. 450-451.

16. Felter, "Pathfinders," p. 20; "Homeopathy in the United States," pp. 451-452.

17. Gray, "Early History of Homeopathy in New York," pp. 336-337; Smith, "Homeopathy in New York," pp. 450-451.

18. Walter Sands Mills, "A Matter of History," *The Chironian,* 29 (1913), 414; Walter Sands Mills, "Historical Sketch of the New York Homeopathic Medical College and Flower Hospital, 1860-1910," *The Chironian,* 26 (1910), 343.

19. Smith, "Homeopathy in New York," pp. 455-456.

20. Smith, "Homeopathy in New York," pp. 457-458. See also Charles Morley, *Elements of Animal Magnetism, or, Process and Application for Relieving Human Suffering* (New York: Fowler and Wells, 1859); "Relations Between the Clerical and Medical Professions," *Boston Medical and Surgical Journal,* 38 (1848), 518.

21. Smith, "Homeopathy in New York," pp. 457-458.

22. I. T. Talbot, "Homeopathy in Massachusetts," *Transactions of the World's Homeopathic Convention, Held at Philadelphia, Under the Auspices of the American Institute of Homeopathy, at Its Twenty-Ninth Session, June 26-July 1, 1876,* Volume II: *History of Homeopathy* (2 volumes) (Philadelphia: Sherman and Company, 1880), p. 641.

23. Talbot, "Homeopathy in Massachusetts," pp. 642-644; "Medical News," *Philadelphia Journal of Homeopathy,* 1 (1852), 95-96; Joseph F. Kett, *The Formation of the American Medical Profession: The Role of Institutions, 1780-1860* (New Haven: Yale University Press, 1968), pp. 154-155; Lamar Riley Murphy, *Enter the Physician: The Transformation of Domestic Medicine, 1760-1860* (Tuscaloosa: University of Alabama Press, 1991), p. 189.

24. Talbot, "Homeopathy in Massachusetts," pp. 644-652.

25. John L. Coffin, "Annual Oration Before the Massachusetts Homeopathic Medical Society, April, 1915," *New England Medical Gazette,* 50 (1915), 277-278; "Proceedings of the American Institute of Homeopathy," *Philadelphia Journal of Homeopathy,* 1 (1852), 140.

26. Coffin, "Annual Oration Before the Massachusetts Homeopathic Medical Society, April, 1915," pp. 280-281.

27. Ibid., pp. 278-279.

28. "Celebration of the Centennial Birthday of Dr. Samuel Hahnemann in Boston," *North American Journal of Homeopathy,* 4 (1855), 150-152.

29. "Boston Homeopathic Fair," *American Homeopathic Review,* 1 (1859), 332-334.

30. "Homeopathy in Rhode Island," *Transactions of the World's Homeopathic Convention,* Volume II: *History of Homeopathy,* pp. 507-518.

31. "Rhode Island Homeopathic Society," *Philadelphia Journal of Homeopathy,* 1 (1852), 240.

32. "Communication," *Philadelphia Journal of Homeopathy,* 3 (1854), 498.

33. G. H. Wilson and N. A. Mosman, "Homeopathy in Connecticut," *Transactions of the World's Homeopathic Convention,* Volume II: *History of Homeopathy,* pp. 487-488.

34. William E. Payne, "Homeopathy in Maine," *Transactions of the World's Homeopathic Convention,* Volume II: *History of Homeopathy,* pp. 549-564.

35. William E. Payne, "History of Homeopathy in Maine," *North American Journal of Homeopathy,* 16 (1867), 210-213.

36. Ibid., pp. 214-215.

37. Ibid., p. 216.

38. Ibid., pp. 217-219.

39. Ibid., p. 223.

40. Ibid., pp. 220-222.

41. J. H. Gallinger and J. F. Whittle, "Homeopathy in New Hampshire," *Transactions of the World's Homeopathic Convention,* Volume II: *History of Homeopathy,* pp. 565-570.

42. C. B. Currier and G. E. Sparhawk, "Homeopathy in Vermont," *Transactions of the World's Homeopathic Convention,* Volume II: *History of Homeopathy,* pp. 493-506.

43. "Historical and Statistical Report of Homeopathy in the United States of America," *Transactions of the World's Homeopathic Convention*, Volume II: *History of Homeopathy*, p. 436.

44. J. C. Guernsey, "Homeopathy in Pennsylvania," *Transactions of the World's Homeopathic Convention*, Volume II: *History of Homeopathy*, pp. 714-715, 719.

45. Ibid., p. 720.

46. "Proceedings of the American Institute of Homeopathy," *Philadelphia Journal of Homeopathy*, 1 (1852), 140.

47. "Proceedings of the 13th Annual Meeting of the Homeopathic Medical Society of the State of New York," *North American Journal of Homeopathy*, 13 (1864), 115.

48. Ibid., pp. 114-115.

49. B. F. Joslin, *Principles of Homeopathy: In a Series of Lectures* (New York: William Radde, 1850), pp. 6-7, 20-23.

50. "Homeopathy in the United States," *Transactions of the World's Homeopathic Convention*, Volume II: *History of Homeopathy*, p. 434.

51. R. J. McClatchey, "Homeopathic Medical Societies," *Transactions of the World's Homeopathic Convention*, Volume II: *History of Homeopathy*, pp. 826-827.

52. Guernsey, "Homeopathy in Pennsylvania," pp. 654-655.

53. Ibid., pp. 655-672.

54. J. C. G., "Homeopathy in New Jersey," *Transactions of the World's Homeopathic Convention*, Volume II: *History of Homeopathy*, pp. 539-548.

55. A. Negendank and Isaiah Lukens, "Homeopathy in Delaware," *Transactions of the World's Homeopathic Convention*, Volume II: *History of Homeopathy*, p. 519; Lewis B. Flinn, "Homeopathic Influence in the Delaware Community: A Retrospective Reassessment," *Delaware Medical Journal*, 48 (1976), 418-419.

56. F. R. McManus, "Homeopathy in Maryland," *Transactions of the World's Homeopathic Convention*, Volume II: *History of Homeopathy*, pp. 489-490, 492.

57. T. S. Verdi, "Homeopathy in the District of Columbia," *Transactions of the World's Homeopathic Convention*, Volume II: *History of Homeopathy*, pp. 594-595.

58. "Washington Homeopathic Medical Society," *American Homeopathic Observer*, 7 (1870), 306.

59. *New York Tribune*, May 9, 1870, p. 3.

60. Joseph V. Hobson, "Homeopathy in Virginia," *Transactions of the World's Homeopathic Convention*, Volume II: *History of Homeopathy*, pp. 765-766; Harris L. Coulter, *Divided Legacy: The Conflict Between Homeopathy and the American Medical Association*, Volume III: *Science and Ethics in American Medicine, 1800-1914* (Washington, DC: Wehawken Book Company, 1973), p. 110.

61. J. P. Dake and L. D. Morse, "Homeopathy in Tennessee," *Transactions of the World's Homeopathic Convention*, Volume II: *History of Homeopathy*, pp. 596-597.

62. I. G. Rosenstein, *Theory and Practice of Homeopathy. First Part, Containing a Theory of Homeopathy, with Dietetic Rules, Etc.* (Louisville: Henkle and Logan, 1840), p. 6.

63. William L. Breyfogle, "Homeopathy in Southern Kentucky," *Transactions of the World's Homeopathic Convention*, Volume II: *History of Homeopathy*, pp. 530-532.

64. William H. Hunt, "Homeopathy in Eastern Kentucky," *Transactions of the World's Homeopathic Convention,* Volume II: *History of Homeopathy,* pp. 532-533, 536.

65. F. H. Orme, "Homeopathy in Georgia," *Transactions of the World's Homeopathic Convention,* Volume II: *History of Homeopathy,* pp. 580-582.

66. F. F. DeDerkey, "Homeopathy in Alabama," *Transactions of the World's Homeopathic Convention,* Volume II: *History of Homeopathy,* pp. 586-589.

67. William H. Holcombe, "Homeopathy in Louisiana," *Transactions of the World's Homeopathic Convention,* Volume II: *History of Homeopathy,* pp. 484-486.

68. John Duffy (ed.), *The Rudolph Matas History of Medicine in Louisiana* (2 volumes) (Baton Rouge: Louisiana State University Press, 1959-1962), Volume II, pp. 35-37.

69. Holcombe, "Homeopathy in Louisiana," pp. 484-486.

70. Valentine, "Homeopathy in Missouri," pp. 618-619.

71. R. J. McClatchey and Joseph C. Guernsey, "Historical and Statistical Report of Homeopathy in the United States of America," *Transactions of the World's Homeopathic Convention,* Volume II: *History of Homeopathy,* p. 766.

72. *Polk's Medical Register and Directory of North America* (Tenth Revised Edition) (Detroit: R.L. Polk and Company Publishers, 1908), p. 91.

73. S. R. Beckwith, D. H. Beckwith, and N. Schneider, "Homeopathy in Ohio," *Transactions of the World's Homeopathic Convention,* Volume II: *History of Homeopathy,* pp. 521, 524-525.

74. Ibid., pp. 528-529.

75. O. P. Baer, "Homeopathy in Indiana," *Transactions of the World's Homeopathic Convention,* Volume II: *History of Homeopathy,* pp. 571-575.

76. A. E. Small and R. Ludlam, "Homeopathy in Illinois," *Transactions of the World's Homeopathic Convention,* Volume II: *History of Homeopathy,* pp. 590-593.

77. "Society of the German Homeopathic Physicians of the Northwest," *American Homeopathic Observer,* 1 (1864), 102.

78. "United States Homeopathic Association," *American Homeopathic Observer,* 2 (1865), 25.

79. Small and Ludlam, "Homeopathy in Illinois," p. 592.

80. "Proceedings of Medical Societies," *United States Journal of Homeopathy,* 1(1860), 574-575.

81. See John S. Haller Jr. and Barbara Mason, *Forging a Medical Practice, 1884-1938. An Illinois Case Study: Wilber Price Armstrong* (Springfield, IL: Pearson Museum, 1997).

82. P. G. Valentine, "Homeopathy in Missouri," *Transactions of the World's Homeopathic Convention,* Volume II: *History of Homeopathy,* pp. 598, 600.

83. Ibid., pp. 604-605.

84. Ibid., pp. 606-617.

85. F. Woodruff, "Homeopathy in Michigan," *Transactions of the World's Homeopathic Convention,* Volume II: *History of Homeopathy,* pp. 576-579.

86. E. B. Keeney, S. E. Lederer, and E. P. Minihan, "Sectarians and Scientists: Alternatives to Orthodox Medicine," in Ronald L. Numbers and Judith W. Leavitt (eds.), *Wisconsin Medicine: Historical Perspectives* (Madison: University of Wisconsin Press, 1981), p. 48.

87. L. E. Ober and T. F. Patchen, "Homeopathy in Wisconsin," *Transactions of the World's Homeopathic Convention*, Volume II: *History of Homeopathy*, pp. 583-585.

88. J. M. Toner, "Tabulated Statistics of the Medical Profession of the United States," *Transactions of the American Medical Association*, 22 (1871), 155-156.

89. Keeney, Lederer, and Minihan, "Sectarians and Scientists," pp. 49-50.

90. G. Neuman Seidlitz, "Homeopathy in Iowa," *Transactions of the World's Homeopathic Convention*, Volume II: *History of Homeopathy*, pp. 635-640.

91. James T. Alley and Albert E. Heybee, "Homeopathy in Minnesota," *Transactions of the World's Homeopathic Convention*, Volume II: *History of Homeopathy*, pp. 623-628.

92. O. S. Wood and A. C. Cowperthwaite, "Homeopathy in Nebraska," *Transactions of the World's Homeopathic Convention*, Volume II: *History of Homeopathy*, pp. 629-632.

93. J. M. Walker, "Homeopathy in Colorado," *Transactions of the World's Homeopathic Convention*, Volume II: *History of Homeopathy*, pp. 633-634; Jean Muirhead, "The Rise and Decline of Homeopathy in Colorado, 1890-1913," unpublished master's thesis, Colorado State University, 1995, pp. 22-65.

94. G. W. Barnes and E. J. Fraser, "Homeopathy in California," *Transactions of the World's Homeopathic Convention*, Volume II: *History of Homeopathy*, pp. 621-622; Josef M. Schmidt, "Homeopathy in the American West: Its German Communities," in Robert Jütte, Guenter B. Risse, and John Woodward (eds.), *Culture, Knowledge, and Healing: Historical Perspectives of Homeopathic Medicine in Europe and North America* (Sheffield: European Association for the History of Medicine and Health Publications, 1998), pp. 142-145.

95. McClatchey and Guernsey, "Historical and Statistical Report of Homeopathy in the United States of America," p. 766.

96. George B. Peck, "1851—Homeopathy—1901," *North American Journal of Homeopathy*, 50 (1902), 60-62; Anne Taylor Kirschmann, "A Vital Force: Women Physicians and Patients in American Homeopathy, 1850-1930," unpublished dissertation, University of Rochester, 1999, p. 151.

97. Peck, "1851—Homeopathy—1901," p. 61.

98. Kett, *The Formation of the American Medical Profession*, pp. 141-142.

99. John D. Davies, *Phrenology, Fad and Science: A Nineteenth Century Crusade* (New Haven: Yale University Press, 1955).

Chapter 3

1. B. F. Joslin, *Principles of Homeopathy. In a Series of Lectures* (New York: William Radde, 1850), p. 30; B. F. Joslin, "Evidences of the Power of Small Doses and Attenuated Medicines, Including the Theory of Potentization," *American Journal of Homeopathy*, 1 (1846-1847), 266.

2. Charles E. Rosenberg, "The Therapeutic Revolution: Medicine, Meaning, and Social Change in Nineteenth-Century America," in Morris J. Vogel and Charles E. Rosenberg (eds.), *The Therapeutic Revolution: Essays in the Social History of American Medicine* (Philadelphia: University of Pennsylvania Press, 1979), pp. 3-25.

3. Quoted in "Teachings of Common Sense," *Philadelphia Journal of Homeopathy,* 3 (1854), 99-100.

4. Samuel Hahnemann, *Materia Medica Pura* (4 volumes) (New York: William Radde, 1846), Volume II, p. v.

5. Samuel Hahnemann, "Remarks on the Extreme Attenuation of Homeopathic Medicines," in Robert E. Dudgeon (trans.), *The Lesser Writings of Samuel Hahnemann* (New York: William Radde, 1852), p. 765.

6. Samuel Hahnemann, "On the Impregnation of the Globules with Medicine," in Dudgeon, *The Lesser Writings of Samuel Hahnemann,* pp. 735-736.

7. James McNaughton, "Annual Address Delivered Before the Medical Society of the State of New York, February 6, 1838," *Transactions of the Medical Society of the State of New York,* 5 (1838), 26.

8. Bernhardt Fincke, "Improved Process of Preparing Homeopathic Medicines," *American Homeopathic Observer,* 9 (1872), 11; "Reviews and Bibliographical Notices," *North American Journal of Homeopathy,* 17 (1869), 554-555.

9. Hahnemann, "Remarks on the Extreme Attenuation of Homeopathic Medicines," pp. 763, 765.

10. James Y. Simpson, *Homeopathy: Its Tenets and Tendencies, Theoretical, Theological, and Therapeutical* (Philadelphia: Lindsay and Blakiston, 1854), p. 55.

11. Simpson, *Homeopathy: Its Tenets and Tendencies,* pp. 68-69; Gustav Puhlman, "The History of Homeopathy in Germany," *Transactions of the World's Homeopathic Convention,* Volume II: *History of Homeopathy,* pp. 32-33.

12. Hahnemann, "Remarks on the Extreme Attenuation of Homeopathic Medicines," p. 765.

13. Gustav Puhlman, "The History of Homeopathy in Germany," *Transactions of the World's Homeopathic Convention, Held at Philadelphia, Under the Auspices of the American Institute of Homeopathy, at Its Twenty-Ninth Session, June 26th-July 1, 1876,* Volume II: *History of Homeopathy* (2 volumes) (Philadelphia: Sherman and Company, 1880), p. 17; Samuel Hahnemann, "How Can Small Doses of Such Very Attenuated Medicine As Homeopathy Employs Still Possess Great Power?" in Dudgeon, *The Lesser Writings of Samuel Hahnemann,* p. 733; Joslin, *Principles of Homeopathy,* pp. 42-43.

14. Hahnemann, *Organon of Homeopathic Medicine* (1836), pp. 210-211.

15. Martin Dinges, "Men's Bodies 'Explained' on a Daily Basis in Letters from Patients to Samuel Hahnemann (1830-35)," in Martin Dinges, *Patients in the History of Homeopathy* (Sheffield: European Association for the History of Medicine and Health, 2002), pp. 85-118. Eventually, this theory was abandoned, and in its place the theory of comminution adopted, which was explained on a less spiritual and more material basis, arguing that grinding or mixing a grain of medicine increased its surface with every fracture and thus increased its distribution through the organism.

16. Anonymous. *The Anatomy of a Humbug, of the Genus Germanicus, Species Homeopathia* (New York: Printed for the Author, 1837), pp. 8, 12-13, 15.

17. J. T. Houghton, "The Question of Doses and Repetition of Medicines," *North American Journal of Homeopathy,* 4 (1856), 327-330.

18. Henry Miller, *An Examination of the Claims of Homeopathy, As a System of Medical Doctrine and Practice: Being a Lecture Delivered Before the Medical Society of Louisville on the 14th December, 1847* (Louisville, Kentucky: G. H.

Monsarrat and Company, 1847), pp. 20-21; Robert L. Park, *Voodoo Science: The Road from Foolishness to Fraud* (New York: Oxford University Press, 2000), p. 74.

19. Samuel Hahnemann, *Organon of Homeopathic Medicine* (Allentown, PA: Academical Bookstore, 1836), pp. ii, x.

20. Constantine Hering, Preface, in Hahnemann, *Organon of Homeopathic Medicine,* pp. xiii, xv.

21. Storm Rosa, "Homeopathy and Eclecticism," *Eclectic Medical Journal,* (1850), 166-167.

22. Ibid., p. 167.

23. E. E. Marcy, "The Homeopathic Law," *North American Homeopathic Journal,* 3 (1853), 24-28.

24. F. A. Espanet, "Some Considerations Upon Dietetics and Posology," *North American Homeopathic Journal,* 3 (1853), 115, 121, 126.

25. John F. Geary, "Our Literature," *North American Journal of Homeopathy,* 6 (1858), 389.

26. S. Remington, "The High Potencies," *Philadelphia Journal of Homeopathy,* 2 (1853), 24-26, 29-31.

27. Curt Pretsch, "Communication," *Philadelphia Journal of Homeopathy,* 3 (1855), 666-669.

28. Hamilton Ring, "A Few Practical Suggestions," *North American Journal of Homeopathy,* 8 (1859), 70.

29. E. W. Jones, "Review of Ring's 'Rational Homeopathy,'" *North American Journal of Homeopathy,* 5 (1856), 284, 287-288 (p. 287).

30. Trinks quoted in "Polemics Among German Homeopathists," *North American Journal of Homeopathy,* 7 (1858), 250-252.

31. I. G. Rosenstein, *Theory and Practice of Homeopathy First Part, Containing a Theory of Homeopathy, with Dietetic Rules, Etc.* (Louisville: Henkle and Logan, 1840), pp. 1-2.

32. Ibid., pp. 84-85.

33. Ibid., p. 104.

34. Ibid., pp. 108, 116.

35. Harris Dunsford, "The Practical Advantages of Homeopathy," *Eclectic Medical Journal,* 1 (1849), 563-564.

36. Ibid., p. 514.

37. Joslin, *Principles of Homeopathy,* pp. 44, 50-51, 58; B. F. Joslin, "Evidences of the Power of Small Doses and Attenuated Medicines, Including a Theory of Potentization," *American Journal of Homeopathy,* 1 (1846-1847), 263-278.

38. Joslin, *Principles of Homeopathy,* pp. 79-80, 82-83.

39. James Kitchen, "The High Dilutions," *Philadelphia Journal of Homeopathy,* 2 (1853-1854), 567.

40. Quoted in "Reviews and Bibliographical Notices," *North American Journal of Homeopathy,* 14 (1866), 437.

41. B. Fincke, "Clinical Cases Treated with High Potencies," *North American Journal of Homeopathy,* 13 (1864), 240-252.

42. "Dr. B. Fincke's High Potencies Before the American Institute of Homeopathy," *North American Journal of Homeopathy,* 16 (1868), 473-474.

43. See B. Fincke, *On High Potencies and Homeopathics, Clinical Cases and Observations* (Philadelphia: A. J. Tafel, 1865).

44. S. A. J., "Od or Odo-Magnetic Force," *American Homeopathic Observer,* 8 (1871), 67-70.

45. "Reviews and Bibliographical Notices," p. 438.

46. "Fincke's High Potencies," *American Homeopathic Observer,* 7 (1870), 197.

47. "Introductory," *American Homeopathic Observer,* 4 (1867), vii.

48. Fincke, "Improved Process of Preparing Homeopathic Medicines," p. 10.

49. Ibid., p. 11.

50. "In Memoriam," *Transactions of the American Institute of Homeopathy,* (1880), 150-151.

51. Charles J. Hempel, *Homeopathy, a Principle in Nature. Its Scientific Universality Unfolded; Its Development and Philosophy Explained; and Its Applicability to the Treatment of Diseases Shown* (New York: C. T. Hurlburt, 1860), pp. 33-37.

52. Hempel, *Homeopathy, a Principle in Nature,* pp. 70-71.

53. Hempel, "Lehrbuck der Homeopathie, by Dr. V. Grauvogl," *American Homeopathic Observer,* 7 (1870), 370-372.

54. Hempel, *Homeopathy, a Principle in Nature,* pp. 116-119 (pp. 118-119).

55. Ibid., p. 128.

56. Ibid., pp. 18-19, 22.

57. Ibid., p. 122.

58. Charles Hempel, "What Might and Should Be the Social and Political Relations of Homeopathy to the Dominant School of Medicine," *American Homeopathic Observer,* 3 (1866), 416-423.

59. C. J. Hempel, "The Dose," *American Homeopathic Observer,* 4 (1867), 361.

60. Ibid., pp. 362-363.

61. Ibid., pp. 363, 366-367.

62. Ibid., p. 371.

63. C. J. Hempel, "Question of Dose," *American Homeopathic Observer,* 1 (1864), 18-19.

64. Hempel, "What Might and Should Be the Social and Political Relations of Homeopathy to the Dominant School of Medicine," pp. 423-424.

65. C. J. Hempel, "Lehrbuck der Homoeopathie, by Dr. V. Grauvogl," *American Homeopathic Observer,* 7 (1870), 362, 381.

66. Carroll Dunham, "Freedom of Medical Opinion and Action: A Vital Necessity, and a Great Responsibility," *North American Journal of Homeopathy,* 19 (1870), 106.

67. H. C. Allen, "The Dilution Question," *American Homeopathic Observer,* 2 (1865), 313-314.

68. J. S. Douglas, "High or Low Dilutions?" *North American Journal of Homeopathy,* 13 (1865), 349.

69. Charles Cropper, "The Mission of Homeopathy," *North American Journal of Homeopathy,* 17 (1868), 1-7.

70. I. S. P. Lord, "Dynamization," *North American Journal of Homeopathy,* 13 (1865), 329-330.

71. Carl Müller, "The Fincke Potencies," *American Homeopathic Observer,* 7 (1870), 402.

72. Carl Müller, "Comments on a Late Reviewer," *American Homeopathic Observer,* 7 (1870), 235.

73. Gustav Puhlman, "The History of Homeopathy in Germany," Volume II, pp. 32-33.

Chapter 4

1. Jakob Bernoulli, *Ars conjectandi* (s.n., 1713); Keith M. Baker, *Condorcet: From Natural Philosophy to Social Mathematics* (Chicago: University of Chicago Press, 1975); Pierre-Simon de Laplace, *Exposition du système du monde* (Paris: J.B.M. Duprat, 1798).

2. Erwin H. Ackerknecht, *Medicine in the Paris Hospital, 1794-1848* (Baltimore, MD: Johns Hopkins Press, 1967); Terrence D. Murphy, "Medical Knowledge and Statistical Methods in Early Nineteenth Century France," *Medical History*, 25 (1981), 301-319.

3. See Michael J. Cullen, *The Statistical Movement in Early Victorian Britain: The Foundations of Empirical Social Research* (Brighton, Sussex: Harvester Press, 1975); Ian Hacking, *The Emergence of Probability. The Philosophical Study of Early Ideas About Probability, Induction, and Statistical Inferences* (Cambridge: University Press, 1975).

4. James Cassedy, *American Medicine and Statistical Thinking, 1800-1860* (Cambridge: Harvard University Press, 1984), Chapters 2 through 5 (pp. 25-119).

5. Jacob Bigelow, "On Self-Limited Diseases," in his *Modern Inquiries: Classical, Professional, and Miscellaneous* (Boston: Little, Brown, 1867), pp. 164-169.

6. Edward Hamilton, "Comparative Results of the Homeopathic and Allopathic Treatment of Asiatic Cholera," *British Journal of Homeopathy*, 3 (1845), 101-105; Dr. Kurtz, "What Is the Inference? Or the Comparative Statistics of Allopathic and Homeopathic Treatment," *British Journal of Homeopathy*, 1 (1843), 260-270.

7. John C. Peters, *A Treatise on the Origin, Nature, Prevention, and Treatment of Asiatic Cholera* (New York; D. Van Nostrand, 1866), p. 40.

8. Ibid., pp. 40-41.

9. "Asiatic Cholera," *American Homeopathic Observer*, 3 (1866), 301-303.

10. Peters, *A Treatise on the Origin, Nature, Prevention, and Treatment of Asiatic Cholera*, pp. 42-43.

11. Daniel Holt, *Views of Homeopathy; with Reasons for Examining and Admitting It As a Principle in Medical Science* (New Haven: J.H. Benham, 1845), pp. 14-15.

12. John Lea, *Cholera, with Reference to the Geological Theory* (Cincinnati: Wright, Ferris and Co., 1850); Margaret Pelling, *Cholera, Fever and English Medicine, 1825-65* (New York: Oxford University Press, 1978).

13. "Asiatic Cholera," pp. 309-312.

14. "Asiatic Cholera," pp. 313-315; Thomas Rowsey, "Asiatic Cholera," *American Homeopathic Observer*, 3 (1866), 454.

15. Peters, *A Treatise on the Origin, Nature, Prevention, and Treatment of Asiatic Cholera*, pp. 130-160.

16. Cassedy, *American Medical and Statistical Thinking*, p. 99.

17. "Asiatic Cholera," pp. 317-318; William Leo-Wolf, *Remarks on the Abracadabra of the Nineteenth Century; or on Dr. Samuel Hahnemann's Homeopathic Medicine, with Particular Reference to Dr. Constantine Hering's Concise View of*

the Rise and Progress of Homeopathic Medicine (New York: Carey, Lea and Blanchard, 1835), p. 2.

18. Thomas Wilson, "Observations on the Pathology and Treatment of Asiatic Cholera," *American Homeopathic Observer,* 3 (1866), 20; "Cholera Treated with Camphor Only," *American Homeopathic Observer,* 3 (1866), 21.

19. According to critic John C. Peters, twenty-two of the thirty-five remedies were not Homeopathic in any sense of the word, but alterative or antagonistic. See Peters, *A Treatise on the Origin, Nature, Prevention, and Treatment of Asiatic Cholera,* pp. 160-161.

20. R. E. Dudgeon, "A Century of Homeopathy," The Lloyd Library and Museum, Eclectic Medical College, Box 37, Folder 1,082, p. 19; Benjamin C. Woodbury Jr., "The Homeopathic School of Medicine," The Lloyd Library and Museum, Eclectic Medical College, Box 37, Folder 1,076, p. 305.

21. Francis Black, "Homeopathic Treatment of Asiatic Cholera," *British Journal of Homeopathy,* 1 (1843), 57-68.

22. Hahnemann quoted in Dr. Escallier, "On the Use of Copper As a Preventive and Cure of Asiatic Cholera," *North American Homeopathic Journal,* 3 (1853), 248-249.

23. "Homeopathy and Cholera," *Eclectic Medical Journal,* 1 (1849), 197-198.

24. J. Gilioli, "On the New Medical School, and the Causes That Prevent Its Being More Generally Adopted by Medical Men," *British Journal of Homeopathy,* 3 (1845), 30-31.

25. "Editorial," *Philadelphia Journal of Homeopathy,* 4 (1855), 116.

26. F. H. Orme, "Homeopathy," *American Homeopathic Observer,* 4 (1867), 467.

27. "Asiatic Cholera," pp. 320-321.

28. "Homeopathy in Europe," *North American Journal of Homeopathy,* 14 (1866), 342.

29. S. A. Merrill, "Homeopathy and Allopathy in the Crucible of Facts and Figures," *American Homeopathic Observer,* 4 (1867), 39; Bernard Leavy, "The Homeopathic Management of Cholera in the Nineteenth Century with Special Reference to the Epidemic in London in 1854," *Medizin Gesellschaft und Geschichte,* 16 (1998), 125-144.

30. "A Panic Among Allopathic Students," *American Homeopathic Observer,* 3 (1866), 528-529.

31. "The Yellow Fever," *North American Homeopathic Journal,* 3 (1853), 418.

32. William H. Holcombe, "Letter to the Editor," *Philadelphia Journal of Homeopathy,* 4 (1855), 459.

33. William H. Holcombe, "Epidemic Yellow-Fever and Its Homeopathic Treatment," *North American Homeopathic Journal,* 3 (1853), 503-504.

34. Holcombe, "Epidemic Yellow-Fever and Its Homeopathic Treatment," pp. 492-494.

35. Ibid., pp. 497-501.

36. Henry D. Paine, "Address Before the Homeopathic Medical Society of the State of New York, Delivered May 10, 1865," *North American Journal of Homeopathy,* 14 (1866), 413.

37. Editorial, *Philadelphia Journal of Homeopathy,* 3 (1854), 251-252.

38. Charles W. Earle, "Homeopathy As It Was and As It Is," *Chicago Medical Examiner,* 12 (1871), 526.

39. Quoted in Worthington Hooker, *Homeopathy: An Examination of Its Doctrines and Evidences* (New York: C. Scribner, 1851), p. 117.

40. Dr. F. W. Irvine, "M. Andral's Homeopathic Experiments at La Pitie," in William Henderson, *Homeopathy Fairly Represented: A Reply to Professor Simpson's "Homeopathy" Misrepresented* (Philadelphia: Lindsay and Blakiston, 1854), Appendix, pp. 289-291, 295-298.

41. E. E. Marcy, *Homeopathy and Allopathy: Reply to an Examination of the Doctrines and Evidences of Homeopathy, by Worthington Hooker, M.D.* (New York: William Radde, 1852), pp. 99-100.

42. Abraham Howard Okie, *Homeopathy: With Particular Reference to a Lecture by O. W. Holmes* (Boston: Otis Clapp, 1842), pp. 23-25 (p. 24).

43. Oliver Wendell Holmes, "Medical Essays. Homeopathy and Its Kindred Delusions," in Oliver Wendell Holmes, *The Complete Writings of Oliver Wendell Holmes* (13 volumes) (New York: Houghton, Mifflin and Company, 1892), pp. ix, 79-80.

44. Holmes, "Medical Essays. Homeopathy and Its Kindred Delusions," pp. 61, 81-82.

45. Rosenstein, *Theory and Practice of Homeopathy*, pp. 267-268; Okie, *Homeopathy: With Particular Reference to a Lecture by O. W. Holmes*, pp. 36-39.

46. Earle, "Homeopathy As It Was and As It Is," pp. 524-525; Anonymous, *The Anatomy of a Humbug, of the Genus Germanicus, Species Homeopathic* (New York: Printed for the Author, 1837), pp. 23-27; "Homeopathy in Military Hospitals," *American Medical Times*, 4 (1862), 42.

47. William Leo-Wolf, *Remarks on the Abracadabra of the Nineteenth Century; or on Dr. Samuel Hahnemann's Homeopathic Medicine, with Particular Reference to Dr. Constantine Hering's Concise View of the Rise and Progress of Homeopathic Medicine* (New York: Carey, Lea and Blanchard, 1835), p. 27.

48. Silas Swift Brooks, "Reasons Why Medicines Should Be Used in Accordance with the Law," *Philadelphia Journal of Homeopathy*, 4 (1855), 225.

49. "Statistics of Homeopathic and Allopathic Hospitals," *North American Journal of Homeopathy*, 13 (1865), 516-521.

50. S. A. Merrill, "Homeopathy and Allopathy in the Crucible of Facts and Figures," *American Homeopathic Observer*, 4 (1867), 40.

51. F. H. Orme, "Homeopathy," *American Homeopathic Observer*, 4 (1867), 466-467.

52. "Hospital Reports," *North American Journal of Homeopathy*, 4 (1855), 293-298.

53. Joseph Hooper, "Homeopathy: What Are Its Claims on Public Confidence?" *American Homeopathic Observer*, 3 (1866), 87; "Homeopathic Statistics," *North American Homeopathic Journal*, 3 (1853), 146.

54. Jean-Paul Tessier, *Clinical Researches Concerning the Homeopathic Treatment of Asiatic Cholera. Preceded by a Review on the Abuse of the Numerical Method in Medicine* (New York: William Radde, 1855); Jean-Paul Tessier, *Clinical Remarks Concerning the Homeopathic Treatment of Pneumonia: Preceded by a Retrospective View of the Allopathic Materia Medica, and an Explanation of the Homeopathic Law of Cure* (New York: William Radde, 1855).

55. Hooker, *Homeopathy: An Examination of Its Doctrines and Evidences*, p. 101.

56. F. H. Orme, "Homeopathy," *American Homeopathic Observer*, 4 (1867), 468.

57. Quoted in Brooks, "Reasons Why Medicines Should Be Used in Accordance with the Law," p. 226.

58. James Y. Simpson, *Homeopathy: Its Tenets and Tendencies, Theoretical, Theological, and Therapeutical* (Philadelphia: Lindsay and Blakiston, 1854), pp. 104-105.

59. Ibid., pp. 111-112.

60. Ibid., pp. 105, 107, 110.

61. Holmes, "Medical Essays. Homeopathy and Its Kindred Delusions," pp. ix, 73.

62. Peters, *A Treatise on the Origin, Nature, Prevention, and Treatment of Asiatic Cholera*, pp. 3-4.

63. "Homeopathic Hospital for Our Sick Troops Engaged in the War," *Philadelphia Journal of Homeopathy*, 4 (1855), 118.

64. See Tessier, *Clinical Researches Concerning the Homeopathic Treatment of Asiatic Cholera;* Tessier, *Clinical Remarks Concerning the Homeopathic Treatment of Pneumonia.*

65. "Homeopathy in England," *Philadelphia Journal of Homeopathy*, 4 (1855), 311-314.

66. Panmure quoted in "Homeopathy in England," p. 315.

67. "Editorial," *Philadelphia Journal of Homeopathy*, 4 (1855), 113-117.

68. Leo-Wolf, *Remarks on the Abracadabra of the Nineteenth Century*, p. 43.

69. E. F. Smith, "Homeopathy Not Recognized in Europe," *St. Louis Medical and Surgical Journal*, 18 (1860), 32-35.

70. Smith, "Homeopathy Not Recognized in Europe," pp. 32-35; H. S. Frieze, "The Position of Homeopathy in Europe and European Medical Schools," *Peninsular Journal of Medicine*, 5 (1857), 290-297.

71. Frieze, "The Position of Homeopathy in Europe and European Medical Schools," p. 293.

72. Ibid., pp. 295-296.

73. William A. Hawley, "Report of Committee on Life Insurance," *North American Journal of Homeopathy*, 14 (1866), 525-527.

74. "A London Life Assurance Office Converted to Homeopathy by the Evidence of Statistics," *American Homeopathic Observer*, 2 (1865), 246-248; "Homeopathic Mutual Life Insurance Company of the City of New York," *North American Journal of Homeopathy*, 17 (1868), 143-144.

75. "Life Insurance for Homeopathists," *North American Journal of Homeopathy*, 14 (1865), 283-284.

76. "A New Feature in Life Insurance," *American Homeopathic Observer*, 2 (1865), 365-368.

77. "Homeopathic Life Insurance Companies," *American Homeopathic Observer*, 8 (1871), 583-584.

78. "Western Institute of Homeopathy," *American Homeopathic Observer*, 3 (1866), 340-341.

79. I. T. Talbot, "Report of the Nineteenth Annual Meeting, Held at Pittsburgh, Pa., June 6th and 7th, 1866," *American Homeopathic Observer*, 3 (1866), 332-333. The Cleveland company, organized in 1865, was sold in 1871 to Republic Life of Chicago. See "Homeopathic Life Insurance Companies," *American Homeopathic Observer*, 8 (1871), 583-584.

80. "Michigan Homeopathic Institute; Eighth Annual Meeting," *American Homeopathic Observer,* 4 (1867), 321.

81. "Second Annual Meeting of the Homeopathic Medical Society of Pennsylvania, Philadelphia, June 3, 1867," *North American Journal of Homeopathy,* 16 (1867), 144.

82. J. A. Cloud, *Homeopathy: Its Difficulties and Some of the Principal Errors Against It, with Hints on Dietetics, Viewed in Relation to the Laws of Digestion; Also the Practice of Homeopathic Medicine Simplified, for the Use of Families and a History of the Cincinnati Homeopathic Medical Dispensary* (Cincinnati: V.C. Tidball, 1869), pp. 16-17.

83. "Homeopathic Mutual Life," *American Homeopathic Observer,* 8 (1871), 259-260.

84. "The Atlantic Mutual Insurance Company of Albany, New York," *American Homeopathic Observer,* 3 (1866), 277.

85. F. H. Orme, "Homeopathy," *American Homeopathic Observer,* 4 (1867), 473-475.

86. "Atlantic Mutual Life Insurance Company," *North American Journal of Homeopathy,* 16 (1867), 624-625.

87. "Atlantic Mutual Life Insurance Company," *American Homeopathic Observer,* 9 (1872), 108.

88. "The Atlantic Mutual Life Insurance Company," *North American Journal of Homeopathy,* 16 (1867), 319.

89. "A New Homeopathic Life Insurance Company," *North American Journal of Homeopathy,* 16 (1867), 472-473; "Homeopathic Mutual Life Insurance Company of the City of New York," *North American Journal of Homeopathy,* 17 (1868), 144.

90. "Homeopathic Mutual Life Insurance Company of the City of New York," *American Homeopathic Observer,* 7 (1870), 583.

91. "American Institute of Homeopathy," *American Homeopathic Observer,* 10 (1873), 384-385; "New York Homeopathic Life Insurance Company of New York City," *American Homeopathic Observer,* 10 (1873), 413.

92. "Miscellaneous," *Transactions of the Thirty-Third Session of the American Institute of Homeopathy* (1880), 665.

93. Neville Wood, "Homeopathy in America," *Monthly Homeopathic Review,* 24 (1880), 54-60.

94. Ibid., p. 57.

95. Ibid., pp. 54-60.

96. Rosenstein, *Theory and Practice of Homeopathy,* pp. 111-112.

97. For interesting insight into this subject, see Glynis Rankin, "Professional Organisation and the Development of Medical Knowledge: Two Interpretations of Homeopathy," in Roger Cooter (ed.), *Studies in the History of Alternative Medicine* (Oxford: MacMillan Press, 1988), pp. 46-62.

98. Cassedy, *American Medicine and Statistical Thinking,* pp. viii, 234.

Chapter 5

1. L. M'Farland, "An Essay on the Moral Obligation of Homeopathists to Sustain and Disseminate Homeopathic Institutes," *Philadelphia Journal of Homeopathy,* 3 (1854), 138-139, 145; A. R. Thomas, "Medical Education and Homeopathic Medical Colleges in the United States," *Transactions of the World's Homeopathic Convention, Held at Philadelphia, Under the Auspices of the American Institute of Homeopathy, at Its Twenty-Ninth Session, June 26-July 1, 1876,* Volume II: *History of Homeopathy* (Philadelphia: Sherman and Company, 1880), p. 769. See also John Harley Warner, *The Therapeutic Perspective: Medical Practice, Knowledge, and Identity in America, 1820-1885* (Cambridge: Harvard University Press, 1986), p. 180.

2. Anonymous, "Homeopathic Medical Education—Present and Future," *North American Journal of Homeopathy,* 8 (1859), 52-54, 57.

3. Ibid., 55-57, 59.

4. E.M. Hale, "Tenth Annual Announcement of the Western Homeopathic College, at Cleveland, Ohio," *North American Journal of Homeopathy,* 8 (1859), 298.

5. E.M. Hale, "Western Homeopathic College," *North American Journal of Homeopathy,* 9 (1861), 529-530.

6. Note that the numbers given for both the Eastern and Western states include reorganizations, mergers, consolidations, and extinct and fraudulent schools.

7. Joseph C. Guernsey, "A Brief Sketch of the Allentown Academy," *Transactions of the World's Homeopathic Convention,* Volume II: *History of Homeopathy,* p. 775.

8. "The First Homeopathic College in the World," The Lloyd Library and Museum, Eclectic Medical College, Box 37, Folder 1,068.

9. Guernsey, "A Brief Sketch of the Allentown Academy," pp. 776-777; "The First Homeopathic College in the World," Folder 1,068; Joseph F. Kett, *The Formation of the American Medical Profession: The Role of Institutions, 1780-1860* (New Haven: Yale University Press, 1968), pp. 135-137.

10. Guernsey, "A Brief Sketch of the Allentown Academy," pp. 776-777, 783; "The First Homeopathic College in the World," Folder 1,068.

11. Guernsey, "A Brief Sketch of the Allentown Academy," pp. 777, 780-781; Frederick C. Waite, "American Sectarian Medical Colleges Before the Civil War," *Bulletin of the History of Medicine,* 19 (1946), 162-163; William Harvey King, *History of Homeopathy and Its Institutions in America* (4 volumes) (New York: Lewis Publishing Company, 1905), Volume II, p. 41.

12. Guernsey, "A Brief Sketch of the Allentown Academy," pp. 783-784; Thomas Lindsay Bradford, *Life and Letters of Dr. Samuel Hahnemann* (Philadelphia: Boericke & Tafel, 1895), pp. 470-471. The academy had sought Hahnemann's advice and support but none was forthcoming.

13. John F. Gray, "Early History of Homeopathy in New York," *North American Journal of Homeopathy,* 12 (1864), 339; King, *History of Homeopathy,* p. 41; Ned D. Heindel and Natalie I. Foster, "The Allentown Academy: America's First German Medical School," *Pennsylvania Folklife,* 30 (1980), 2-8.

14. [William A. Gardiner], "Homeopathic Medical College of Pennsylvania," *Philadelphia Journal of Homeopathy,* 1 (1852), 330.

15. A. R. Thomas, "Homeopathic Medical College of Pennsylvania," *Transactions of the World's Homeopathic Convention,* Volume II: *History of Homeopathy,* pp. 786-787.

16. William A. Gardiner, "Introductory Lecture," *Philadelphia Journal of Homeopathy,* 2 (1853), 414.

17. Thomas, "Homeopathic Medical College of Pennsylvania," pp. 787-788.

18. Gardiner, "Homeopathic Medical College of Pennsylvania," p. 239.

19. "Medical Colleges of Philadelphia," *Philadelphia Journal of Homeopathy,* 2 (1853), 128.

20. Naomi Rogers, *An Alternative Path: The Making and Remaking of Hahnemann Medical College and Hospital of Philadelphia* (New Brunswick, NJ: Rutgers University Press, 1998), pp. 41-42. See also *Humphreys' Homeopathic Directory for the Use of Humphreys' Pharmaceutical Preparations* (New York: Humphreys' Homeopathic Medicine Company, 1900). Humphreys' Specific Homeopathic Medical Company, at 109 Fulton Street, New York City, supplied books, medicine cases, Humphreys' Homeopathic Specifics, Humphreys' Veterinary Specifics, Witch Hazel Oil, and Marvel of Healing, a patent medicine taken internally and externally for bruises, corns, diarrhea, earache, neuralgia, rheumatism, shaving, sunburn, toothache, varicose veins, and vomiting.

21. Adolphus Lippe, "My Review of the Complete Repertory of C. Hempel, M.D., and His Answers," *Philadelphia Journal of Homeopathy,* 2 (1853), 60-61; Charles J. Hempel, "Communication," *Philadelphia Journal of Homeopathy,* 3 (1854), 535.

22. Hempel, "Communication," p. 534.

23. C. J. Hempel, "Modern Teachings," *American Homeopathic Observer,* 4 (1867), 126.

24. Ibid., pp. 128, 131.

25. Charles J. Hempel, "Letter to Editor," *American Homeopathic Observer,* 4 (1867), 380.

26. Charles J. Hempel, *Homeopathy, a Principle in Nature; Its Scientific Universality Unfolded; Its Development and Philosophy Explained; and Its Applicability to the Treatment of Disease Shown* (New York: C.T. Hurlburt, 1860), pp. vi, x.

27. Ibid., pp. viii, xii.

28. Ibid., pp. 138-139.

29. Ibid., p. 112.

30. Ibid., pp. 7, 10-11.

31. Thomas, "Homeopathic Medical College of Pennsylvania," p. 792.

32. "Homeopathic Medical College of Pennsylvania. Thirteenth Annual Announcement, 1860-61," *North American Journal of Homeopathy,* 9 (1860), 163.

33. Thomas, "Homeopathic Medical College of Pennsylvania," pp. 793-796.

34. "The Hahnemann Medical College of Philadelphia: Session of 1867-68," *North American Journal of Homeopathy,* 16 (1867), 160.

35. "A New College," *American Homeopathic Observer,* 4 (1867), 304.

36. Rogers, *An Alternative Path,* p. 44; King, *History of Homeopathy,* Volume II, pp. 63-64, 70-71.

37. Thomas, "Homeopathic Medical College of Pennsylvania," pp. 796-798.

38. Thomas, "Medical Education and Homeopathic Medical Colleges in the United States," pp. 771-773; King, *History of Homeopathy,* Volume II, pp. 71-72.

39. "Hahnemann Medical College of Philadelphia," *American Homeopathic Observer,* 9 (1872), 443.

40. See Thomas Lindsley Bradford, *History of the Homeopathic Medical College of Pennsylvania; the Hahnemann Medical College and Hospital of Philadelphia* (Philadelphia: Boericke & Tafel, 1898).

41. C. S. Cameran, "Hahnemann Yesterday—Its Spirit Lives," *Pennsylvania Medicine,* 76 (1973), 38-39.

42. "Proceedings of the Homeopathic Medical Society of the State of New York," *North American Homeopathic Journal,* 3 (1853), 142.

43. James W. Cox, "Annual Meeting of the Homeopathic Medical Society of the State of New York," *Philadelphia Journal of Homeopathy,* 1 (1853), 557-558; "Report of the Special Committee Appointed by the Homeopathic Medical Society of the State of New York, to Consider the Expediency of Establishing a Homeopathic Medical College," *North American Homeopathic Journal,* 3 (1853), 186-187, 191.

44. W. C. Bryant, *Popular Considerations on Homeopathia* (New York: William Radde, 1841); *New York Evening Post,* October 31, November 1, and November 6, 1854.

45. Edward Bayard, "Homeopathia and Nature against Allopathia and Art," *North American Journal of Homeopathy,* 7 (1858), 1.

46. "Report of the Minority of the Select Committee in Favor of Introducing Homeopathy into Bellevue Hospital," *North American Journal of Homeopathy,* 6 (1858), 435.

47. "Report of the Minority of the Select Committee in Favor of Introducing Homeopathy into Bellevue Hospital," p. 436.

48. "Proceedings of Medical Societies," *United States Journal of Homeopathy,* 1 (1860), 355.

49. Thomas, "Homeopathic Medical College of Pennsylvania," p. 790.

50. *Sixth Annual Prospectus and Announcement for 1865-66, of the New York Homeopathic Medical College* (New York City: n.p., 1865), pp. 10, 13-14; Franklin B. Hough, *Historical and Statistical Record of the University of the State of New York During the Century from 1784 to 1884* (Albany: Weed, Parsons, Printers, 1885), p. 397.

51. Walter S. Mills, "Historical Sketch of the New York Homeopathic Medical College and Flower Hospital, 1860-1910," pp. 347-350; Walter Sands Mills, "A Matter of History," *The Chironian,* 29 (1913), 415-416; "Opening of the New Medical College in New York City," *United States Journal of Homeopathy,* 1 (1860), 589-591.

52. Mills, "Historical Sketch of the New York Homeopathic Medical College and Flower Hospital, 1860-1910," p. 350.

53. Mills, "A Matter of History," p. 417.

54. Mills, "Historical Sketch of the New York Homeopathic Medical College and Flower Hospital, 1860-1910," pp. 351-352.

55. King, *History of Homeopathy,* Volume II, pp. 281-282; S. J. Greenberg, "On the History of the New York Medical College," *New York Medical Quarterly,* 6 (1986), 118.

56. Mills, "Historical Sketch of the New York Homeopathic Medical College and Flower Hospital, 1860-1910," pp. 352-354; King, *History of Homeopathy,* Volume II, p. 290.

57. S. J. Greenberg, "On the History of New York Medical College," *New York Medical Quarterly,* 6 (1986), 119.

58. Kenneth M. Ludmerer, *Learning to Heal: The Development of American Medical Education* (Baltimore: Johns Hopkins Press, 1985), pp. 201-202. See also E. Richard Brown, *Rockefeller Medicine Men: Medicine and Capitalism in America* (Berkeley: University of California Press, 1979), pp. 109-111.

59. "Homeopathic Association of Boston University Organized," *American Homeopathic Observer,* 10 (1873), 341-342.

60. John L. Coffin, "Annual Oration Before the Massachusetts Homeopathic Medical Society, April 1915," *New England Medical Gazette,* 50 (1915), 279; I. T. Talbot, "Boston University School of Medicine," *Transactions of the World's Homeopathic Convention,* Volume II: *History of Homeopathy,* pp. 809-811; "American Institute of Homeopathy," *American Homeopathic Observer,* 10 (1873), 387.

61. "Editorial," *Journal of the American Institute of Homeopathy,* 11 (1918-19), 581-583.

62. Dean Cornelia C. Brant, "The New York Medical College and Hospital for Women," *The Chironian,* The Lloyd Library and Museum, Special Collections, Box 38, Folder 1,90, pp. 280-282.

63. Jay Yasgur, "Lozier's School: A Brief Historical Sketch of the New York Medical College and Hospital for Women," *The American Homeopath,* 4 (1998), 42.

64. Yasgur, "Lozier's School: A Brief Historical Sketch of the New York Medical College and Hospital for Women," pp. 43-45.

65. Ibid., pp. 43, 45.

66. William Barlow and David O. Powell, "Homeopathy and Sexual Equality: The Controversy Over Coeducation at Cincinnati's Pulte Medical College, 1873-1879," *Ohio History,* 90 (1891), 102-113; Kirschmann, *A Vital Force: Women Physicians and Patients in American Homeopathy,* pp. 56-71.

67. Kirschmann, *A Vital Force: Women Physicians and Patients in American Homeopathy,* pp. 169, 182, 191-192; Phillip A. Nicholls, "Class, Status and Gender: Toward a Sociology of the Homeopathic Patient in Nineteenth Century Britain," in Martin Dinges (ed.), *Patients in the History of Homeopathy* (Sheffield: European Association for the History of Medicine and Health, 2002), pp. 141-156; Naomi Rogers, "The Public Face of Homeopathy: Politics, the Public and Alternative Medicine in the United States in 1900-1940," in Dinges (ed.), *Patients in the History of Homeopathy,* pp. 351-371; Iris Ritzmann, "Children As Patients in Early Homeopathy," in Dinges (ed.), *Patients in the History of Homeopathy,* pp. 119-140.

68. Thomas Nichol, "A Homily for the Homeopaths," *American Homeopathic Observer,* 8 (1871), 390.

69. Samuel Dickson, *Fallacies of the Faculty; with the Principles of the Chronothermal System of Medicine* (London: Simpkin, Marshall, 1841).

70. Harold J. Abrahams, *Extinct Medical Schools of Nineteenth-Century Philadelphia* (Philadelphia: University of Pennsylvania Press, 1966), pp. 195-198, 200; William F. Norwood, *Medical Education in the United States Before the Civil War* (Philadelphia: University of Pennsylvania Press, 1944), p. 101.

71. A. R. Thomas, "The Penn Medical University," *Transactions of the World's Homeopathic Convention,* Volume II: *History of Homeopathy,* pp. 801-802.

72. Abrahams, *Extinct Medical Schools of Nineteenth-Century Philadelphia,* pp. 183-184.

73. John S. Haller Jr., *Medical Protestants: The Eclectics in American Medicine, 1825-1939* (Carbondale: Southern Illinois University Press, 1994), pp. 75-83.

74. Resolution quoted in "To the Homeopathic Physicians of the United States," *Eclectic Medical Journal,* 1 (1849), 308.

75. "Obituary," *North American Journal of Homeopathy,* 13 (1864), 139-140.

76. "To the Homeopathic Physicians of the United States," pp. 309-310.

77. Ibid., p. 312.

78. Joseph R. Buchanan, "Homeopathy," *Eclectic Medical Journal,* 1 (1849), 478-479.

79. Storm Rosa, "The History of Medical Science," *Eclectic Medical Journal,* 2 (1850), 86.

80. S. R. Beckwith, D. H. Beckwith, and N. Schneider, "Homeopathy in Ohio," *Transactions of the World's Homeopathic Convention, Held at Philadelphia, Under the Auspices of the American Institute of Homeopathy, at Its Twenty-Ninth Session, June 26-July 1, 1876,* Volume II: *History of Homeopathy* (Philadelphia: Sherman and Company, 1880), pp. 526-527.

81. D. B., "Homeopathy," *Eclectic Medical Journal,* 2 (1850), 36-37.

82. Quoted in D. H. Beckwith, "The History of the Western College of Homeopathic Medicine from 1850 to 1860," *Cleveland Homeopathic Reporter,* 1 (1900), 9.

83. "Storm Rosa," *American Homeopathic Observer,* 1 (1864), 128.

84. S. R. Beckwith, D. H. Beckwith, and N. Schneider, "Homeopathy in Ohio," *Transactions of the World's Homeopathic Convention,* Volume II: *History of Homeopathy,* pp. 527-528.

85. D. H. Beckwith, "The History of the Western College of Homeopathic Medicine from 1850 to 1860," *Cleveland Homeopathic Reporter,* 1 (1900), 12-13.

86. D. H. Beckwith, "Cleveland Homeopathic Hospital College," *Transactions of the World's Homeopathic Convention,* Volume II: *History of Homeopathy,* pp. 798-799.

87. Beckwith, "The History of the Western College of Homeopathic Medicine from 1850 to 1860," pp. 13-14.

88. Beckwith, "Cleveland Homeopathic Hospital College," p. 800.

89. "Announcement," *North American Journal of Homeopathy,* 9 (1860), 160-161; "Reports of Homeopathic Colleges," *United States Journal of Homeopathy,* 1 (1860), 589-591; Frederick C. Waite, *Western Reserve University, Centennial History of the School of Medicine* (Cleveland, 1946), pp. 310-315.

90. "Western Homeopathic College," *American Homeopathic Observer,* 1 (1864), 65.

91. *Annual Announcement and Catalogue of the Cleveland Homeopathic College, Cleveland, Ohio, for the Session of 1865-6* (Cleveland, OH: Sanford and Hayward, 1865), pp. 3-4.

92. "Western Homeopathic College," *American Homeopathic Observer,* 1 (1864), 30-31.

93. Beckwith, "Cleveland Homeopathic Hospital College," p. 800; "The Homeopathic Hospital College, Cleveland, Ohio," *American Homeopathic Observer,* 8 (1871), 152-153.

94. "The Homeopathic Hospital College, Cleveland, Ohio," pp. 152-153.

95. Beckwith, "The History of the Western College of Homeopathic Medicine from 1850 to 1860," p. 20.

96. Ibid., p. 16.

97. "Pulte Medical College," *American Homeopathic Observer,* 10 (1873), 231; "Pulte Medical College of Cincinnati," *Transactions of the World's Homeopathic Convention,* Volume II: *History of Homeopathy,* pp. 813-814.

98. Henry Ford, *History of Cincinnati, Ohio, with Illustrations and Biographical Sketches* (Cleveland: L.A. Williams, 1881), p. 306.

99. William H. Roberts, "Orthodoxy vs. Homeopathy: Ironic Developments Following the Flexner Report at the Ohio State University," *Bulletin of the History of Medicine,* 60 (1986), 73-87.

100. A. Leight Monroe, "Southwestern Homeopathic Medical College and Hospital," in King, *History of Homeopathy,* Volume II, pp. 318-320, 322, 325.

101. A. Leight Monroe, "Southwestern Homeopathic Medical College and Hospital," in King, *History of Homeopathy,* Volume II, pp. 318-320, 322, 325; "Kentucky," *Journal of the American Institute of Homeopathy,* 3 (1910), 307.

102. "Chicago Hospital," *North American Journal of Homeopathy,* 6 (1857), 276-277.

103. Martin Kaufman, *Homeopathy in America: The Rise and Fall of a Medical Heresy* (Baltimore: Johns Hopkins University Press, 1971), pp. 64-65.

104. A. E. Small, "Hahnemann Medical College and Hospital of Chicago," *Transactions of the World's Homeopathic Convention,* Volume II: *History of Homeopathy,* pp. 802-803.

105. "First Annual Announcement of the Hahnemann Medical College, Chicago, Illinois," *North American Journal of Homeopathy,* 8 (1860), 688; "The Hahnemann Medical College of Chicago," *North American Journal of Homeopathy,* 9 (1860), 351; Clifford Mitchell, "Homeopathy in Illinois," Special Collections, Illinois State Historical Library, p. 1.

106. "Our Colleges," *American Homeopathic Observer,* 6 (1870), 158; Mitchell, "Homeopathy in Illinois," p. 1; Otto F. Kampmeier, "Other Medical Schools in Illinois Established During the 19th Century," in David J. Davis (ed.), *History of Medical Practice in Illinois,* Volume II: *1850-1900* (Chicago: Illinois State Medical Society, 1955), p. 450.

107. "Hahnemann Medical College of Chicago," *American Homeopathic Observer,* 9 (1872), 253; Mitchell, "Homeopathy in Illinois," p. 1.

108. R. Ludlam, "The Annual Report," *Hoyne's Homeopathic Directory,* 1882 (Chicago: T. S. Hoyne, 1882), p. 17; Frederick Karst, "Homeopathy in Illinois," *Caduceus,* 4 (1988), 1-30.

109. "About Valparaiso University," *Journal of the American Institute of Homeopathy,* 13 (1920-1921), 884-885; "Hahnemann of Chicago: Progress of Reorganization," *Journal of the American Institute of Homeopathy,* 14 (1921-1922), 104; "The Education Number," *Journal of the American Institute of Homeopathy,* 14 (1921-1922), 294.

110. "Hahnemann College, Chicago," *Journal of the American Institute of Homeopathy,* 14 (1921-1922), 2-4.

111. Clifford Mitchell, "Homeopathy in Illinois," Special Collections, Illinois State Historical Society, p. 3.

112. Thomas, "Medical Education and Homeopathic Medical Colleges in the United States," p. 822; Mitchell, "Homeopathy in Illinois," p. 2.

113. Nux, "Our Chicago Letter," *American Homeopathic Observer,* 2 (1865), 306-307.

114. Mitchell, "Homeopathy in Illinois," p. 2.

115. King, *History of Homeopathy,* Volume II, pp. 424-425.

116. A.G. Allan, "Post-Graduate School of Homeopathics," *Medical Advance,* 27 (1891), 371-374.

117. Julian Winston, *The Faces of Homeopathy* (Tawa, New Zealand: Great Auk Publishing, 1999), pp. 190-191, 528-533.

118. "Annual Announcement, 1901-1902," *Medical Advance,* 39 (1901), 342-343.

119. King, *History of Homeopathy,* Volume II, pp. 429-430.

120. Anne Taylor Kirschmann, "A Vital Force: Women Physicians and Patients in American Homeopathy, 1850-1930" (Rochester, NY: Doctoral dissertation, University of Rochester, 1999), p. 231.

121. Guernsey P. Waring, "Dunham Medical College of Chicago," in King, *History of Homeopathy,* Volume II, pp. 118-119.

122. Waring, "Dunham Medical College of Chicago," p. 120.

123. Ibid., pp. 120-121; Julian Winston, *The Faces of Homeopathy* (Tawa, New Zealand: Great Auk Publishing, 1999), pp. 528-533.

124. Flexner, *Medical Education in the United States and Canada,* pp. 213-214.

125. Philo G. Valentine, "Homeopathic Medical College of Missouri, St. Louis," *Transactions of the World's Homeopathic Convention,* Volume II: *History of Homeopathy,* p. 804; "First Annual Announcement of the Western Homeopathic Medical College, at St. Louis, Missouri," *North American Journal of Homeopathy,* 8 (1859), 132; David J. Davis and Lucius H. Zeuch, *History of Medical Practice in Illinois* (Chicago: Book Press, 1927), pp. 242-243.

126. William Tod Helmuth, "Homeopathic Medical College of Missouri," *American Homeopathic Review,* 1 (1858), 139-140.

127. Philo G. Valentine, "Homeopathy in Missouri," pp. 602-603.

128. Valentine, "Homeopathic Medical College of Missouri, St. Louis," p. 805.

129. "Colleges, Societies, etc.," *American Homeopathic Observer,* 3 (1866), 97; "The Homeopathic Medical College of Missouri," *American Homeopathic Observer,* 3 (1866), 482.

130. "Homeopathic College of Missouri," *American Homeopathic Observer,* 8 (1871), 203.

131. Valentine, "Homeopathic Medical College of Missouri," pp. 806-807.

132. Ibid., pp. 806-807; "Report of the Council on Medical Education," *Journal of the American Institute of Homeopathy,* 11 (1919), 361. See also *Polk's Medical Registrar and Directory of North America* (Tenth edition) (Detroit: R.L. Polk and Co., 1908).

133. Monroe, "Southwestern Homeopathic Medical College and Hospital," in King, *History of Homeopathy,* Volume II, pp. 331-333, 335-336.

134. William F. Norwood, *Medical Education in the United States Before the Civil War* (Philadelphia: University of Pennsylvania Press, 1944), pp. 350-352.

135. Quoted in "A Case of Medical Jurisprudence: Homeopathy in University of Michigan," *American Homeopathic Observer,* 8 (1871), 209, emphasis added.

136. John C. Morgan, "The University of Michigan; The Homeopathic Medical College," *Transactions of the World's Homeopathic Convention, Held at Philadelphia, Under the Auspices of the American Institute of Homeopathy, at Its Twenty-Ninth Session, June 26-July 1, 1876,* Volume II: *History of Homeopathy* (Philadelphia: Sherman and Company, 1880), pp. 814-815.

137. "Homeopathy in the University of Michigan," *American Homeopathic Observer,* 8 (1871), 140.

138. Ibid., pp. 143-144.

139. "Michigan Homeopathic Institute; Eighth Annual Meeting," p. 314.

140. Resolution quoted in "Michigan Homeopathic Institute; Eighth Annual Meeting," pp. 315-316.

141. Morgan, "The University of Michigan; The Homeopathic Medical College," p. 817.

142. Quoted in "Homeopathy in University of Michigan," p. 493.

143. The college held four sessions of medical lectures and graduated a total of eighty-four students. "Detroit Homeopathic College," *Transactions of the World's Homeopathic Convention,* pp. 812-813; Daniel A. MacLachlan, "The Detroit Homeopathic College," in William Harvey King, *History of Homeopathy and Its Institutions in America: their Founders, Benefactors, Faculties, Officers, Hospitals, Alumni, etc., With a Record of Achievement of Its Representatives in the World of Medicine* (4 volumes) (New York: Lewis Publishing Company, 1905), Volume II, pp. 173-175.

144. "Lansing Homeopathic College," *American Homeopathic Observer,* 8 (1871), 539.

145. "Homeopathic Medical College of Detroit," *Transactions of the World's Homeopathic Convention,* Volume III: *History of Homeopathy,* pp. 811-812.

146. E. H. Drake, "Homeopathy in University of Michigan," *American Homeopathic Observer,* 8 (1871), 565-566.

147. Thomas F. Pomeroy, C. Hastings, E. H. Drake, and William R. Grorton, "Detroit Homeopathic College—A Protest," *American Homeopathic Observer,* 9 (1872), 250-251.

148. "Homeopathy in Michigan," pp. 56, 58.

149. William Gallupe quoted in Edwin A. Lodge, "Homeopathy in Michigan," *American Homeopathic Observer,* 10 (1873), 116.

150. "Another Explanation," *American Homeopathic Observer,* 10 (1873), 174.

151. Quoted in "Detroit Homeopathic College," *American Homeopathic Observer,* 9 (1872), 597.

152. Quoted in "Detroit Homeopathic College," p. 598.

153. "Explanations—Drs. Younghusband and Frost," *American Homeopathic Observer,* 10 (1873), 172-174; Jane B. Donegan, *Hydropathic Highway to Health: Women and Water-Cure in Antebellum America* (New York: Greenwood Press, 1986), pp. 24-27.

154. Quoted in Edwin A. Lodge, "Diplomas, Regular and Irregular," *American Homeopathic Observer,* 9 (1872), 536.

155. "Detroit Homeopathic College," p. 599.

156. Morgan, "The University of Michigan; The Homeopathic Medical College," p. 819; MacLachlan, "The Detroit Homeopathic College," p. 176.

157. E. A. Lodge, "University of Michigan," *American Homeopathic Observer,* 12 (1875), 329-334.

158. Ibid., p. 384.

159. "Letter of A. Sager to James B. Angell, June 3, 1875," *American Homeopathic Observer,* 12 (1875), 385-386.

160. Gross quoted in "University of Michigan," p. 480.

161. E. S. Dunster, "Communication," *American Homeopathic Observer,* 12 (1875), 477.

162. J. C. M., "University of Michigan," *American Homeopathic Observer,* 12 (1875), 578-579.

163. Morgan, "The University of Michigan; The Homeopathic Medical College," p. 820.

164. Homoeopathist, "Michigan Homeopathic College," *American Homeopathic Observer,* 12 (1875), 579.

165. "Special Meeting of the Michigan Society," *Journal of the American Institute of Homeopathy,* 14 (1921-1922), 655; "Summer Course in Homeopathy in Michigan," *Journal of the American Institute of Homeopathy,* 15 (1922-1923), 961-962.

166. "Homeopathy in the University of Iowa," *American Homeopathic Observer,* 10 (1873), 494.

167. Stow Persons, "The Decline of Homeopathy—The University of Iowa, 1876-1919," *Bulletin of the History of Medicine,* 65 (1991), 74-75.

168. King, *History of Homeopathy,* Volume II, pp. 187-190; Persons, "The Decline of Homeopathy—The University of Iowa, 1876-1919," p. 76.

169. Quoted in King, *History of Homeopathy,* Volume II, pp. 208-209.

170. Ibid., pp. 190-191.

171. Ibid., pp. 193-95, 207.

172. Persons, "The Decline of Homeopathy—The University of Iowa, 1876-1919," pp. 81-83.

173. King, *History of Homeopathy,* Volume II, pp. 210-211.

174. Persons, "The Decline of Homeopathy—The University of Iowa, 1876-1919," pp. 79-80.

175. Stow Persons, "The Decline of Homeopathy—The University of Iowa, 1876-1919," *Bulletin of the History of Medicine,* 65 (1991), 84-86; "Department of Homeopathic Materia Medica and Therapeutics," *Journal of the American Institute of Homeopathy,* 11 (1918-1919), 1302.

176. King, *History of Homeopathy,* Volume III, pp. 240-241, 243-244.

177. Ibid., pp. 245-246.

178. Ibid., pp. 247.

179. Ibid., pp. 251.

180. King, *History of Homeopathy,* Volume III, p. 251; Flexner, *Medical Education in the United States and Canada,* pp. 247-248.

181. George T. Shower, "The Southern Homeopathic Medical College and Hospital of Baltimore," in King, *History of Homeopathy,* Volume III, pp. 142, 144.

182. Shower, "The Southern Homeopathic Medical College and Hospital of Baltimore," pp. 145-147, 149-150.

183. Ibid., p. 151.

184. Flexner, *Medical Education in the United States and Canada,* p. 238.

185. James William Ward, "Hahnemann Medical College of the Pacific," in King, *History of Homeopathy,* Volume III, pp. 214, 217-220; Josef M. Schmidt, "Homeopathy in the American West: Its German Connections," in Robert Jütte, Guenter B. Risse, and John Woodward, (eds), *Culture, Knowledge, and Healing: Historical Perspectives of Homeopathic Medicine in Europe and North America* (Sheffield: European Association for the History of Medicine and Health Publications, 1998), pp. 148, 160-161.

186. Ward, "Hahnemann Medical College of the Pacific," pp. 224-225; "Editorial," *Hahnemannian Monthly,* 29 (1894), 294-295; Schmidt, "Homeopathy in the American West," p. 161.

187. Ward, "Hahnemann Medical College of the Pacific," pp. 226-227, 230-233.

188. Schmidt, "Homeopathy in the American West," p. 162; James W. Ward, "University of California: Report of the Committee on Homeopathic Instruction," *Journal of the American Institute of Homeopathy,* 12 (1919-1920), 367-370; Winston, *Faces of Homeopathy,* p. 224.

189. B, "Homeopathy, Hunkerism and Progress," *Eclectic Medical Journal,* 11 (1854), 328-329. The author of this article was probably John Rodes Buchanan; King, *History of Homeopathy,* Volume II, pp. 46-47.

Chapter 6

1. James McNaughton, "Annual Address Delivered Before the Medical Society of the State of New York, February 6, 1838," *Transactions of the Medical Society of the State of New York,* 4 (1838), 10-11.

2. Ibid., pp. 17-18.

3. Ibid., pp. 20-22.

4. Henry M. Smith, "Homeopathy in New York," *Transactions of the World's Homeopathic Convention, Held at Philadelphia, Under the Auspices of the American Institute of Homeopathy, at Its Twenty-Ninth Session, June 26-July 1, 1876,* Volume II: *History of Homeopathy* (Philadelphia: Sherman and Company, 1880), p. 449; John F. Gray, "Early History of Homeopathy in New York," *North American Journal of Homeopathy,* 12 (1864), 333-334.

5. Gray, "Early History of Homeopathy in New York," pp. 334-335.

6. William Channing, *The Reformation of Medical Science, Demanded by Inductive Philosophy: A Discourse Delivered Before the New-York Physicians' Society, on Their Anniversary, November 21, 1838* (Second Edition) (New York: Wiley and Putnam, 1839), pp. 14, 17.

7. Ibid., pp. 48, 58.

8. Ibid., pp. 34, 46.

9. "The American Institute of Homeopathy," *North American Journal of Homeopathy,* 16 (1867), 145; "American Institute of Homeopathy," *Transactions of the American Institute of Homeopathy,* (1880), 679.

10. "Proceedings of the American Institute of Homeopathy," *Philadelphia Journal of Homeopathy,* 2 (1853), 267-268.

11. "Medical News," *Philadelphia Journal of Homeopathy,* 1 (1852), 95-96.

12. Martin Kaufman, *Homeopathy in America: The Rise and Fall of a Medical Heresy* (Baltimore: Johns Hopkins University Press, 1971), p. 55.

13. William A. Gardiner, "The American Institute of Homeopathy," *Philadelphia Journal of Homeopathy,* 1 (1853), 523-524.

14. "Historical and Statistical Report of Homeopathy in the United States of America," *Transactions of the World's Homeopathic Convention,* Volume II: *History of Homeopathy,* p. 438.

15. "Proceedings of the American Institute of Homeopathy," *North American Homeopathic Journal,* 3 (1853), 412, 416; "Proceedings of the American Institute of Homeopathy," *Philadelphia Journal of Homeopathy,* 2 (1853), 290.

16. "Proceedings of the Eleventh Annual Session of the American Institute of Homeopathy," *Philadelphia Journal of Homeopathy,* 3 (1854), 248.

17. "Proceedings of the 12th Session of the American Institute of Homeopathy, Buffalo, New York, June 6th and 7th, 1855," *Philadelphia Journal of Homeopathy,* 4 (1855), 169.

18. "Proceedings of the 12th Session of the American Institute of Homeopathy, Buffalo, New York, June 6th and 7th, 1855," p. 170. Humphreys' Homeopathic Medicine Company continues today as Humphreys' Pharmacal and his *Humphreys' Manual of Specific Homeopathy* (First Edition, 1858) went through ten different editions. See Jay Yasgur, *Yasgur's Homeopathic Dictionary and Holistic Health Reference* (Fourth Edition) (Greenville, PA: Van Hoy Publishers, 1998), p. 379.

19. "Illinois State Homeopathic Medical Association," *North American Journal of Homeopathy,* 13 (1864), 131-132.

20. "Proceedings of the Fifteenth Annual Meeting of the American Institute of Homeopathy," *North American Journal of Homeopathy,* 7 (1859), 502.

21. "Proceedings of the American Institute of Homeopathy—Sixteenth Annual Session," *American Homeopathic Review,* 1 (1859), 467-468.

22. E. M. Hale, "Correspondence," *North American Journal of Homeopathy,* 8 (1859), 303.

23. John F. Geary, "Medical Creeds," *North American Journal of Homeopathy,* 9 (1861), 644-645.

24. Quoted in Geary, "Medical Creeds," pp. 645-646.

25. Geary, "Medical Creeds," pp. 644-646, 649, 652.

26. "Proceedings of Medical Societies," *United States Journal of Homeopathy,* 1 (1860), 574-575.

27. Kaufman, *Homeopathy in America: The Rise and Fall of a Medical Heresy,* p. 54.

28. Samuel Jackson, *An Introductory Address, Delivered Before the Medical Class of the University of Pennsylvania* (Philadelphia, William S. Young, 1846), pp. 10-11.

29. Ibid., pp. 12-13.

30. Quoted in John Fitzgibbon Geary, "Remarks on a Resolution," *Philadelphia Journal of Homeopathy,* 4 (1855), 106.

31. Geary, "Remarks on a Resolution," pp. 106-107.

32. Ibid., pp. 154-158.

33. Quoted in Henry I. Bowditch, "The Past, Present, and Future Treatment of Homeopathy, Eclecticism, and Kindred Delusions," *Transactions of the Rhode Island Medical Society,* 3 (1877), 295-296.

34. Quoted in "The Past—The Present," *Philadelphia Journal of Homeopathy,* 2 (1853), 508-512.

35. J. G. C., "Legislation," *Transactions of the World's Homeopathic Convention, Held at Philadelphia, Under the Auspices of the American Institute of Homeopathy, at Its Twenty-Ninth Session, June 26th-July 1, 1870,* Volume II: *History of Homeopathy* (Philadelphia: Sherman and Company, 1880), pp. 997-998.

36. I. T. Talbot, "Legislation," *Transactions of the World's Homeopathic Convention,* Volume II: *History of Homeopathy,* pp. 1012-1013.

37. Ibid., pp. 1014-1015,

38. William A. Gardiner, "The Value of Allopathic Testimony," *Philadelphia Journal of Homeopathy,* 1 (1852), 89-90.

39. "Strange Medical Inquest," *Philadelphia Journal of Homeopathy,* 3 (1854), 537-562. Additional testimony was given by numerous allopaths, each of whom gave their diagnoses—from marsh miasm, meningitis, to intermittent fever induced by malaria.

40. Silas S. Brooks, "Philadelphia County Medical Society," *Philadelphia Journal of Homeopathy,* 4 (1856), 729-735.

41. "War Among the Regulars," *American Homeopathic Review,* 1 (1859), 478-479.

42. "The Hahnemannian Institute," *Philadelphia Journal of Homeopathy,* 2 (1853-1854), 628-630.

43. E. J. Fraser, "Defence of Homeopathy," *North American Journal of Homeopathy,* 16 (1867), 318.

44. B. F. Bowers, "The Relation of Homeopathy to Surgery," *North American Journal of Homeopathy,* 12 (1863), 92.

45. Edwin A. Lodge, "Annual Address, Delivered Before the Michigan Homeopathic Institute, at Jackson, June 19, 1867," *American Homeopathic Observer,* 4 (1867), 334.

46. T. P. Wilson, "Medical Reform and Medical Monopoly in the Army," *American Homeopathic Observer,* 2 (1865), 131, 133.

47. T. P. Wilson, "Medical Reform and Medical Monopoly in the Army," *North American Journal of Homeopathy,* 14 (1866), 357.

48. Wilson, "Medical Reform and Medical Monopoly in the Army," (1865), p. 130.

49. Wilson, "Medical Reform and medical Monopoly in the Army," (1866), p. 357.

50. "Editorial—Let Us Have Peace," *North American Journal of Homeopathy,* 19 (1871), 574.

51. "Homeopathy in Military Hospitals," *American Medical Times,* 4 (1862), 42.

52. T. R. Nute, "Preamble and Resolutions Concerning the Introduction of Homeopathy into the United States Military Hospitals," *American Homeopathic Observer,* 1 (1864), 140-141.

53. Quoted in "Proceedings of the 13th Annual Meeting of the Homeopathic Medical Society of the State of New York," *North American Journal of Homeopathy,* 13 (1864), 127.

54. "Exclusion of Homeopathic Physicians from the Army," *American Homeopathic Observer,* 1 (1864), 86; "Proceedings of the 13th Annual Meeting of the Homeopathic Medical Society of the State of New York," p. 115.

55. B. F. Bowers, "The Relation of Homeopathy to Surgery," *North American Journal of Homeopathy,* 12 (1863), 83.

56. George Worthington Adams, *Doctors in Blue; The Medical History of the Union Army in the Civil War* (New York: Collier Books, 1961), pp. 46-47.

57. Michael A. Flannery, "Another House Divided: Union Medical Service and Sectarians During the Civil War," *Journal of the History of Medicine* 54 (1999), 486-487.

58. John King, "Army Surgeons," *Eclectic Medical Journal,* 21 (1862), 44-45; John King, "Eclectics in the Army," *Eclectic Medical Journal,* 22 (1863), 247; Flannery, "Another House Divided," pp. 492-494.

59. E. C. Franklin, "Homeopathy in the Army," *North American Journal of Homeopathy,* 12 (1863), 267-268.

60. E. C. Franklin, "Homeopathy in the Army," *North American Journal of Homeopathy,* 12 (1864), 417-418.

61. Ibid., pp. 420-421.

62. Hammond quoted in B. F. Bowers, "The Relation of Homeopathy to Surgery," *North American Journal of Homeopathy,* 12 (1863), 93.

63. Quoted in Editor, "Surgeon-General Hammond's Order, Prohibiting Calomel and Tartar-Emetic in the Army," *North American Journal of Homeopathy,* 12 (1863), 150.

64. Ibid., p. 151.

65. Ibid., p. 148.

66. Editors, "Gangrene of the North," *North American Journal of Homeopathy,* 12 (1863), 124-133. See also John S. Haller Jr., "Samson of the Materia Medica: Medical Theory and the Use and Abuse of Calomel in 19th Century America," *Pharmacy in History,* 13 (1971), 27-34, 67-76.

67. "Calomel in the Army; the Surgeon-General's Order," *Chicago Medical Journal and Examiner,* 6 (1863), 316-320.

68. "American Medical Profession," *American Homeopathic Observer,* 2 (1865), 275-276; Martin Kaufman, *Homeopathy in America: The Rise and Fall of a Medical Heresy* (Baltimore: Johns Hopkins Press, 1971), pp. 86-87.

69. N. F. Cooke, "Veriphobia medicorum," *American Homeopathic Observer,* 2 (1865), 79, 81. Not until 1879 did Congress and President Rutherford B. Hayes annul the court martial of Hammond. See Alex Zeidenfelt, "The Embattled Surgeon, General William A. Hammond," *Civil War Times,* 17 (1978), 24-32; Louis C. Duncan, "The Strange Case of Surgeon General Hammond," *Military Surgeon,* 64 (1929), 98-110, 252-262; Harvey C. Greisman, "William Hammond and His Enemies," *Medical Heritage,* 2 (1986), 322-331.

70. Quoted in "Eighteenth Annual Meeting of the New York State Homeopathic Medical Society," *North American Journal of Homeopathy,* 17 (1869), 565.

71. W. H. Watson, "The Future of Homeopathy," *American Homeopathic Observer,* 9 (1872), 170-171.

72. Quoted in "Van Aernam Exit," *American Homeopathic Observer,* 8 (1871), 255.

73. Quoted in Alexander Wilder, "Defeat of the Medical Proscriptionists," *American Homeopathic Observer,* 8 (1871), 446-447.

74. Ibid., pp. 445, 447.

75. J. G. C., "Legislation," pp. 998-999.

76. "Van Aernam Exit," p. 255; Kaufman, *Homeopathy in America,* pp. 72-73.

77. William E. Payne, "Legislation," *Transactions of the World's Homeopathic Convention,* Volume II: *History of Homeopathy,* p. 1002.

78. Quoted in "Homeopathy in Massachusetts," *American Homeopathic Observer,* 8 (1871), 568-569.

79. Walter L. Burrage, *History of the Massachusetts Medical Society* (Boston: Plimpton Press, 1923), pp. 127-131; Samuel L. Baker, "A Strange Case: The Physician Licensure Campaign in Massachusetts in 1880," *Journal of the History of Medicine,* 40 (1985), 286-308.

80. Talbot, "Legislation," pp. 1016-1017.

81. "Homeopathy in Boston," *American Homeopathic Observer,* 9 (1872), 60-61.

82. Talbot, "Legislation," pp. 1018-1019.

83. Quoted in Talbot, "Legislation," p. 1017.

84. William Tod Helmuth, "A.D. 1851—Reminiscences of the Year of Its Birth," *North American Journal of Homeopathy,* 50 (1902), 5.

85. John Harley Warner, *The Therapeutic Perspective: Medical Practice, Knowledge, and Identity in America, 1820-1885* (Cambridge: Harvard University Press, 1986), p. 176.

Chapter 7

1. Oliver Wendell Holmes, "Medical Essays. Homeopathy and Its Kindred Delusions," in Oliver Wendell Holmes, *The Complete Writings of Oliver Wendell Holmes* (13 volumes) (New York: Houghton, Mifflin and Company, 1892), Volume IX, pp. 1-2.

2. Ibid., pp. 39-40.

3. Ibid., pp. 46-47.

4. Ibid., pp. 52, 62-63.

5. Ibid., pp. 53-54.

6. Ibid., pp. 58-59.

7. Ibid., pp. 60-62, 81-82.

8. Ibid., pp. 64-65, 100-101.

9. Ibid., pp. 83-84.

10. Ibid., pp. 98-99.

11. See Dr. Okie, *Homeopathy, with Particular Reference to a Lecture by O. W. Holmes, M.D.* (Boston: Otis Clapp, 1842); Dr. Charles Neidhard, *Answer to the Homeopathic Delusions, of Dr. O. W. Holmes* (Philadelphia: J. Dobson, 1842); and Robert Wesselhoeft, *Some Remarks on Dr. O. W. Holmes's Lectures on Homeopathy and Its Kindred Delusions; Communicated to a Friend* (Boston: Otis Clapp, 1842).

12. Neidhard, *Answer to the Homeopathic Delusions,* pp. 4-5. See Caleb Bingham Ticknor, *Letter to the Hon.—, with Reasons for Examining and Believing the Fundamental Principles of Homeopathy* (New York: H. Ludwig, 1840).

13. Neidhard, *Answer to the Homeopathic Delusions,* p. 6.

14. Ibid., pp. 11-12.

15. Ibid., pp. 14-15, 19.

16. Ibid., p. 7.

17. Wesselhoeft, *Some Remarks,* pp. 5, 8-9.

18. Ibid., pp. 12, 39.

19. Ibid., p. 16.

20. Ibid., pp. 10-11.

21. Okie, *Homeopathy: With Particular Reference to a Lecture by O. W. Holmes,* pp. 10, 12-13.

22. Oliver Wendell Holmes, "Some More Recent Views on Homeopathy," *Atlantic Monthly* 1 (1857), 187.

23. Quoted in Carl Müller, "Introductory," *American Homeopathic Observer,* 7 (1870), 4.

24. John Forbes, *Homeopathy, Allopathy, and "Young Physic"* (Philadelphia: Lindsay and Blakiston, 1846), pp. 6-9.

25. Ibid., pp. 21-24.

26. Ibid., pp. 30-42.

27. Ibid., pp. 43, 46.

28. Ibid., pp. 82-84, 90. See also John Forbes, *Of Nature and Art in the Cure of Disease* (New York: S.S. and W. Wood, 1858).

29. Forbes, *Homeopathy, Allopathy, and "Young Physic,"* pp. 94-96, 98.

30. Ibid., pp. 101-107.

31. Ibid., pp. 111-120.

32. William Henderson, *Letter to John Forbes, M.D., F.R.S., Editor of the "British and Foreign Medical Review," on his Article titled "Homeopathy, Allopathy, and Young Physic"* (New York: William Radde, 1846), pp. 3, 11-13.

33. Ibid., pp. 23, 28-29.

34. Ibid., pp. 36-42.

35. Worthington Hooker, *Homeopathy: An Examination of Its Doctrines and Evidences* (New York: Charles Scribner, 1851), in passim.

36. Ibid., pp. v, ix.

37. Ibid., p. 20.

38. Poem quoted in Hooker, *Homeopathy: An Examination of Its Doctrines and Evidences,* p. 25.

39. Hooker, *Homeopathy: An Examination of Its Doctrines and Evidences,* pp. 27, 36.

40. Ibid., pp. 54-57.

41. Ibid., p. 93.

42. Ibid., pp. 136-137.

43. Ibid., p. 121.

44. Ibid., pp. 138-140.

45. Ibid., pp. 138-140.

46. Ibid., p. 143.

47. Ibid., p. 145.

48. Editor, "Review of *Homeopathy; An Examination of Its Doctrines and Evidences.* By Worthington Hooker, M.D., author of 'Physician and Patient,' and 'Medical Delusions.'" *The Philadelphia Journal of Homeopathy,* 1 (1852), 37.

49. Erastus E. Marcy, *Homeopathy and Allopathy: Reply to an Examination of the Doctrines and Evidences of Homeopathy,* by Worthington Hooker, M.D. (New York: William Radde, 1852), pp. 20, 102-103, 130.

50. Ibid., pp. 21, 23, 37.

51. Ibid., pp. 63-65.

52. William Tod Helmuth, "A.D. 1851—Reminiscences of the Year of Its Birth," *North American Journal of Homeopathy,* 50 (1902), 108.

53. Marcy, *Homeopathy and Allopathy,* pp. 42-43, 71-72.

54. Editor, "Bibliographia," *North American Homeopathic Journal,* 3 (1853), 536-537.

55. James Y. Simpson, *Homeopathy: Its Tenets and Tendencies, Theoretical, Theological, and Therapeutical* (Philadelphia: Lindsay and Blakiston, 1854), p. iii.

56. Ibid., pp. 13-14, 16.

57. Hahnemann quoted in Simpson, *Homeopathy: Its Tenets and Tendencies,* p. 185.

58. Simpson, *Homeopathy: Its Tenets and Tendencies,* pp. 183-184.

59. Ibid., pp. 249-256, 259.

60. Editor, "Bibliographia," pp. 536-537.

61. William Henderson, *Homeopathy Fairly Represented. A Reply to Professor Simpson's "Homeopathy" Misrepresented* (Philadelphia: Lindsay and Blakiston, 1854), pp. 27, 55.

62. Editor, "Bibliographia," pp. 536-537.

63. Henderson, *Homeopathy Fairly Represented,* pp. 61-63.

64. Ibid., pp. 88, 106-108.

65. Ibid., pp. 178, 180.

66. Ibid., pp. 260, 262.

67. Ibid., pp. 233, 235-236.

68. William T. Helmuth, "Homeopathic Convention—The Western Institute of Homeopathy," *North American Journal of Homeopathy,* 14 (1865), 112-210.

Chapter 8

1. Dr. George W. Perine, "Address Before the New York State Homeopathic Society," *North American Journal of Homeopathy,* 4 (1855), 178. See also J. P. Dake, "Pseudo-Homeopathists," *Philadelphia Journal of Homeopathy,* 1 (1852), 62-63; I. G. Rosenstein, *Theory and Practice of Homeopathy. First Part, Containing a Theory of Homeopathy, with Dietetic Rules, etc.* (Louisville: Henkle and Logan, 1840), p. 134.

2. Lamar Riley Murphy, *Enter the Physician; The Transformation of Domestic Medicine, 1760-1860* (Tuscaloosa: University of Alabama Press, 1991, pp. xiii, xv.

3. Gustav Puhlman, "The History of Homeopathy in Germany," *Transactions of the World's Homeopathic Convention, Held at Philadelphia, Under the Auspices of the American Institute of Homeopathy, at Its Twenty-Ninth Session, June 26-July 1, 1876,* Volume II: *History of Homeopathy* (2 volumes) (Philadelphia: Sherman and Company, 1880), pp. 50-51.

4. John S. Haller Jr., *The People's Doctors: Samuel Thomson and the American Botanical Movement, 1790-1860* (Carbondale, IL: Southern Illinois University Press, 2000), Chapters 1 and 2.

5. John F. Geary, "Our Literature—A Review," *Philadelphia Journal of Homeopathy,* 4 (1855), 266.

6. Constantine Hering, *The Homoeopathist, or Domestic Physician* (Philadelphia: Jacob Behlert and J. N. Bauersachs, 1844), pp. iii-iv, vi-x.

7. Howard A. Okie (ed.), *Bönninghausen's Therapeutic Pocket-Book for Homeopathists; To Be Used at the Bedside of the Patient and in the Study of the Materia Medica* (Boston: Otis Clapp, 1847), pp. xiii-xxiii.

8. Joseph Laurie, *Homeopathic Domestic Medicine* (Fourth Edition) (New York: William Radde, 1848), p. 9.

9. Hull quoted in Laurie, *Homeopathic Domestic Medicine,* pp. iii-iv.

10. H. C. Allen, "Domestic Medicine," *American Homeopathic Observer,* 2 (1865), 359.

11. J. H. Pulte, *Homeopathic Domestic Physician, Containing the Treatment of Diseases; Popular Explanations of Anatomy, Physiology, Hygiene and Hydropathy: Also an Abridged Materia Medica* (Second Edition) (Cincinnati: D. W. Derby and Company, 1851), pp. xvi-xix.

12. Pulte, *Homeopathic Domestic Physician,* pp. 27-29, 34-35, 38.

13. Benjamin L. Hill, *An Epitome of the Homeopathic Healing Art, Containing the New Discoveries and Improvements to the Present Time; Designed for the Use of Families, for Travelers on their Journey, and as a Pocket Companion for the Physician* (Cleveland, Ohio: Hohn Hall, 1859), pp. vi-viii.

14. Ludlam, "Reviews and Bibliographical Notices," *North American Journal of Homeopathy,* 13 (1864), 261.

15. Christopher Hoolihan (compiler and annotator), *An Annotated Catalogue of the Edward C. Atwater Collection of American Popular Medicine and Health Reform* (2 volumes) (Rochester, NY: University of Rochester Press, 2001), Volume I, p. 289.

16. R. L. Robb, J. V. Bean, and S. Lucretia Robb, *Robb and Co's Family Physician. A Work on Domestic Medicines, Designed to Show the Causes, Symptoms and Treatment of Disease. For the Use of the People* (Burlington, Iowa: Robb and Co., 1880).

17. Puhlman, "The History of Homeopathy in Germany," p. 50.

18. Advertisement in J. A. Cloud, *Homeopathy: Its Difficulties and Some of the Principal Errors Against It, with Hints on Dietetics, Viewed in Relation to the Laws of Digestion; Also the Practice of Homeopathic Medicine Simplified, for the Use of Families and a History of the Cincinnati Homeopathic Medical Dispensary* (Cincinnati: V. C. Tidball, 1869), n.p.

19. Allen, "Domestic Medicine," pp. 361-362; Dr. Lodge, *Detroit Homeopathic Pharmacy. Price Lists* (Detroit: Homeopathic Pharmacy, 1865), n.p.

20. Samuel Hahnemann, *The Chronic Diseases: Their Specific Nature and Homeopathic Treatment* (5 volumes) (New York: William Radde, 1845-1846), Volume I, advertisement, p. xii; Charles J. Hempel (trans. and ed.), *Materia Medica Pura by Samuel Hahnemann* (Volume II) (New York: William Radde, 1846), p. xi.

21. Allen, "Domestic Medicine," pp. 357-358.

22. An American Physician, "Homeopathic Medical Education—Present and Future," *North American Journal of Homeopathy,* 8 (1859), 53.

23. T. F. Pomeroy, "Hering's Homeopathic Domestic Physician," *North American Journal of Homeopathy,* 7 (1858), 108.

24. J. W. Metcalf, "Dr. Pulte's Domestic Physician," *North American Journal of Homeopathy,* 1 (1851), 266-277.

25. William H. Holcombe, "A Few Words About Our Domestic Treatises," *North American Journal of Homeopathy,* 6 (1857), 102.

26. J. R. Coxe Jr., "Review," *American Homeopathic Review,* 1 (1858), 84-85.

27. Edward P. Fowler, "Letter," *American Homeopathic Review,* 1 (1859), 180.

28. T. C. Duncan, "Proceedings of the Cook County Medical Society," *North American Journal of Homeopathy,* 16 (1868), 619.

29. Okie, *Homeopathy: With Particular Reference to a Lecture by O. W. Holmes,* p. 27.

30. John S. Haller Jr., *Medical Protestants: The Eclectics in American Medicine, 1825-1939* (Carbondale, IL: Southern Illinois University Press, 1994), p. 16; Thomas Nichol, "A Homily for the Homeopaths," *American Homeopathic Observer,* 8 (1871), 390.

31. Rev. Dr. William Hunter, "Speech of Rev. Dr. William Hunter," *Philadelphia Journal of Homeopathy,* 4 (1855), 303-309.

32. "Physicians Who Are Episcopal Preachers," *American Homeopathic Observer,* 12 (1875), 339.

33. "Homeopathic Physicians Who Are Preachers of Churches," *American Homeopathic Observer,* 7 (1870), 202.

34. "Editorial—Let Us Have Peace," *North American Journal of Homeopathy,* 19 (1871), 429.

35. Sermon of Rev. Thomas R. Everest preached in the Church of St. Augustin, Cheapside, April 9, 1851, quoted in Simpson, *Homeopathy: Its Tenets and Tendencies,* pp. 39, 42. See also M. Stolberg, "Homeopathy and the Clergy: The Portrait of a Relationship," *Medizin Gesellschaft und Geschichte,* 17 (1998), 131-148; A. Kotok, "Homeopathy and the Russian Orthodox Clergy: Russian Homeopathy in Search of Allies in the Second Part of the Nineteenth and Beginning of the Twentieth Centuries," *Medizin Gesellschaft und Geschichte,* 16 (1997), 171-193.

36. Jahr quoted in Simpson, *Homeopathy: Its Tenets and Tendencies,* p. 42.

37. John Gilchrist, *A Practical Appeal to the Public, Through a Series of Letters, in Defence of the New System of Physic by the Illustrious Hahnemann* (London: Parbury, Allen and Co., 1833), title page.

38. George Bush, *Mesmer and Swedenborg; Or the Relation of the Developments of Mesmerism to the Doctrines and Disclosures of Swedenborg* (New York: J. Allen, 1847); Charles J. Hempel, *The True Organization of the New Church As Indicated in the Writings of Emanuel Swedenborg and Demonstrated by Charles Fourier* (New York: William Radde, 1848); Joseph F. Kett, *The Formation of the American Medical Profession: The Role of Institutions, 1780-1860* (New Haven: Yale University Press, 1968), Chapter 5.

39. Charles A. Lee, "Homeopathy," *New Church Messenger,* 23 (1854), 365.

40. E. H. D., "The Question 'Why Are so Many Homeopathic Physicians Swedenborgians?' answered," *American Homeopathic Observer,* 8 (1871), 164-165. See also Catherine L. Albanese, "Physic and Metaphysic in Nineteenth-Cen-

tury America: Medical Sectarians and Religious Healing," *Church History,* 55 (1986), 489-502.

41. William A. Gardiner, "Provings of Remedies—Influence of Temperaments," *Philadelphia Journal of Homeopathy,* 1 (1852), 128-129; George Bancroft, "Temperaments," *Philadelphia Journal of Homeopathy,* 4 (1855), 130-139; "Massachusetts Homeopathic Society," *American Homeopathic Observer,* 2 (1865), 351.

42. Logie Barrow, "An Imponderable Liberator: J. J. Garth Wilkinson," *Society for the Social History of Medicine,* 36 (1985), 29-31; Josef M. Schmidt, "Homeopathy in the American West: The German Connections," in Robert Jütte, Guenter B. Risse, and John Woodward (eds.), *Culture, Knowledge, and Healing: Historical Perspectives of Homeopathic Medicine in Europe and America* (Sheffield: European Association for the History of Medicine and Health Professions, 1998), pp. 157-158; Robert C. Fuller, *Alternative Medicine and American Religious Life* (New York: Oxford University Press, 1989), pp. 22-26, 59-53; John Ellis, *Personal Experience of a Physician, with an Appeal to the Medical and Clerical Professions* (Philadelphia: Hahnemann Publishing House, 1892).

43. Hempel quoted in Samuel Hahnemann, *The Chronic Diseases: Their Specific Nature and Homeopathic Treatment* (5 volumes) (New York: William Radde, 1845-1846), Volume I, p. iv.

44. Hempel quoted in Hahnemann, *The Chronic Diseases: Their Specific Nature and Homeopathic Treatment,* Volume I, pp. iv-x.

45. Ibid.

46. Hempel, "Lehrbuck der Homeopathie, by Dr. V. Grauvogl," p. 369. See also Charles J. Hempel, *The True Organization of the New Church, As Indicated in the Writings of Emanuel Swedenborg, and Demonstrated by Charles Fourier* (New York: William Radde, 1848).

47. "Personal," *American Homeopathic Observer,* 1 (1864), 96. See also William H. Holcombe, *Our Children in Heaven* (Philadelphia: J. B. Lippencott and Company, 1875); and William H. Holcombe, *The Other Life* (London: P. Pitman, 1871).

48. "Reviews and Book Notices," *American Homeopathic Observer,* 8 (1871), 72-73. See also Immanuel Swedenborg, *True Christian Religion* (New York: American Swedenborg Printing and Publishing Company, 1853).

49. Editor, "Review of *The Scientific Basis of Homeopathy* by William H. Holcombe, M.D.," *Philadelphia Journal of Homeopathy,* 1 (1852), 40.

50. E. A. L., "Reviews and Book Notices," *American Homeopathic Observer,* 8 (1871), 73.

51. Josef M. Schmidt, "Homeopathy in the American West: The German Connections," in Robert Jütte, Guenter B. Risse, and John Woodward (eds.), *Culture, Knowledge, and Healing,* pp. 157-158; John Tebbell, *A History of Book Publishing in the United States* (2 volumes) (New York: R.R. Bowker, 1975), Volume I, p. 427.

52. Quoted in Alexander Wilder, History of Medicine: *A Brief Outline of Medical History from the Earliest Historic Period with an Extended Account of the Various Sects of Physicians and New Schools of Medicines in Later Centuries* (Augusta, ME: Maine Farmer Publishing Company, 1904), p. 681.

53. Campbell, "The Origins of Classical Homeopathy?" pp. 79-80.

54. James Tyler Kent, *Lectures on Homeopathic Philosophy* (Chicago: Ehrhart and Karl, 1919); James Tyler Kent, *Kent's Minor Writings on Homeopathy* (Heidel-

berg: Karl F. Haug, 1987); Winston, *The Faces of Homeopathy*, pp. 166-167, 190-195.

55. Gustav Puhlman, "The History of Homeopathy in Germany," *Transactions of the World's Homeopathic Convention, Held at Philadelphia, Under the Auspices of the American Institute of Homeopathy, at Its Twenty-Ninth Session, June 26-July 1, 1876*, Volume II: *History of Homeopathy* (2 volumes) (Philadelphia: Sherman and Co., 1880), pp. 33-35.

56. John Fitzgibbon Geary, "Our Literature—A Review," *Philadelphia Journal of Homeopathy*, 4 (1856), 646-647, 649.

57. Prof. Bamberger, "Varieties of Syphilization," *United States Journal of Homeopathy*, 1 (1860), 335-339. See William Boeck, *Recherches dur la syphilis appuyées de tableaux de statistique tirés des archives de hôpitaux de Christiana* (Jensen; Christiania, 1862); Casimiro Sperino, *La syphilisation étudiée comme méthode curative et comme moyen prophylactique des maladies vénériennes* (Turin: Bocca, 1853).

58. "Michigan Homeopathic Institute; Eighth Annual Meeting," *American Homeopathic Observer*, 4 (1867), 325.

59. Samuel Hahnemann, *Organon of Homeopathic Medicine* (Allentown, PA: Academical Bookstore: 1836), p. 62.

60. S. L., "Vaccination," *American Homeopathic Observer*, 7 (1870), 421.

61. "Reviews and Bibliographical Notices," *North American Journal of Homeopathy*, 9 (1860), 326-327.

62. Henry C. Preston, "Vaccination," *Philadelphia Journal of Homeopathy*, 1 (1852), 98.

63. Preston, "Vaccination," pp. 103-104.

64. Dr. J. Bryant, "Vaccination," *Philadelphia Journal of Homeopathy*, 1 (1852), 275-276.

65. "Reviews and Bibliographical Notices," pp. 326-328.

66. Ibid.

67. T. S. Verdi, "Suggestive Facts Concerning Vaccination and Small-Pox in Washington," *American Homeopathic Observer*, 10 (1873), 258-260.

68. Article by Benjamin C. Woodbury Jr., "The Homeopathic School of Medicine," in The Lloyd Library and Museum, Eclectic Medical College, Box 37, Folder 1,076, p. 308.

69. W. H. Galt, "The Lost Art of Acupuncture," *Louisville Medical News*, 7 (1879), 88; John Linden, *Manual of the Exanthematic Method of Cure Also Known As Bauncheidtism* (Cleveland: Evangelical Association, 1875), p. v; G. F. C. "Baunscheidtism," *University of Texas Medical Journal*, 4 (1898-1899), 54; L. Dodge and J. Firmenich, *Dermapathic Treatment of Acute and Chronic Diseases* (Buffalo: Rockwell and Baker, 1861), p. 14.

70. W. J. Midelton, "The Pyonex Treatment," *Medical Times*, 38 (1910), 989; Car. Baunscheidt, *Der Baunscheidtismus* (Bonn: J. Wittman, 1858), p. 42.

71. Midelton, "The Pyonex Treatment," p. 989; Carl Baunscheidt, *Der Baunscheidtismus by the Inventor of the New Curing Method* (Bonn: J. Wittman, 1858), p. 42.

72. "Baunscheidtismus," *American Homeopathic Observer*, 1 (1864), 31, 93, 118.

73. J. H. Pulte, *Homeopathic Domestic Physician, Containing the Treatment of Diseases; Popular Explanations of Anatomy, Physiology, Hygiene and Hydropathy, a Treatise on Domestic Surgery, and an Abridged Materia Medica* (Ninth Edition) (Cincinnati: Smith and Worthington, 1868 [1857]), pp. 609-626.

74. J. A. Cloud, *Homeopathy: Its Difficulties and Some of the Principal Errors Against It, with Hints on Dietetics, Viewed in Relation to the Laws of Digestion; Also the Practice of Homeopathic Medicine Simplified, for the Use of Families and a History of the Cincinnati Homeopathic Medical Dispensary* (Cincinnati: V. C. Tidball, 1869), pp. 28-31.

75. Sylvester Graham, *A Treatise on Bread and Bread-Making* (Payson, Arizona: Leaves-Of-Autumn Books, 1991 [1837]); Sylvester Graham, *Sylvester Graham's Lectures on the Science of Human Life* (Manchester: Vegetarian Society, 1887); Sylvester Graham, *Review of Beaumont's Experiments* (Boston: Cambell, 1838); Stephen Nissenbaum, *Sex, Diet, and Debility in Jacksonian America: Sylvester Graham and Health Reform* (Chicago: Dorsey Press, 1980).

76. Rosenstein, *Theory and Practice of Homeopathy*, pp. 181-183.

77. Charles F. Taylor, "The Movement Cure," *North American Journal of Homeopathy*, 6 (1857), 177-192.

78. Charles F. Taylor, *Exposition of the Swedish Movement-Cure, Embracing the History and Philosophy of This System of Medical Treatment, With Examples of Single Movements, and Directions for Their Use in Various Forms of Chronic Disease, Forming a Complete Manual of Exercises; Together With a Summary of the Principles of General Hygiene* (New York: S. R. Wells, and Company, 1876), p. 50.

79. Ibid., pp. 52, 55-57.

80. Ibid., p. ix.

81. Ibid., p. 29.

82. Ibid., p. 24.

83. William A. Gardiner, "Progressive Homeopathy," *Philadelphia Journal of Homeopathy*, 1 (1852), 236; Pulte, *Homeopathic Domestic Physician*, pp. 628-630.

84. [William A. Gardiner], "Hydropathy," *Philadelphia Journal of Homeopathy*, 1 (1852), 58, 61.

85. Ibid., p. 281.

86. William A. Gardiner, "To Contributors and Subscribers," *Philadelphia Journal of Homeopathy*, 1 (1852), 328.

87. J. Davies, "Cold As a Therapeutic Agent," *North American Journal of Homeopathy*, 16 (1868), 371-375.

88. Samuel Gregg, "On Water As an Adjuvant in Homeopathic Treatment," *North American Journal of Homeopathy*, 16 (1868), 366-370.

89. E. B. Keeney, S. E. Lederer, and E. P. Minihan, "Sectarians and Scientists: Alternatives to Orthodox Medicine," in Ronald L. Numbers and Judith W. Leavitt (eds.), *Wisconsin Medicine: Historical Perspectives* (Madison: University of Wisconsin Press, 1981), p. 55.

90. "Honor to Whom Honor," *Philadelphia Journal of Homeopathy*, 4 (1855), 380-381.

91. "Miscellaneous Items," *North American Journal of Homeopathy*, 4 (1856), 440-441.

92. B. F. Joslin, *Principles of Homeopathy. In a Series of Lectures* (New York: William Radde, 1850), p. 33.

93. Quoted in James Y. Simpson, *Homeopathy: Its Tenets and Tendencies, Theoretical, Theological, and Therapeutical* (Philadelphia: Lindsay and Blakiston, 1854), pp. 134-137.

94. Ibid., p. 141.

95. Ibid., p. 143.

96. Ibid., pp. 144-145, 148.

97. William J. Maynard, "Cases in Electro-Therapeutics," *American Homeopathic Observer,* 8 (1871), 183-184; W. R. McLaren, "Electricity As a Therapeutic Agent," *American Homeopathic Observer,* 8 (1871), 184-185. See also Julius Althaus, *A Treatise on Medical Electricity: Theoretical and Practical and Its Use in the Treatment of Paralysis, Neuralgia and other Diseases* (Philadelphia: Lindsay and Blakiston, 1873); Sir J. Russell Reynolds, *Lectures on the Clinical Uses of Electricity: Delivered in University College Hospital* (Lancet London: J.J. Croft, 1870); William A. Hammond, *A Treatise on Diseases of the Nervous System* (New York: D. Appleton and Company, 1873); and Moritz Meyer and William A. Hammond, *Electricity in Its Relations to Practical Medicine* (New York: D. Appleton and Company, 1869).

98. E. E. Marcy, "The Homeopathic Law," *North American Homeopathic Journal,* 3 (1853), 22.

99. "Proceedings of the Fourteenth Annual Meeting of the American Institute of Homeopathy," *North American Journal of Homeopathy,* 7 (1859), 500.

100. J. P. Dake, "Pseudo-Homeopathists," *Philadelphia Journal of Homeopathy,* 1 (1852), 64.

101. W. Paine, "Eclecticism and Homeopathy," *Eclectic Medical Journal,* Vol. 2, (1852), 208-209.

102. "Colleges, Societies, etc.," *American Homeopathic Observer,* 3 (1866), 193-196.

103. "Medical Union," *American Homeopathic Observer,* 10 (1873), 149-151.

104. "Editorial—Let Us Have Peace," *North American Journal of Homeopathy,* 19 (1871), 573-574.

105. "Medical Union," *American Homeopathic Observer,* 10 (1873), 273-274.

106. Alfred Hughes, "Some Absurdities of Homeopathic Practitioners," *American Homeopathic Observer,* 7 (1870), 268-273.

Chapter 9

1. Naomi Rogers, "American Homeopathy Confronts Scientific Medicine," in Robert Jütte, Guenter B. Risse, and John Woodward, *Culture, Knowledge, and Healing: Historical Perspectives of Homeopathic Medicine in Europe and North America* (Sheffield: European Association for the History of Medicine and Health Publications, 1998), p. 31.

2. Henry M. Smith, "Present Position of Medical Science," *American Homeopathic Review,* 1 (1858), 2-4.

3. John C. Peters, "Reviews and Bibliographical Notices," *North American Journal of Homeopathy,* 8 (1859), 272-275.

4. Ludlam, "Reviews and Bibliographical Notices," *North American Journal of Homeopathy,* 9 (1860), 318-319; John S. Haller Jr., "Decline of Bloodletting: A

Study in Nineteenth Century Ratiocinations," *Southern Medical Journal,* 79 (1986), 469-475; David J. Davis (ed.), *History of Medical Practice in Illinois,* Volume II: *1850-1900* (Chicago: Illinois Medical Association, 1955), pp. 451-452.

5. Peters, "Reviews and Bibliographical Notices," pp. 504-505.

6. S. M. Gale, "Irregular Regulars—Homeopathic Allopathists," *American Homeopathic Observer,* 7 (1870), 359-360.

7. J. A. Cloud, *Homeopathy: Its Difficulties and Some of the Principal Errors Against It, with Hints on Dietetics, Viewed in Relation to the Laws of Digestion; Also the Practice of Homeopathic Medicine Simplified, for the Use of Families and a History of the Cincinnati Homeopathic Medical Dispensary* (Cincinnati: V. C. Tindball, 1869), p. 25.

8. Lewis Dodge, "On Venesection in Puerperal Convulsions," *North American Journal of Homeopathy,* 6 (1858), 358-360.

9. James T. Alley, "Adjuvants to Medical Treatment," *North American Journal of Homeopathy,* 8 (1859), 19-20.

10. William H. Holcombe, "What Is Homeopathy?" *North American Journal of Homeopathy,* 13 (1865), 332-334. See also William H. Holcombe, *The Scientific Basis of Homeopathy* (Cincinnati: H.W. Derby, 1852).

11. Holcombe, "What Is Homeopathy?" pp. 334-335.

12. Ibid., pp. 335-338.

13. Ibid., pp. 341-342.

14. J. C. Peterson, "On the Dissensions Between the Schools," *North American Journal of Homeopathy,* 9 (1860), 308-309.

15. Ibid., pp. 311-312.

16. H. B. Clarke, "Annual Address, Delivered Before the Massachusetts Homeopathic Medical Society, April 12, 1865," *American Homeopathic Observer,* 4 (1867), 264-265.

17. Reuben Ludlam, "Medical Toleration," *North American Journal of Homeopathy,* 16 (1868), 340-342.

18. Quoted in Charles W. Earle, "Homeopathy As It Was and As It Is," *Chicago Medical Examiner,* 12 (1871), 539-540.

19. Thomas Nichol, "A Homily for the Homoeopaths," *American Homeopathic Observer,* 8 (1871), 308-309.

20. "Homeopathy, Allopathy, and Expectancy," *North American Journal of Homeopathy,* 9 (1860), 322-326.

21. J. C. Peters, "Our Journal," *North American Journal of Homeopathy,* 6 (1858), 418-420.

22. J. C. Peters, *American Medical Times,* 3 (1861), 108-109.

23. John C. Peters, *On Sects in Medicine* (New York: J. R. McDivitt, 1874), p. 1.

24. Ibid., pp. 1-2.

25. Ibid., pp. 2-3.

26. Ibid., pp. 4-5.

27. Quoted in William Harvey King, *History of Homeopathy and Its Institutions in America: Their Founders, Benefactors, Faculties, Officers, Hospitals, Alumni, etc., With a Record of Achievement of Its Representatives in the World of Medicine* (4 volumes) (New York: Lewis Publishing Company, 1905), Volume II, p. 423.

28. Ibid., p. 424.

29. *Polk's Medical Register and Directory of North America* (Tenth Revised Edition) (Detroit: R.L. Polk and Company Publishers, 1908), p. 84.

30. William Tod Helmuth, "Sectarianism in Medicine," in Lloyd Library and Museum, Special Collections, Box 38, Folder 1,100, pp. 105-106.

31. Ibid.

32. Ibid.

33. Ibid.

34. John H. Warner, "Orthodoxy and Otherness: Homeopathy and Regular Medicine in Nineteenth Century America," in Robert Jütte, Guenter B. Risse, and John Woodward (eds.), *Culture, Knowledge, and Healing: Historical Perspectives of Homeopathic Medicine in Europe and North America* (Sheffield: European Association for the History of Medicine and Health Publications, 1998), p. 17; John H. Warner, "The 1880s Rebellion Against the AMA Code of Ethics," in Robert B. Baker, Arthur L. Caplan, Linda L. Emanuel, and Stephen R. Latham (eds.), *The American Medical Ethics Revolution* (Baltimore: Johns Hopkins University Press, 1999), pp. 52-69; Paul R. Walpe, "Alternative Medicine and the American Medical Association," in Baker et al., *The American Medical Ethics Revolution*, pp. 218-239.

35. Bowditch, "The Past, Present, and Future Treatment of Homeopathy, Eclecticism and Kindred Delusions," pp. 288, 298-301.

36. R. E. Dudgeon, "A Century of Homeopathy," The Lloyd Library and Museum, Special Collections, Box 37, Folder 1,082, p. 25; Naomi Rogers, "American Homeopathy Confronts Scientific Medicine," in Jütte et al. (eds.), *Culture, Knowledge, and Healing*, p. 35.

37. Edward C. Atwater, "The Physicians of Rochester, New York, 1860-1910: A Study in Professional History, II," *Bulletin of the History of Medicine*, 51 (1977), 93-106.

38. William G. Rothstein, *American Physicians in the Nineteenth Century: From Sects to Science* (Baltimore: Johns Hopkins University Press, 1972), pp. 236-237, 245; Julian Winston, *The Faces of Homeopathy* (Tawa, New Zealand: Great Auk Publishing, 1999), pp. 215-216.

39. William L. Morgan, "How to Train a Physician to Practice Homeopathy," *Homeopathic Recorder*, 18 (1903), 433-434.

40. Ibid., p. 436.

41. Ibid.

42. Stuart Close, "The Hahnemannian as a Specialist," *Medical Advance*, 42 (1904), 671-677.

43. "Miscellany," *The Medical Advance*, 30 (1893), 26.

44. "Editorial," *The Medical Advance*, 35 (1898), 180.

45. "Resolutions of the A.I.H. Regulating the Conduct of Its Affiliated Colleges," *Medical Advance*, 40 (1902), 402-403.

46. "Editorial," *Medical Advance*, 43 (1905), 54-55.

47. Abraham Flexner, *Medical Education in the United States and Canada; A Report to the Carnegie Foundation on the Advancement of Teaching* (New York: The Carnegie Foundation, 1910), pp. 158-159. The five schools that required a high school education were the state universities of Iowa and Michigan, Detroit Homeopathic, and the two New York schools.

48. Ibid., p. 159.

49. Ibid., pp. 160-161.

50. Ibid., pp. 159-160.

51. Ibid., p. 161.

52. Ibid., pp. 156-157.

53. "New York," *Journal of the American Institute of Homeopathy,* 3 (1910), 310.

54. G. R., "Editorial," *Journal of the American Institute of Homeopathy,* 3 (1910), 751.

55. "Michigan," *Journal of the American Institute of Homeopathy,* 3 (1910), 552.

56. W. John Harris, "Our Colleges, the Outlook," *Journal of the American Institute of Homeopathy,* 3 (1910), 178-180.

57. J. R. H., "The Carnegie Foundation Report," *Journal of the American Institute of Homeopathy,* 3 (1910), 225-227.

58. "The Hahnemann Medical College of Philadelphia," *Journal of the American Institute of Homeopathy,* 3 (1910), 289.

59. "Massachusetts," *Journal of the American Institute of Homeopathy,* 3 (1910), 434.

60. "State Board of Statistics for 1912," *Journal of the American Medical Association,* 60 (1913), 1638-1639.

61. "Statistics 1912-1913," *Journal of the American Medical Association,* 61 (1913), 585-587.

62. "Medical Education in the United States," (1914), p. 584.

63. "Medical Education in the United States," *Journal of the American Medical Association,* 64 (1915), 687.

64. "Medical Education in 1911-12," *Journal of the American Institute of Homeopathy,* 5 (1912-1913), 280-281.

65. "Annual Statistics," *Journal of the American Institute of Homeopathy,* 6 (1913), 1001-1003.

66. Stuart Close, "A Century of Homeopathy in America," *Homeopathic Recorder,* 40 (1925), 510.

67. R. F. Rabe, "President's Address," *Homeopathic Recorder,* 40 (1925), 282.

68. Willis Alonzo, "Medical Education in the Homeopathic School of Medicine," *Report, U.S. Bureau of Education,* 1 (1914), 219-222.

69. "Symposium—The Individual College and Its Appeal to the Student," *Journal of the American Institute of Homeopathy,* 9 (1916-1917), 814-831.

70. George L. LeFevre, "Report of the Committee on Medical Examining Boards," *Journal of the American Institute of Homeopathy,* 10 (1917-1918), 353.

71. G. M. Cushing, "Taking Stock of Our Homeopathic Colleges," *Journal of the American Institute of Homeopathy,* 11 (1918-1919), 89-90.

72. Ralph R. Mellon, "The Vital Necessity of a Research Institute in the Homeopathic School and Its Probably Scope," *Journal of the American Institute of Homeopathy,* 11 (1918-1919), 117, 120.

73. Ibid., p. 120.

74. Thomas J. Preston, "The College Situation and Prospects," *Journal of the American Institute of Homeopathy,* 12 (1919-1920), 473, 477.

75. R. F. Rabe, "Some Causes of Disintegration," *Homeopathic Recorder,* 37 (1922), 427-428.

76. R. F. Rabe, "Homeopathy—A Review of Its Condition at the Present Time," 35 (1920), 237-238.

77. Ibid., pp. 238-239.
78. Ibid., p. 239.
79. "Report of the Council on Medical Education," *Journal of the American Institute of Homeopathy,* 15 (1922-1923), 251-253.
80. Stuart Close, "Incentives to Industry in Homeopathy," *Homeopathic Recorder,* 40 (1925), 416-418.
81. Alfred Pulford, "What Ever Homoeopath Needs," *Homeopathic Recorder,* 41 (1926), 113-115.
82. H.A. Roberts, "Post-Graduate School of the American Foundation for Homeopathy," *Homeopathic Recorder,* 47 (1932), 361-362; "The Summer Session of the Post-Graduate School of the American Foundation for Homeopathy," *Homeopathic Recorder,* 50 (1935), 264-265; "Editorial," *Homeopathic Recorder,* 51 (1936), 470-478.
83. "Homeopathy in New York," *Homeopathic Recorder,* 40 (1925), 230-231.
84. "Quoted in "Editorial," *Homeopathic Recorder,* 50 (1935), 47.
85. "Editorial," *Homeopathic Recorder,* 50 (1935), 48.
86. John S. Haller Jr., *A Profile in Alternative Medicine: The Eclectic Medical College of Cincinnati, 1845-1942* (Kent, OH: Kent State University Press, 1999).
87. Morris Fishbein, *The Medical Follies* (New York: Boni and Liverwright, 1925).
88. W. A. Dewey, "Propagantism of Homeopathy in Universities," *Transactions of the American Institute of Homeopathy,* (1905), pp. 118-126; John Benjamin Nichols, "Medical Sectarianism," *Journal of the American Medical Association,* 60 (1913), 331-337.

Index

Ackerknecht, Erwin, 37
Aconite
    effects of, 26, 236-237
    as homeopathic medicine, 18, 20, 103,
        104, 173, 204, 229, 260, 261
Adams, Dr. R. E. W., 60, 61
Aesculapius in the Balance, 17-18
African-American homeopaths, 56-57
Agnew, Cornelius R., 272
Ague, 221, 223
Alabama, homeopathy in, 58
Albany Medical College, 140
Albertson, Dr. J. A., 169
Alcohol, dangers of, 24, 75
Alcott, Louisa May, 199
Allen, Dr. Henry C., 89, 150, 232, 270
Allen, Timothy F., 137, 138
Allentown Academy. *See* North
        American Academy of the
        Homeopathic Healing Art
Alley, Dr. James T., 262
Allopathy. *See* Regular medicine
Allshorn, George E., 226
Althaus, Julius, 253
American Association of Medical
        Colleges, 123
American College of Medical Science,
        359
American Foundation for Homeopathy,
        288, 289, 290
American Homeopathic Observer, 83,
        90, 100, 160, 256, 296-297
    on eclectics, 255
    feuds reported in, 128
    on religion and homeopathy, 238
    Swedenborgianism and, 240

American Institute of Homeopathy
        (AIH), 45, 62, 65, 83, 84, 114,
        155, 175
    Council on Medical Education
        (Intercollegiate Committee)
        of, 157, 276-277, 285, 288
    dissension in, 177, 178-180, 268-269,
        270
    on drug provings, 176
    establishes pharmacy, 176
    examines medical students, 134
    and Flexner Report, 280, 281, 286
    on higher potencies, 269
    and hydropathy, 249
    journal of, 149, 176, 280, 281, 328
    on law of similars, 177
    on medical education, 134, 150,
        157, 169, 177, 276-277, 280,
        281, 286, 288
    membership requirements for, 176,
        269
    reorganized, 274
American Journal of Homeopathia, 41,
        42, 43, 298
American Journal of Materia Medica,
        52, 299-300
American Magazine, 249, 300
American Medical Association
    Code of Ethics of, 181, 183, 185,
        272-273, 274
    on consultation, 181-182, 192,
        272-273, 274
    defines doctor's qualifications, 194
    on Hammond's Circular Order No.
        6, 191, 192

Index 433

Homeopathic Medical College of
Missouri, 62, 63, 153, 155,
156, 284, 366
Homeopathic Medical College of
Pennsylvania, 52, 54, 87, 131,
142, 153, 161, 366
feuds in, 126-130
Homeopathic Medical College of St.
Louis, 155, 366
Homeopathic Medical College of the
State of New York, 133, 366
Homeopathic Medical Dispensary, 46
Homeopathic Medical Dispensary of
Washington, DC, 55
Homeopathic Medical Society of
Pennsylvania, 54, 114
Homeopathic Medical Society of
Philadelphia, 54
Homeopathic Mutual Life Insurance
Company, 115, 116
Homeopathic Recorder, 287-288, 322
Homeopathic State Medical Society of
New York, 132, 195, 271
Homeopathic Times, 253, 323
Homopathic, 378 n. 45
Hooker, Worthington, 108, 218
on curative power of nature, 215,
216
on dynamization, 215
on homeopathy as quackery, 214,
216-217
on infinitesimal doses, 214-215, 262
on law of similars, 215-216
on provings, 219
on spirituality in homeopathy, 216
Hoppin, Courtland, 195
Hosack, David, 40, 41, 42
Hospitals, 7, 65-66, 109, 165, 201
in Crimean War, 110
in Europe, 104, 105, 108, 110-111,
112
in Illinois, 147, 189, 190
in Maine, 196
in Massachusetts, 45-46, 47, 197

Hospitals *(continued)*
for medical schools, 121, 134-135,
146-147, 149, 151, 155, 278,
285
military, 187
in Missouri, 107
in New York, 107, 133, 134
in Ohio, 110
in Pennsylvania, 110
recordkeeping in, 94
Houghton, J. T., 75
Howe, Julia Ward, 137
Hubbard, Dr. Elizabeth Wright, 289
Hufeland, Christoph Wilhelm, 10, 233,
267-268
Journal of Practical Medicine of,
13, 16-17
Hughes, Alfred, 256
Hull, Amos Gerald, 41, 42-43, 183, 229
Humphreys, Dr. Frederick, 126, 177
Humphreys, Dr. Gideon, 52
Humphreys' Specific Homeopathic
Medical Company, 396 n. 20
Hungary, homeopathy in, 111
Hunter, John, 21
Hunter, Rev. Dr. William, 235
Huss, John, 19
Hydropathy, 46, 161, 169, 225
in cholera epidemic, 98, 110
eclectics on, 254
and homeopathy, 249-251, 256
law of similars negated by, 250, 251
women prefer, 251
Hydrophobia, 243

Ihm, Dr. Carl, 51, 53
Iidem iisdem curanture. See Isopathy
Illinois
homeopathy in, 60-62, 147
hospitals in, 147, 189, 190
licensing in, 165
medical education in, 137, 141,
148-153, 360, 362, 363, 364,
367-368
medical societies in, 61-62, 180, 234

Illinois State Homeopathic Medical
   Association, 61-62, 180
Independent Medical School of
   Philadelphia, 366-367
Indiana, homeopathy in, 60
Ingalls, Dr. William, 46
Ingersol, Dr. Luther J., 64
International Hahnemannian
   Association, 83-84, 150, 289
   founding of, 127, 269-270
International Homeopathic Congress,
   150
Iowa
   homeopathy in, 64, 164, 165
   medical education in, 141, 164-166,
      276, 278, 282-283, 371
Ipecacuanha, 18, 99, 260
Ironside, A. S., 151
Irving, Washington, 67
Isopathy, 225, 242-243, 276
Italy, homeopathy in, 105-106, 111
Itch. *See* Psora

Jackson, H. R., 112
Jackson, Dr. James, 182, 260, 272
Jackson, James, Jr., 94, 105
Jackson, Samuel, 175, 180, 181
Jacobi, Abraham, 272
Jahr, Gottlieb H. G., 84
   Manual of Homeopathic Medicine
      of, 43, 66, 203, 228, 233,
      236-237
   Symptomen Codex of, 41, 43, 49
James, William, 199
Jeanes, Dr. Jacob, 52, 125
Jefferson, Joseph, 67
Jenichen, Julius Caspar, 73
Johns Hopkins University, 282
Jones, E. W., 79
Jones, Dr. Samuel A., 162
Joslin, Benjamin F., 42, 52-53, 69
   on electricity, 252
   on high dilutions, 81-82
Jourdan, A. J. L., 25

Journal of Practical Medicine, 13
*Journal of the American Institute of
   Homeopathy,* 149, 176, 280,
   281, 328
Journals. *See also* individual journals
   by name
   homeopathic, 7, 66, 266, 295-297
   regular, 5, 201

Kafka, Dr. F., 65
Kanosh, Rev. Mr., 63
Kansas City Hahnemann Medical
   College, 157, 283, 284, 367
Kansas City Homeopathic Medical
   College, 157, 279, 367
Kant, Immanuel, 83
Kaufman, Martin, 176, 180
Kellogg, Dr. E. M., 115, 117
Kellogg, George, 57
Kellogg, John Harvey, 251
Kent, James Tyler, 150, 151, 153, 289
   on Swedenborgianism, 239, 241-242
Kentucky
   homeopathy in, 57-58
   licensing in, 147
   medical education in, 141, 146-147,
      371
Kett, Joseph F., 66
King, John, 189
Kirby, Stephen R., 43, 175
Kirschmann, Anne Taylor, 65, 151
Kitchen, James, 52
Kits, homeopathic, 186, 226, 228-229,
   230. *See also* Domestic
   medicine
Kneipp, Father Sebastian, 251
Knight, Hon. H. C., 63
Koch, Dr. Richard, 130
Koller, Francis, 28
Korsakov, Semen Nikolaievitch, 72, 83

La Berge, Ann, 37
Lachesis, 103, 206

Pinel, Philippe, 93
Piorry, Pierre Adolphe, 36
Piper, Dr. J. R., 55
Pitcairn, John, 150
Pitney, Dr. Aaron, 60
Pittard, Henry G., 272
Placebos, 212
Plympton, A., 142
Pneumonia
    mortality rates in, 106-107, 115
    treatments for, 49, 107, 108, 246
Polk, James K., 96
Pomeroy, Dr. Thomas F., 270
Porter, Roy, 3
Post-Graduate School of Homeopathics,
    150-151, 153, 370
Potentization. *See* Dynamization
Poulson, Dr. T. Wilhelm, 270
Preston, Dr. Henry C., 48, 244
Preston, Thomas J., 286
Pretsch, Curt, 79
Priessnitz, Vincenz, 249
Prover's Union, 73, 86
Provings, 2, 40, 83, 176, 218, 262
    Andral on, 104-105, 204, 206
    Hahnemann's, 12-13, 15, 18, 19-20,
        26, 86, 206, 210
    Hempel on, 86-87
    Hooker on, 219
    and symptomatology, 236
Psora (the itch), 32
    Hahnemann on, 74, 202-203, 204,
        207, 208, 213
Psychometry, 237
Pulsatilla, 236
Pulte, Dr. Joseph H., 57, 60, 123, 142,
    146
    on dilutions, 229-230
    domestic text of, 226, 229-230, 233
    on Hahnemann, 230
    on hydropathy, 250
Pulte Medical College, 139, 146, 278,
    279, 370
Pyonex, 245

Quackery, 44, 202
Quin, Dr. Frederick H. F., 18, 28,
    252-253
Quinine, 101

Rabe, R. F., 284, 287-288
Radde, William, 127, 212, 231
Rau, Gottlieb M. W. L., 25, 213, 241
Raue, Charles G., 130, 161
Rayer, Pierre François O., 36
Rea, Dr. Albert, 49
Reed, Dr. C. A. L., 284
Reed, Rev. J. N., 63
Reed, Dr. Marco, 61
Reformed Medical School of New
    York, 57
Regular medicine
    and biomedicine, 5, 7, 259, 262-264,
        265
    bleeding used in, 20, 101, 211
    calomel used in, 191
    cholera treated by, 98, 99-100, 115
    consultation in, 181-182, 192,
        272-273, 274
    conversion to homeopathy in, 41, 43,
        46, 49, 50, 51, 52-53, 54-55,
        57, 58, 59, 60, 63, 100-101,
        108, 174, 184, 185
    eclecticism and, 254
    embraces all systems, 267-268
    as exclusive, 184, 186-187, 193
    expectant medicine of, 261
    Hahnemann criticized by, 18,
        263-264
    Hahnemann on, 6, 10-11, 17-18,
        20-21, 69, 202, 220
    heroic system of, 3, 101, 107, 115,
        212, 259, 261
    homeopathy criticized by, *xi,* 7, 18,
        69, 74, 79, 99, 108-110,
        182-193, 198, 199, 201-223,
        274-275